HIV-INFECTION – IMPACT, AWARENESS AND SOCIAL IMPLICATIONS OF LIVING WITH HIV/AIDS

Edited by **Eugenia Barros**

HIV-Infection – Impact, Awareness and Social Implications of Living with HIV/AIDS
Edited by Eugenia Barros

Published by InTech
Janeza Trdine 9, 51000 Rijeka, Croatia

Publishing Process Manager Silvia Vlase

Technical Editor Teodora Smiljanic

Cover Designer InTech Design Team

Additional hard copies can be obtained from orders@intechopen.com

HIV-Infection – Impact, Awareness and Social Implications of Living with HIV/AIDS,
Edited by Eugenia Barros
p. cm.
ISBN 978-953-307-343-9

Meet the editor

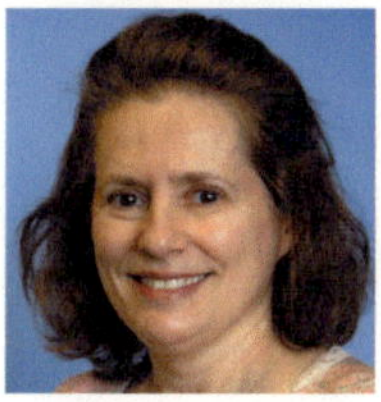

Eugenia Barros has a PhD in Microbiology from the University of Cape Town, South Africa and she is a Principal Researcher in the Biosciences Unit of CSIR (Council for Scientific and Industrial Research) in Pretoria, South Africa. She has led many scientific projects in the areas of Molecular Biology and has been instrumental in applying some of her research outcomes in the agricultural and food sectors. She has also been in the forefront of plant-made therapeutic antibodies through a collaborative project with European laboratories and has scaled-up the production of an HIV-AIDS monoclonal antibody. Living in South Africa she is very aware of the impact of HIV-AIDS in society and in the most vulnerable communities in rural Africa.

Contents

Preface

HIV/AIDS is a disease that has had a huge impact on the lives of people all over the world, as well as on the economies of many countries. The African continent, as well as other third world countries, is the most affected. As new drugs are being developed to slow down the progress of this disease, other interventions have proved to be successful in preventing new HIV infections. This book aims to give an update on the initiatives that have been used to combat this 'pandemic' in a more holistic manner, where the treatment with ARVs is not the only solution, but the whole well being of the person is considered. To facilitate the reading of this book, chapters written by different contributors, were organized according to their subject area. The first section gives an overview of the disease, the description of the drugs that are available, and how better targeted drugs are being developed for more efficient treatment, taking into consideration the rapid mutation of the virus. The second section deals with a variety of secondary effects and conditions that have been observed in people taking ARVs; in some cases the side effects can be quite severe and unpleasant and could present possible reasons for treatment failure due to non-adherence to treatment. This brings us to the third section in which education plays a pivotal role in bringing awareness to the different communities, both directly - and indirectly - affected by HIV/AIDS. Community involvement is crucial in alleviating the impact that the disease can have on the affected families with serious socio-economic consequences. Culture and gender are also important social factors that cannot be overlooked in the management of this disease. The impact of HIV/AIDS on the daily lives of those people affected by the disease is discussed in section four. The ethical aspects of HIV infection and the acceptability of an HIV vaccine are discussed in section five. I trust that after reading this brief account of what this book is all about, you will be eager to read the different chapters in order to gain a better insight of the plight of the people living with HIV/AIDS, and that you, the reader, might come up with new suggestions on how to improve the communication and awareness campaigns as well as better ways and new medicines to alleviate the undesirable consequences of some of the existing ARVs. I would like to acknowledge all the authors who have contributed to this book.

Dr. Eugenia Barros
CSIR Biosciences, Meiring Naudee Road, Brummeria
Pretoria, South Africa

Part 1

Overview of the Evolving HIV Pandemic - Prevention and Treatment

1

HIV Epidemiology and Prevention

Ayesha B.M. Kharsany[1] and Quarraisha Abdool Karim[1,2]
[1]*Centre for the AIDS Programme of Research in South Africa, University of KwaZulu-Natal, Durban*
[2]*Department of Epidemiology, Mailman School of Public Health, Columbia University, New York*
[1]*South Africa*
[2]*USA*

1. Introduction

Three decades after the discovery of the Human Immuno deficiency Virus (HIV) and its causal relationship with Acquired Immune Deficiency Syndrome (AIDS), HIV/AIDS continues to be a global burden, with more than 60 million people being infected resulting in approximately 25 million deaths. The devastating impact of the HIV/AIDS pandemic on morbidity and premature mortality on families, communities and societies is most noticeable in resource limited countries that bear the brunt of the disease burden.

By the mid-1990s, following the introduction and success of the life prolonging combination of antiretroviral (ARV) treatment (ART), also known as Highly Active Anti-Retroviral Therapy (HAART), transformed HIV-1 from being an "inherently untreatable" (Broder, 2010) infectious agent to one highly susceptible to a range of therapies. Through global solidarity, political will, effective government and private agency partnerships, ART has become increasing accessible in resource constrained settings, significantly reducing AIDS-related morbidity and mortality. Despite these major advances in the scale-up of ART provision, the continued spread of HIV remains a challenge in many resource-rich and poor countries, and preventing sexual transmission of HIV remains a public health priority.

A key lesson in terms of altering pandemic trajectories at a country level and globally has been the importance of understanding the local epidemic with regard to the virus, modes of transmission and populations most impacted. This will provide information to customize targeted interventions. Recent research on HIV prevention strategies highlights the increasing opportunities available and progress made to prevent HIV transmission, however, implementing these interventions remain a challenge.

This chapter reviews the complex diversity of the evolving HIV pandemic, and potential interventions, strategies and challenges in planning access to prevention programmes to alter the course of the disease worldwide.

2. Epidemiology of HIV/AIDS: Recent trends

Current estimates by the Joint United Nations Program on HIV/AIDS (UNAIDS) suggest a declining trend in the number of new infections due to a combination of factors, including HIV prevention efforts and the natural course of the epidemic. By the end of 2009, globally an estimated 33.3 million (range 31.4 million–35.3 million) people were living with HIV, with 2.6 million (range 2.3 million–2.8 million) new HIV infections and 1.8 million (range 1.6 million–2.1 million) deaths from AIDS occurred. However, in several regions and countries new HIV infections increased by more than 25% (Eastern Europe and Central Asia) or has remained stable (Western, Central and North America). In some countries there is evidence of a resurgence of HIV in men who have sex with men (MSM), and high rates of HIV transmission continue to occur in networks of people who inject drugs through shared needles and their sexual partners. Worldwide majority of all new HIV infections occur in women and account for more than 45% in the 15–24 year age groups each year.

Sub-Saharan Africa is home to approximately 10% of the world's population, yet bears a disproportionate burden of the disease, accounting for 67% of the global HIV infections, with over 80% occurring in women. While there has been some decline in the recent number of new HIV infections, HIV incidence and mortality rates remain unacceptably high, with more than 75% of global AIDS related deaths occurring in this region. Despite the much later appearance of the epidemic in Asia, the region home to approximately 60% of the world's population, the epidemic patterns vary between and within countries. HIV prevalence is increasing in low-prevalence countries such as the Philippines, Bangladesh and Pakistan where injecting drug use (IDU) is the main mode of HIV transmission. In Thailand the prevalence is close to 1% and the epidemic appears to be stable, while in China five provinces account for more than 50% of infections. In India the prevalence has remained below 1% and remains concentrated in IDU's, sex workers and their clients. Although the numbers of new HIV infections are increasing in certain parts of South-East Asia, the national adult HIV prevalence is likely to mask growing local concentrated epidemics. In many eastern European countries and in central Asia, the number of HIV/AIDS cases is rapidly increasing, with an estimated 70% of those infected live in the Russian Federation. The trends in HIV infections in Latin America have changed little in the past decade, with the largest epidemic being in Brazil (adult prevalence 2%), which, due to widespread access to ART, has seen a decline in the number of deaths. Throughout North America, Western and Central Europe, the HIV epidemic has remained stable for several years, as access to life-prolonging ART has led to an increase in the number of people living with the disease. However, recent data suggests that new epidemics are emerging among young women 15 to 24 years of age and in minority ethnic groups. Of concern are the growing epidemics in the Oceania region, where the number of new infections has doubled, and over 70% of HIV infected people live in Papua New Guinea. In Australia and New Zealand, the HIV prevalence has remained below 1% and is concentrated among MSM. While the epidemic in the Caribbean region appears to have stabilized, the majority of people living with HIV are concentrated in the Dominican Republic and Haiti, with MSM accounting for more than 80% of all reported HIV cases. The epidemics in the Middle East and North Africa regions have not been well characterized, as there is a paucity of surveillance data, with adult HIV prevalence not exceeding 0.3%. Figure 1 shows the current worldwide burden of HIV infection (Joint United Nations Programme on HIV/AIDS (UNAIDS) and World Health Organization (WHO). 2010).

Considerable progress has been made towards the Millennium Development Goal (MDG) 6, "to halt and begin to reverse the HIV epidemic" (United Nations Millennium Development

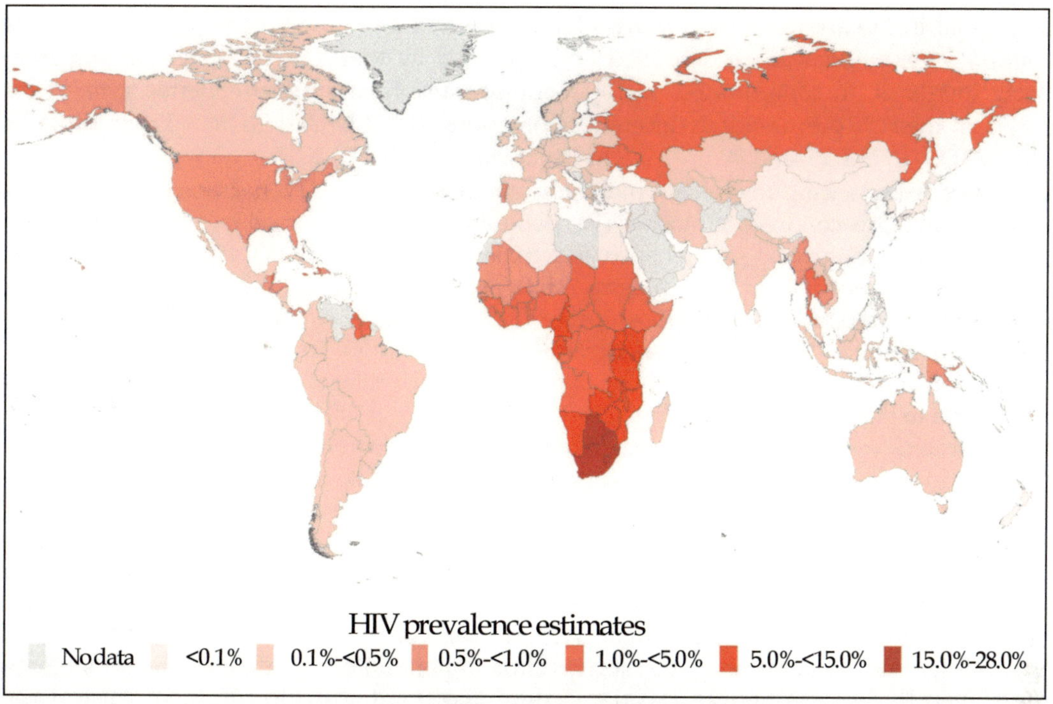

Fig. 1. Worldwide burden of HIV infection (Joint United Nations Programme on HIV/AIDS (UNAIDS) and World Health Organization (WHO). 2010)

Goals., 2000) through the Declaration of Commitment made in the 2001 United Nations General Assembly Special Session on HIV/AIDS (UNGASS) where member states committed to enhance, co-ordinate and intensify regional, national and international efforts to comprehensively address the problem of HIV/AIDS in all its aspects (United Nations General Assembly., 2001). This commitment was intensified more recently through the 2006 United Nations Political Declaration on HIV/AIDS. Prevalence appears to have stabilized or show a downward trend in many countries, yet worldwide, HIV continues to disproportionately affect women and young girls. For example in southern Africa, where more women than men are living with HIV, young women aged 15-24 years are as much as eight times more likely than men to be HIV positive (Gouws, Stanecki, Lyerla, & Ghys, 2008). Therefore, any decline in new infections in young women in this age group will significantly impact the epidemic globally.

3. Know your HIV epidemiological typology and modes of transmission

The HIV epidemic has evolved differently around the world, and it is important to understand the evolving transmission dynamics at country, regional and local level to prioritize and tailor appropriate prevention interventions. Epidemics are highly dependent on when the virus was introduced into a community, the sexual networks, risk behaviours of partner change, concurrent or overlapping sexual relationships, bridging populations, mobile populations through migratory work systems and gender imbalances. In addition, poor infrastructure development, poorly skilled populations, poverty, widespread hunger and social instability in many countries have impacted and aided the spread of HIV. The country level epidemics are described and classified by their current state, ranging from being low-level, to concentrated, then generalised and finally hyper-endemic generalised based on the HIV prevalence in different populations (Joint United Nations Programme on HIV/AIDS (UNAIDS) and World Health Organization (WHO), 2007a).

Countries experiencing low-level epidemics are those where HIV has been prevalent for many years but is confined to most-at risk populations, often amongst individual with high risk behaviour in specific groups such as female sex workers (FSW), IDU and MSM. The sexual networks of risk in this epidemic state are not diffuse, with low levels of partner change or concurrent sexual relationships, or the virus may have been introduced only very recently. Generally, the HIV prevalence does not exceed 5% in any defined most-at-risk population and 1% in pregnant women, and this type of epidemic is seen in Senegal in West Africa and in parts of central Europe.

Concentrated epidemics are characterized by HIV spreading within a defined sub-population such as MSM, IDU or sex workers and their clients. HIV remains at high levels in these sub-populations and is not well established in the general population, suggesting active networks of risk are within a defined sub-population that do not bridge or cross into other populations. The disease burden and infection rates vary substantially between countries, and HIV prevalence is consistently above 5% in most-at risk populations, yet remains below 1% in pregnant women. Within these concentrated epidemics, the mode of transmission may change as epidemics within sub-populations continue. The epidemic in the United States of America, Canada, Central and South America, Europe, Australasia, China, many countries of South East Asia and parts of Africa (Ghana) represent this type of epidemic. Most countries have geographical and regional variations in their HIV epidemics and can experiences a mix of epidemics which evolve over time from low level epidemics to concentrated epidemics.

In generalized epidemics, such as in most countries in sub-Saharan African, HIV is firmly established in the general population and not dependent on the most-at-risk groups. The epidemic is sustained through heterosexual transmission; countries report an HIV prevalence of about 5% in adults and in excess of 5% among pregnant women with a concomitant epidemic of perinatally acquired infections. Southern Africa remains at the epicentre of the global AIDS epidemic and has the characteristic of a hyper-endemic generalized epidemic, with an adult HIV prevalence exceeding 15% in the general population [Swaziland (25.9%), Botswana (24.8%), Lesotho (23.6%), Mozambique (16.1%), South Africa (17.8%), Zambia (13.5%) and Zimbabwe (14.3%)] (Joint United Nations Programme on HIV/AIDS (UNAIDS) and World Health Organization (WHO). 2010). New infection rates are higher than 5% per year despite high and increasing morbidity and mortality rates, with all sexually active persons having an elevated risk of acquiring HIV infection. These epidemics are driven through extensive heterosexual multiple concurrent partner relationships, specifically when young women have sexual relationships with men who are older through intergenerational or cross-generational relationships which often involves the exchange of goods or money through transactional sex.

4. Principles for HIV prevention

As the HIV epidemics within countries and regions may not be homogeneous in typology, may evolve over time from a low level scenario through concentrated and generalized phases to a hyper-endemic scenario, or remain relatively stable or decline, the design of HIV programs must be tailored to shape the course of the epidemic. To ensure an effective national HIV prevention response, "strong, informed and committed leadership, coordination and accountability" are required to include the most vulnerable and to meaningfully include those living with HIV. UNAIDS guidelines encourage countries to "know your epidemic and your current response", which requires identifying the key drivers of the epidemic, focusing on the relationship between the epidemiology of HIV infection and the behaviours and social conditions that impede their ability to access, as well as to use HIV information and services. Knowledge of the epidemic provides the basis for determining the response, and enables countries to "match and prioritize your response" by identifying, selecting and funding those HIV prevention measures that are most appropriate and effective for the country in relation to its specific epidemic scenario. The key to this response must enable countries to "set ambitious, realistic and measurable prevention targets" in relation to the epidemic scenario, to synthesize essential prevention measures required to "tailor your prevention plans" and "utilize and analyse strategic information" to modify, enhance or strengthen the HIV prevention measures that are likely to produce the greatest impact in each setting by promoting access to HIV prevention, treatment, care and support.

5. Preventing sexual transmission of HIV

Despite the many diverse HIV epidemics globally, each with its own dynamic characteristic, young women continue to be at considerable risk of infection. Sexual transmission remains the primary route of infection worldwide, accounting for approximately 80% of all cases. Transmission occurs through any unprotected penetrative sex act where one partner is infected with HIV (discordant sex acts), with the risk of becoming infected being dependent on the background prevalence in the population, the number of concurrent partnerships, the frequency of change of sex partners, the frequency of unprotected sex acts, the type of sex act (receptive anal versus receptive vaginal), and the amount of virus (viral dose) present in the semen, vaginal, or cervical secretions of the infected partner. The viral dose is dependent on the stage of HIV infection, with individuals who have recently been infected having the highest virus load, followed by those with a concomitant sexually transmitted disease, followed by those with advancing HIV disease, having a high concentration of HIV receptor cells at the site of infection, which increases the risk of acquiring and transmitting HIV (Abu-Raddad & Longini, 2008; Gray, et al., 2001; Pettifor, Macphail, Rees, & Cohen, 2008; Pilcher, et al., 2007; Pilcher, et al., 2004; Quinn, et al., 2000).

In generalized hyper-endemic epidemics, HIV infection extends beyond discrete populations of MSM, IDU and sex workers; the background prevalence of HIV is a significant risk factor for HIV acquisition. The majority of HIV-infected individuals are unaware of their HIV status which remains a barrier for both treatment access and prevention. For many women, being married is the single biggest risk factor for HIV acquisition. Concurrent and multiple sexual partnerships, low condom use, low levels of male circumcision, early sexual debut, transactional sex, age disparate or intergenerational sex relationships, anal sex, non-injecting drug use, alcohol use, and sexual violence increase HIV risk disproportionately in women and help sustain high rates of HIV infection in these settings. (Dunkle, et al., 2007; Harrison, Cleland, & Frohlich, 2008; Jewkes, et al., 2006; Kalichman, et al., 2007; Kenyon C & Badri M, 2009; Leclerc-Madlala, 2008; Lurie, Williams, & Gouws, 1997; A. E. Pettifor, van der Straten, Dunbar, Shiboski, & Padian, 2004; Sikweyiya & Jewkes, 2009; Van Tieua & Koblina, 2009; Zablotska, et al., 2009). To appreciate the complexities of HIV transmission, it is important to better understand individual behaviours and sexual networks within a broader context of political, economic, and social forces that enable or serve as barriers to HIV risk (Rothenberg 2009). While there are a number of issues that need to be addressed in order to prevent the spread of HIV infection, developing promising new preventative technologies could directly benefit young girls and women who account for more than 50% of new infections worldwide.

5.1 Health sector interventions

In many health care settings, HIV counselling and testing, peer education, treatment of sexually transmitted infections (STIs) as well as condom promotion and provision are delivered as integrated HIV prevention packages. Despite the 90% clinical effectiveness of preventing HIV transmission, the public health use of condoms is confined predominantly to FSW and MSM. Patterns of male condom use as a barrier method are heavily influenced by the form of partnerships. Condom use is generally highest in commercial sex work and lower in non-commercial and regular partnerships. In long-term or regular partnerships, condom use is often inconsistent and low among those at highest risk where the partner is not monogamous (Moyo, Levandowski, MacPhail, Rees, & Pettifor, 2008). In many relationships, women's inability to influence men reflects the fact that men usually dominate women's sexual lives and often impose whether intercourse will take place or not, and whether a condom will be used. As male condom use is largely dependent on male partners, the female condom, a female-initiated HIV prevention method if used correctly and consistently, can potentially help women to protect themselves from becoming infected with HIV. However, although the female condom allows partners to share the responsibility of condom use, it still requires some degree of male co-operation. As men are involved in sexual transmission of HIV either through heterosexual transmission or through MSM, men's behaviour is strongly influenced by concepts of masculinity. It is important that programs are designed to influence and persuade men to be responsible and protective to themselves and their partners.

The sexual transmission of HIV infection within partnerships seems to be facilitated by several STIs. Epidemiological studies suggest a synergistic bidirectional relationship between STIs and HIV. STIs in HIV-uninfected men and women increases their susceptibility to HIV infection and similarly in infected individuals with HIV and STIs there is enhanced shedding of HIV in genital secretions (Rottingen, Cameron, & Garnett, 2001). Thus far only one community based randomised trial conducted in Mwanza demonstrated the effectiveness of enhanced case detection and treatment of symptomatic curable STI's (chancroid, syphilis, gonorrhoea, chlamydial infection, and trichomoniasis) in primary health-care services to impact on HIV incidence. The Mwanza trial demonstrated a significant 42% reduction in HIV acquisition in intervention communities (Hayes, et al., 1995), while no effect of an STI intervention on HIV incidence was reported from other trials (Ghys, et al., 2001; Kamali, et al., 2002; Kaul, et al., 2004; Wawer, et al., 1998). The recently reported trials on herpes simplex virus type 2 (HSV-2) suppressive therapy for preventing HIV acquisition also failed to demonstrate effectiveness (Celum, et al., 2008; Celum, et al., 2010; Watson-Jones, et al., 2008). While several factors may have contributed to these contrasting results, treatment of STIs remains a public health priority.

5.2 HIV counselling and testing

HIV counselling and testing (HCT) has been an important prevention tool, and has been hypothesized that knowing one's status allows positive people to protect others from being infected and those who are negative to protect themselves from infection (The Voluntary HIV-1 Counseling and Testing Efficacy Study Group., 2000). As HIV is predominantly transmitted sexually and linked to MSM's, it has been surrounded by stigma and discrimination. Paradoxically, HIV testing, counselling and social support has provided limited confidentiality to those accessing these services and testing positive. A major hurdle for HIV infected young women to access prevention of mother to child transmission services following HIV counselling and testing is fear of stigma, discrimination and violence, further stigmatizing this age group. More recent studies have demonstrated that lack of access to HIV counselling and testing services remains a significant barrier to expanding access to treatment, particularly in developing countries. Efforts are under way in many countries to enhance acceptability, increase uptake, widen accessibility and provide an entry point to care and support for HIV positive individuals. The innovative approaches of provider-initiated HCT in health care settings (Joint United Nations Programme on HIV and AIDS and World Health Organization., 2007), and the client-initiated community based approaches (Coates, Richter, & Caceres, 2008; Khumalo-Sakutukwa, et al., 2008) are likely to promote knowledge of HIV status fundamental to accessing treatment, preventing onward transmission and promoting prevention. Despite the expansion of services, knowledge of HIV status remains low.

5.3 Microbicides and Pre-exposure prophylaxis (PrEP)

Female-controlled methods of HIV prevention are urgently needed, as the only proven method of consistent male or female condom use is dependent on male co-operation and compliance. Research into the development of microbicides (gel or cream) that could be applied to the vagina without a partner knowing, and which would prevent HIV infection, has received unprecedented attention and support. The over 60 candidate microbicides in development and 11 clinical trials testing six non-virus specific products have produced disappointing results, with none demonstrating a protective effect for HIV. The six candidate microbicides include nonoxynol-9 (N9) (Van Damme, et al., 2002), SAVVY® (C31G; Cellegy Pharmaceuticals, USA) (Feldblum, et al., 2008; Peterson, et al., 2007), cellulose sulfate (CS) (Van Damme, et al., 2008), Carraguard® (PC-515; Clean Chemical Sweden) (Skoler-Karpoff, et al., 2008), PRO 2000 (Endo Pharamceuticals, USA) (Abdool Karim, et al., 2011; Kamali, et al., 2010) and BufferGel® (ReProtect LLC, USA)(Abdool Karim, et al., 2011).

Based on pre-clinical studies in different animal models, multiple studies have established tenofovir (antiretroviral, a nucleotide reverse transcriptase inhibitor) as a promising antiretroviral agent whether administered as pre-exposure or post-exposure prophylaxis to prevent simian immunodeficiency virus (SIV) (Tsai, et al., 2000; Van Rompay, 2010; Van

Rompay, et al., 2004), The recent major breakthrough and promising results from the CAPRISA 004 trial of 1% tenofovir gel used intravaginally to prevent HIV acquisition in women are welcomed (Abdool Karim, et al., 2010). The trial was the first phase 11B proof-of-concept study of an ARV in which 889 HIV uninfected; sexually active 18-40 year old, urban and rural women were randomly assigned to receive either placebo or tenofovir containing gel for the study duration. Women were prescribed to insert gel vaginally within 12 hours before and after having sex, and to use not more two gels within 24 hours. Of the 444 women on the placebo gel, 60 women became HIV infected while 38 of the 445 women in the tenofovir gel arm became HIV infected. The overall effectiveness was 39%, while 54% were protected when they adhered to using the gel as prescribed, covering more than 80% of sex acts, and 28% were protected when fewer than 50% of sex acts were covered. The added important finding of this trial was the absence of viral resistance, its safety and more importantly, the effectiveness of tenofovir gel to reduce the acquisition of HSV-2 infections by 51%. This finding is important as the risk of HIV acquisition increases to a large extent in women who are HSV-2 infected (Tobian & Quinn, 2009; Wald & Link, 2002).

Shortly after the release of the CAPRISA 004 trial results, the iPrEx (Pre-exposure Prophylaxis Initiative) trial demonstrated a 44% protection against HIV acquisition among MSM following the daily single oral dose of the ARV drug of Truvada® which contains two drugs : tenofovir disoproxil fumarate (TDF-300 mg) and emtricitabine (FTC-200 mg) (Grant, et al., 2010). The iPrEx study was a double-blind, placebo-controlled, Phase III clinical trial which enrolled 2,499 HIV-negative male volunteers and took place at 11 research sites in Brazil, Ecuador, Peru, South Africa, Thailand and the United States. There were 64 HIV infections among the 1,248 participants who received a placebo pill, while 36 HIV infections among those who received Truvada®. Among participants who used the pill more than 90 percent of days, protection against HIV acquisition was over 72%. However, the iPrEX study found no evidence that Truvada® taken orally provided protection against HSV-2 infection.

The success of these two trials provides growing evidence of the potential of ARV's to prevent sexual transmission of HIV. The efficacy and safety of ARV's are being tested in several oral and topical PrEP clinical trials. The FEM PrEP trial tested a daily single oral dose of Truvada® for heterosexual HIV prevention in 3900 high risk HIV uninfected women, 18-35 years of age in Kenya, Malawi, Tanzania, Zambia and South Africa. However, an interim review of the results of the FEM PrEP trial has established that Truvada® tablets taken orally was not able to demonstrate a protective effect in women against HIV infection, thus Truvada® may not be as effective in preventing HIV in women compared to its proven effectiveness in preventing HIV infection in MSM.

The Centre for Disease Control (CDC) BangkokTenofovir Study is testing the daily single oral dose of tenofovir in approximately 2400 HIV uninfected IDU in Thailand. Despite the disappointing FEM PrEP trial results, the CDC TDF2 PrEP study, a randomised, placebo controlled trial examined the safety and effectiveness of a daily single oral dose of Truvada® for reducing the risk of HIV acquisition among 1200 heterosexual men and women at two sites in Botswana. The study enrolled approximately 1200 participants and randomly assigned to one of two arms: 601 were assigned to take Truvada® tablet and 599 were assigned to receive a placebo. In the primary trial analysis there were nine HIV infections among the participants assigned to Truvada® compared to 24 infections among those assigned to placebo, translating to a 62.6% (95% CI, 21.5 to 83.4; P= 0.0133) reduction in the risk of HIV infection among those receiving Truvada® .

Similarly the University of Washington 's Partners PrEP Study was a randomised, placebo controlled trial of daily single oral dose of tenofovir or Truvada® for the prevention of HIV-1 acquisition among HIV-1 seronegative partners in heterosexual HIV-1 sero-discordant partnerships. In the 4758 sero-discordant heterosexual couples in Kenya and Uganda, a total of 78 HIV infections occurred in the study: 18 among those assigned to tenofovir, 13 among those assigned to Truvada® , and 47 among those assigned to the placebo. Thus, those who received tenofovir had an average of 62% fewer HIV infections (95% CI 34 to 78%, P=0.0003) and those who received Truvada® had 73% fewer HIV infections (95% CI 49 to 85%, P<0.0001) than those who received placebo.

In 5029 sexually active, HIV uninfected women, 18-40 years of age in Malawi, Zambia, Zimbabwe, Uganda and South Africa the VOICE (Vaginal and Oral Interventions to Control the Epidemic) trial is not only testing the daily single oral dose of tenofovir or Truvada® but also the vaginal tenofovir gel formulation. The trial design is important for determining how each product works compared to its control and which approach women may prefer. The trial is expected to complete follow-up in June 2012, by which time women would have used the assigned allocation for at least one year and some for nearly three years. The trial results are expected to be available in early 2013. More importantly, the development of HIV prevention products in the form of vaginal rings and injections may provide alternate modes of delivery possibly providing protection for longer duration. The planned Phase III Dapivirine ring study will expand the spectrum of ARV's available, with an alternate delivery mode for HIV prevention. The diverse populations, including heterosexual men and women in the ongoing clinical trials, would provide further evidence for HIV protection in different at-risk groups, although a key question to be addressed is whether the optimal drug level would be achieved if ARV's taken orally or inserted vaginally to provide maximum protection .

Both tenofovir and Truvada® are approved by the United States Food and Drug Administration (FDA) to treat HIV infection, and following long-term use, there have been no safety concerns. More importantly, these ARV microbicides provide hope to millions of women, and enables them to take responsibility and initiate its use as a female-controlled method to protect them from acquiring HIV. Adapting different forms of ARV's for HIV prevention, whether taken orally or inserted vaginally, either daily or coitally, has a great potential to transform the global response to the HIV/AIDS epidemic. The confirmation of these innovative scientific approaches from the proof-of-concept trials using ARVs for HIV prevention, suggest that new HIV prevention tools are attainable, but need to be easily accessible and affordable to potentially alter the epidemic trajectory which remains a global public health priority.

5.4 Medical male circumcision

The biological plausibility that HIV-1 targets cells in the inner mucosal surface of the male human foreskin which makes it highly susceptible to HIV infection has been tested through three randomized controlled trials. To evaluate the effect of medical male circumcision (MMC), i.e. partial or complete surgical removal of the foreskin on HIV prevention, the trials enrolled more than 10,000 HIV uninfected men from South Africa (Auvert, et al., 2005),

Kenya (Bailey, et al., 2007), and Uganda (Gray, et al., 2007). After 21 to 24 months of follow-up, all three trials demonstrated that MMC significantly decreased male heterosexual HIV acquisition by 41% to 66%, despite differences in age eligibility criteria, urban or rural settings, and surgical procedure (Auvert, et al., 2005; Bailey, et al., 2007; Gray, et al., 2007; Siegfried, Muller, Deeks, & Volmink, 2009).

Based on the compelling evidence from clinical trials and modelling of data (Hallett, et al., 2008; Williams, et al., 2006), UNAIDS and WHO have recommended that MMC be provided as an important intervention to reduce heterosexually acquired HIV in men, and that it be part of a comprehensive HIV prevention package which includes HIV testing and counselling services, treatment for STIs, male and female condom provision (Joint United Nations Programme on HIV/AIDS (UNAIDS) and World Health Organization (WHO), 2007b).

In countries with generalised heterosexual HIV epidemics with high incidence rates, male circumcision rates are generally low, and for any significant public health benefit to be achieved, urgent scale up of MMC services should be considered (Lissouba, et al., 2010). A rapid public health impact would be achieved if MMC services are prioritised to age groups at highest risk of acquiring HIV. Nevertheless, providing MMC services to younger age groups will also have public health impact over the longer term. In countries with concentrated HIV epidemics, specific high risk populations of IDU's and MSM should be targeted to achieve an individual benefit for men at high risk of sexually acquired infection. While the scale-up of MMC programmes has the potential to lower HIV prevalence among the male population, in the long term women would benefit from reducing their risk of exposure.

Mathematical modelling suggests that in high burden countries in sub-Saharan Africa, with maximum coverage of male circumcision over a ten year period, it could avert 2 million new HIV-infections and 0.3 million deaths. In the 10 years thereafter, it could avert a further 3.7 million new infections and 2.7 million deaths, demonstrating the substantial public health benefits of male circumcision to lessen the transmission of HIV (Williams, et al., 2006).

Many sub-Saharan African countries have begun taking steps to increase the availability of MMC services, with set targets of maximum coverage to be achieved over the next five years despite the concerns of risk compensation, the challenges of cultural and social acceptability, limited financial and human resources, poor infrastructure and systems for monitoring and evaluating circumcision programmes (Kim & Goldstein, 2009; Weiss, Dickson, Agot, & Hankins, 2010). Additionally, more research is needed to determine the side effects of poorly performed circumcision with a risk HIV acquisition from poorly healed procedures, serious bleeding, risk of cross infection and damage to the penis (Lagarde, Taljaard, Puren, & Auvert, 2009; Schackman, 2010). As MMC provides partial protection, such programmes must be part of the comprehensive HIV prevention package (Hallett, et al., 2008; Joint United Nations Programme on HIV/AIDS (UNAIDS) and World Health Organization (WHO), 2007b).

5.5 Antiretroviral treatment for HIV prevention

The transmission probability of HIV is dependent on the viral load, and there is a substantial reduction in HIV viral load following ART initiation, with simultaneous improvement in the general health of the person being treated. Increasing evidence from several studies suggest that following the introduction of ART, transmission of HIV declines at the individual level. Amongst IDU's on ART in Vancouver, British Columbia, a decrease in the median plasma HIV-1 RNA concentration correlated with a decline in the incidence of HIV-1 infection. In a cohort study, HIV-1 transmission was 92% lower among couples in whom the index partner was taking ART (Donnell, et al., 2010). Extensive experience on the role of ART has been amongst pregnant and breastfeeding HIV positive women, with maternal ART having been highly successful as a prevention strategy for lowering the risk of mother to child transmission. Ongoing studies among sero-discordant couples will provide evidence of ART to lower the viral load and decreasing the risk of HIV transmission among adults.

The potential impact of ART to significantly impact on new HIV infection rates has recently been modelled on data from South Africa. Mathematical modelling suggests that wider HIV testing, and immediate ART for those testing positive, will significantly impact on new infection rates (Granich, Gilks, Dye, De Cock, & Williams, 2009). While the model assumes that individuals will test annually for HIV, persons testing positive, commencing ART immediately and maintain it for life will significantly reduce the new infection from 17 per 100 people per year (Joint United Nations Programme on HIV/AIDS (UNAIDS) and World Health Organization (WHO), 2008) to 1 per 1000 people per year over the next 10 years, leading to eventual elimination of the epidemic. The model however, does not include the timing between infection, diagnosis and the introduction of ART, the acceptability of HCT, the need for high adherence to ART, risk behaviours of people undergoing treatment, as well as low level of transmission and an emerging drug-resistant virus. The risk of HIV transmission is generally highest during acute infection and the later stages of infection, providing some indication of where treatment might have its biggest prevention effect, thereby fitting into a comprehensive prevention approach. While the model is optimistic, it may be unattainable in real-world settings, as the effectiveness of ART, behavioural risk factors, HIV testing coverage, reluctance to commence ART for fear of stigma and discrimination and epidemiological scenario could have a major influence on the overall impact of HIV testing and treatment programs. Furthermore, more than 50% of HIV infected persons worldwide are unaware of their HIV status, and these figures are much higher in high burden countries. In many resource-poor countries, the existing strain on health care services is a major obstacle to initiation of ART, while in many well resourced countries, the HIV-linkage to care and treatment cascade dramatically declines, with many individuals requiring ART not being on treatment. Nevertheless there are numerous programmatic issues that need addressing prior to implementation of the wider HIV testing and immediate ART for those testing positive strategy. Research on each component will guide the programmes roll-out including providing evidence of the risk and benefits of early ART to individuals.

The most convincing results and significant findings of HIV treatment as prevention come from the HPTN 052 study which took place at 13 sites in Botswana, Brazil, India, Kenya, Malawi, South Africa, Thailand, the United States and Zimbabwe. The randomised controlled trial enrolled 1,763 serodiscordant couples to test the effectiveness of currently licensed regimens of ART whether delivered early or delayed to reduce the risk of HIV transmission. At the time of enrolment, the HIV-infected partners (890 men, 873 women) had a median CD4+ T-cell count of 436 cells/mm^3, ranging from 350 and 550 cells per mm^3, while the HIV-uninfected partners tested negative for the virus. Participating couples were randomly assigned to one of two treatment arms. In the first group, the HIV-infected partners immediately began taking a combination of three ARV drugs. In the second group, the HIV-infected partners delayed taking ARV drugs until their CD4+ T-cell counts fell below 250 cells/mm^3, or an AIDS-related illness as defined by World Health Organization guidelines occurred. Following a scheduled interim review of the study's safety and effectiveness data by the independent data and safety monitoring board (DSMB), the DSMB found that 28 of the HIV infections were linked through genetic testing to the HIV-infected partner as the source of infection. Of the 28 cases of linked HIV infection that occurred, 27 infections were among the 877 couples in which the HIV-infected partner delayed antiretroviral treatment. Only one case of HIV infection occurred among the 886 couples in which the HIV-infected partner began immediate antiretroviral treatment. This means that earlier initiation of ARV drugs led to a 96% reduction in HIV transmission to the HIV-uninfected partner ($P \leq 0.0001$). The added therapeutic benefit was the decline in the morbidity and mortality events; 40 events occurred in the early treatment arm compared to the 65 in the delayed treatment arm. There were 17 cases of extrapulmonary tuberculosis among HIV-infected participants in the delayed treatment arm compared with three cases in the early treatment arm ($P=0.0013$). There were 23 deaths during the study: 10 in the early treatment group and 13 in the delayed treatment group, a difference that did not reach statistical significance (National Institute of Allergy and Infectious Diseases., 2011).

While the initial WHO treatment guidelines of November 2003 recommended that anyone with advanced clinical HIV disease or those with CD4+ T-cell counts less than 200 cells/mm^3 begin ART, the follow-up revision over time recommended that ART be considered between 200 and 350 cells/mm^3. The most recent guidelines of November 2009 recommend the initiation of ART in all patients who have a CD4+ T-cell count of less than 350 cells/mm^3, irrespective of clinical symptoms. Though several countries have adopted the new guidelines, most have not primarily due to cost constraints and a lack of drug supply (World Health Organization., 2009).

If ART is to be considered as part of the HIV prevention program, programmatic scaling up of services will be required. Identifying appropriate target population; educating health workers; a wider availability of ART; regular HCT services; education and counselling of all people who test positive for HIV are key to ART initiation. Adherence counselling for people who agree to treatment; and regular follow-up, including ART safety assessment, ongoing adherence counselling, ongoing risk behaviour counselling, and testing for viral load rebounds and resistant virus are vital to sustaining the programme. While the roll-out and maintenance of such programmes pose numerous challenges, these are highly dependent on the commitment of ministries of health, donors, provider organizations and community groups. Preliminary studies from Côte d'Ivoire, San Francisco, Spain, and Taiwan, indicate that wider treatment is associated with fewer new HIV infections where ART-as-prevention occurs. In developing countries, expanding HCT services are offered by mobile testing units, mainly as part of provider initiated routine health care services, as an opportunity to rapidly identify persons to be linked to care and ART as prevention. The scale-up of ART provision requires critical evaluation to expand the evidence base. More data are needed through monitoring and evaluation that ART provides potential gains in preventing new HIV infections.

5.6 Behaviour change programmes for HIV prevention

Population based surveys have shown that young people 15 to 24 years of age are at a considerable risk for HIV acquisition, and account for almost 50% of new HIV infections worldwide. Early age of sexual debut, inconsistent or incorrect use of condoms, and experimentation with alcohol and other substances, multiple, frequent and concurrent sexual partners significantly increase the risk of HIV acquisition.

To reduce the incidence of HIV, behavioural change interventions have been developed and implemented to reduce sexual risk (Coates, et al., 2008). These approaches include broad and diffused dissemination of factual information about HIV, frank discussions about condom use, and small-group interventions following interaction and role playing to enhance motivation and relevant knowledge and skills. School based HIV intervention programmes generally provide young learners with basic knowledge and are limited to being informational on how to prevent being infected. In a recent meta-analysis of sexual risk reduction interventions that have been successful at modifying behaviours more broadly delaying sexual debut, increasing condom use, abstinence or reducing or delaying frequencies of penetrative sex, and increasing skills to negotiate safer sex and acquire condoms have shown to be effective. Although intervention success varied across studies, the benefits were evidence sustained for up to three years post intervention, across gender and geographic region (Johnson, Scott-Sheldon, Huedo-Medina, & Carey, 2011). HIV intervention programmes amongst couples and families attempt to promote risk reduction through innovative strategies that include motivational behaviour change.

Behavioural science theories of using informational, motivational, and skills-based content to deliver interventions confirm that the efficacy of behavioural strategies together with motivational training providing greater condom skills training thereby encouraging condom use, and were more successful at decreasing the frequency of sex in younger rather than older adolescents. Effective behaviour change programs with comprehensive information on reducing HIV risk must be designed, tailored and implemented with informational, motivational, and skills-based content. They should be customised to address the needs and values of the groups they are designed to reach which will make them more likely to be effective at preventing HIV acquisition.

5.7 Structural interventions for HIV prevention

Insights into the variation in levels of risk in populations, as well as the biological and socioeconomic factors, are key to understanding risk of HIV acquisition and the speed at which HIV spreads through a population. This is dependent on a combination of structural, social, and political factors that shape behaviour, vulnerability, and risk. Sexual and ethnic practices, marginalised populations, women's status, restrictive national policies, restricted access to health care, fear of stigma and discrimination are important structural 'drivers', increasing vulnerability and contributing to HIV transmission. In many countries, HIV prevention efforts have not succeeded, as the underlying social and structural drivers of HIV risk and vulnerability have not been addressed.

Stigma and discrimination, gender inequalities, gender-based violence, human rights violations, mobility and economic power are the major structural drivers that hamper HIV prevention efforts and impede progress towards universal access to prevention and treatment programmes. HIV prevention efforts need to be adapted to change the root causes or structures that affect individual risk and vulnerability to HIV, ensuring that resources are targeted where they could have the greatest impact. While in many settings, structural interventions have addressed access to health care, sexuality and gender relations, stigma and discrimination; these have not been adequately evaluated at the programmatic level.

6. Combination HIV prevention programmes

The diversity and complexity of epidemics that make up the HIV pandemic underscores the importance of a diverse set of responses rather than a single solution for all settings. The UNAIDS "know your epidemic, know your response" provides a strategic, intensified framework for understanding the local epidemic in terms of prevalence and what is contributing to its spread (Wilson & Halperin, 2008). The proficient and competent planning of effective customized HIV prevention programs and monitoring their impact relies on strong health information systems as well as good local and national surveillance. The exact mix of HIV prevention, treatment, care, support strategies, and structural interventions is determined by this data (Horton & Das, 2008).

While several HIV prevention interventions appear promising with mathematical modelling providing further optism for the intervention, no single intervention is likely to be sufficient to prevent transmission of HIV on a global scale. Each intervention has its strengths and limitations, yet the current HIV prevention landscape consists of several important but partially effective interventions, none having been shown to be fully protective. The appropriate mix for each epidemic, to identify the target populations and establish what coverage and saturation levels are required remain challenges for effective approaches to alter the current epidemic trajectories The role of combination prevention programmes includes multi-level and multi-component interventions that incorporate biomedical, behavioural, and structural approaches which are considered highly active HIV prevention strategies and has been gaining increasing attention (figure 2).

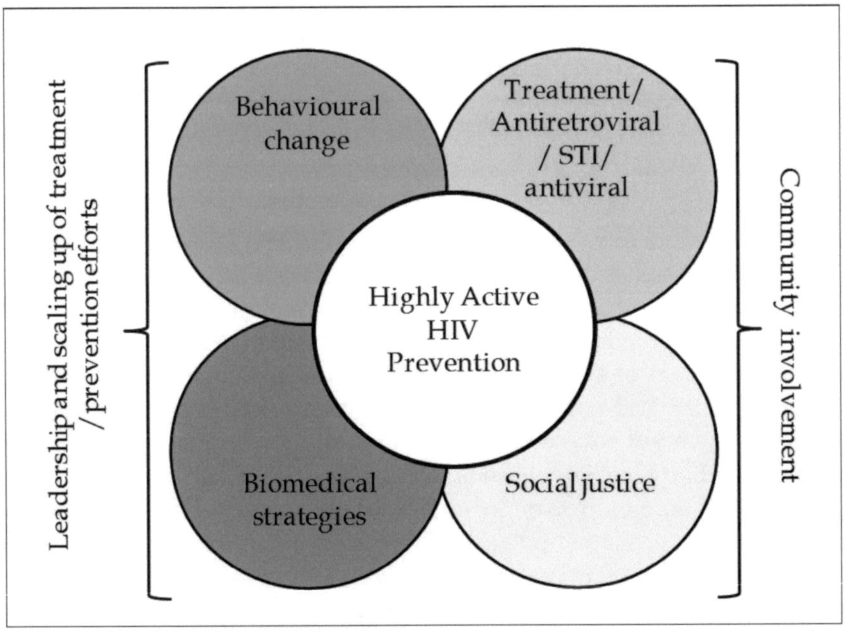

Fig. 2. Highly active HIV prevention Programme (Coates, et al., 2008)

The multilevel approach of combination behaviour change interventions is included into the HCT programme. The programmes are designed to include a range of activities to encourage people to reduce their risk of being infected with HIV and to increase their protective behaviour. The approach aims to delay sexual debut, reduce sexual partnerships, reduce age-disparate relationships, encourage mutual monogamy, promote correct and consistent condom use, and increase the frequency of HCT. The messaging at different levels is to promote individual behaviour change and to encourage families, communities and social networks to adopt and maintain healthy norms and a supportive environment. In this context, at the individual level, educational, skills building and counselling can be delivered through small groups or schools-based HIV prevention programmes, and while these may be informational, they should be followed up with motivational skills-based programmes. Among couples, the HCT programme attempts to motivate behaviour change within primary and secondary relationships, and to focus on factors that are critical drivers of the epidemic. Concordant HIV positive couples have the advantage of joint referral for care, support and treatment. HCT, through a family-centred approach, has the advantage of easy access, reduces stigma and facilitating disclosure.

Behaviour change can be facilitated through education programmes delivered by peer groups, community leadership or through networks. Involving peers groups in vulnerable populations of FSW, MSM, IDU, high risk men at truck stops and transport workers has been effective in increasing condom use and reducing STIs. Peer education programmes have been highly successful in increasing condom use among secondary school students. The involvement of community leaders to initiate HIV prevention and risk reduction messages, and to sustain risk reduction conversations, has been an innovative method of diffusing information through communities. Network-based interventions are particularly important in disseminating HIV risk reduction messages, as social networks have played a role in the transmission of HIV. Intervention information delivered through workplace programmes not only provide an opportunity to reach large numbers of often high risk individuals, but take advantage of motivational approaches and peer network support.

In the absence of an HIV vaccine, recent evidence from biomedical interventions appears to be promising, although the levels of evidence have been inconsistent. While male and female condoms, if used correctly and consistently, have proven to be very effective in blocking HIV transmission during sexual intercourse, the challenges of access, availability, lack of negotiating skills, co-operation of male partner and gender related violence have been major obstacles to their use. Despite their ability to prevent transmission of HIV by more than 80%, there has been no impact on HIV incidence rates. The inconclusive results from the STI treatment trials on HIV acquisition make them difficult to interpret and to translate from research to policy. However, treatment of STIs remains an important public health benefit. The results from the three randomised trials on MMC, demonstrating the protective effect against HIV acquisition among men, provides sufficient available evidence to consider it as a public health intervention and calls for the its urgent scale up.

The two trials of topical and oral antiretroviral compounds demonstrate the potential of methods that could be used for protection from HIV acquisition during sexual intercourse. However, research on biomedical interventions poses formidable challenges and concerns with implementation; product adherence and the possibility of sexual disinhibition. While expanding ART for HIV infected individuals to reduce infectiousness, expanding the wider HIV testing, and immediate ART for those testing positive strategy could have a major impact on HIV transmission and HIV-1 incidence. Nevertheless, strengthening and expanding the HIV treatment programme is expected to have substantial benefits in reducing morbidity, mortality and infectiousness.

In countries where HIV prevalence remain disturbingly high, there have been calls for prevention programmes to fully address social and economic factors that increase vulnerability, and to focus on high impact interventions. Currently, there are no research studies which best address the role of combination HIV prevention programmes to determine the appropriate mix of interventions. At the individual level, it is not clear whether there might be personal preferences for a particular intervention, whether choices might be available, individuals may require customised risk reduction options or the intervention may need to be tailored to different times in their lives. Even more difficult is the role of health care planners who have difficulty in prioritising interventions and whether to target specific groups or the general population, and then implementing those programmes.

Within the context of a combination HIV prevention strategies, structural approaches that address social, economic, and political factors are deeply entrenched and difficult to change. However, interventions to combat gender violence, gender or income inequality and the social marginalisation of risk groups are long-term intervention initiatives that need to be supported through community and leadership involvement within the broader economic and social development. Structural interventions of facilitating microcredit programmes, involving women in opportunities to improve household economic wellbeing, their social capital, and reduce their vulnerability to intimate partner violence and therefore to HIV. Furthermore, attempts to address structural factors to reduce HIV risk are promoted through partnerships with non-governmental organisations, community groups and government agencies, but their value has been difficult to measure. Access to broader family planning and reproductive health care services may further empower women to take control of their live and reduce their vulnerability to HIV.

7. Conclusions

HIV prevention interventions need to be appropriate to the epidemic context and to address the right population groups with co-ordinated evidence and informed strategies that work toward shared prevention goals. This means prioritising scale-up, quality delivery and close monitoring and evaluation of prevention strategies of those that have the best chance of success within the background on the epidemic scenario. Combination HIV prevention programmes need to include strategies that address socio-cultural and behavioural communication issues relating to sexual partnerships. They also need to provide safe biomedical interventions for MMC as well as topical microbicides and PrEP within the context of wider sexual and reproductive health services. This needs to include strategic condom programming, risk perceptions and awareness integrated through easily and widely available HCT services to ensure that the majority of person in need of treatment are supported and rapidly initiated on ART for maximum coverage. Optimistically, with an integrated combined response of HIV treatment and prevention, the benefits are expected to be substantial, particularly in high burden settings such as sub-Saharan Africa (figure 3) (Salomon, et al., 2005). An impact on HIV acquisition in a region with the highest burden of infection will impact on the disease globally. As agreed by the member states at the United Nations General Assembly Special Session on HIV/AIDS, countries need to continue with their efforts and scale up towards the goal of "universal access to comprehensive prevention programmes, treatment, care and support" which complement the United Nations Millennium Development Goals to reduce child mortality, improve maternal health and combat HIV/AIDS, malaria and other major diseases.

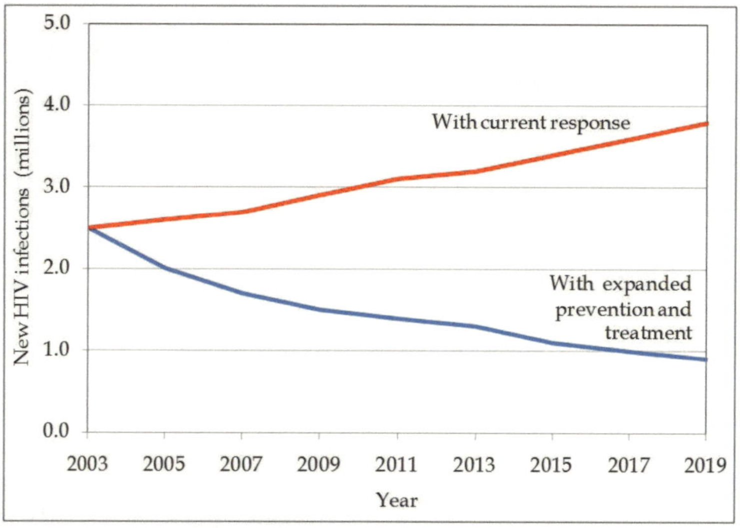

Fig. 3. Impact of treatment and prevention on new HIV infections in Africa (Salomon, et al., 2005).

8. References

Abdool Karim, Q., Abdool Karim, S. S., Frohlich, J. A., Grobler, A. C., Baxter, C., Mansoor, L. E., et al. (2010). Effectiveness and safety of tenofovir gel, an antiretroviral microbicide, for the prevention of HIV infection in women. *Science, 329*(5996), 1168-1174.

Abdool Karim, S. S., Richardson, B. A., Ramjee, G., Hoffman, I. F., Chirenje, Z. M., Taha, T., et al. (2011). Safety and effectiveness of BufferGel and 0.5% PRO2000 gel for the prevention of HIV infection in women. *AIDS*.

Abu-Raddad, L. J., & Longini, I. M., Jr. (2008). No HIV stage is dominant in driving the HIV epidemic in sub-Saharan Africa. *AIDS, 22*(9), 1055-1061.

Auvert, B., Taljaard, D., Lagarde, E., Sobngwi-Tambekou, J., Sitta, R., & Puren, A. (2005). Randomized, controlled intervention trial of male circumcision for reduction of HIV infection risk: the ANRS 1265 Trial. *PLoS Med, 2*(11), e298.

Bailey, R. C., Moses, S., Parker, C. B., Agot, K., Maclean, I., Krieger, J. N., et al. (2007). Male circumcision for HIV prevention in young men in Kisumu, Kenya: a randomised controlled trial. *Lancet, 369*(9562), 643-656.

Broder, S. (2010). The development of antiretroviral therapy and its impact on the HIV-1/AIDS pandemic. *Antiviral Res, 85*(1), 1-18.

Celum, C., Wald, A., Hughes, J., Sanchez, J., Reid, S., Delany-Moretlwe, S., et al. (2008). Effect of aciclovir on HIV-1 acquisition in herpes simplex virus 2 seropositive women and men who have sex with men: a randomised, double-blind, placebo-controlled trial. *Lancet, 371*(9630), 2109-2119.

Celum, C., Wald, A., Lingappa, J. R., Magaret, A. S., Wang, R. S., Mugo, N., et al. (2010). Acyclovir and transmission of HIV-1 from persons infected with HIV-1 and HSV-2. *N Engl J Med, 362*(5), 427-439.

Coates, T. J., Richter, L., & Caceres, C. (2008). Behavioural strategies to reduce HIV transmission: how to make them work better. *Lancet, 372*(9639), 669-684.

Donnell, D., Baeten, J. M., Kiarie, J., Thomas, K. K., Stevens, W., Cohen, C. R., et al. (2010). Heterosexual HIV-1 transmission after initiation of antiretroviral therapy: a prospective cohort analysis. *Lancet, 375*(9731), 2092-2098.

Dunkle, K. L., Jewkes, R., Nduna, M., Jama, N., Levin, J., Sikweyiya, Y., et al. (2007). Transactional sex with casual and main partners among young South African men in the rural Eastern Cape: prevalence, predictors, and associations with gender-based violence. *Soc Sci Med, 65*(6), 1235-1248.

Feldblum, P. J., Adeiga, A., Bakare, R., Wevill, S., Lendvay, A., Obadaki, F., et al. (2008). SAVVY vaginal gel (C31G) for prevention of HIV infection: a randomized controlled trial in Nigeria. *PLoS One, 3*(1), e1474.

Ghys, P. D., Diallo, M. O., Ettiegne-Traore, V., Satten, G. A., Anoma, C. K., Maurice, C., et al. (2001). Effect of interventions to control sexually transmitted disease on the incidence of HIV infection in female sex workers. *AIDS, 15*(11), 1421-1431.

Gouws, E., Stanecki, K. A., Lyerla, R., & Ghys, P. D. (2008). The epidemiology of HIV infection among young people aged 15-24 years in southern Africa. *AIDS, 22 Suppl 4*, S5-16.

Granich, R. M., Gilks, C. F., Dye, C., De Cock, K. M., & Williams, B. G. (2009). Universal voluntary HIV testing with immediate antiretroviral therapy as a strategy for elimination of HIV transmission: a mathematical model. *Lancet, 373*(9657), 48-57.

Grant, R. M., Lama, J. R., Anderson, P. L., McMahan, V., Liu, A. Y., Vargas, L., et al. (2010). Preexposure chemoprophylaxis for HIV prevention in men who have sex with men. *N Engl J Med, 363*(27), 2587-2599.

Gray, R. H., Kigozi, G., Serwadda, D., Makumbi, F., Watya, S., Nalugoda, F., et al. (2007). Male circumcision for HIV prevention in men in Rakai, Uganda: a randomised trial. *Lancet, 369*(9562), 657-666.

Gray, R. H., Wawer, M. J., Brookmeyer, R., Sewankambo, N. K., Serwadda, D., Wabwire-Mangen, F., et al. (2001). Probability of HIV-1 transmission per coital act in monogamous, heterosexual, HIV-1-discordant couples in Rakai, Uganda. *Lancet, 357*(9263), 1149-1153.

Hallett, T. B., Singh, K., Smith, J. A., White, R. G., Abu-Raddad, L. J., & Garnett, G. P. (2008). Understanding the impact of male circumcision interventions on the spread of HIV in southern Africa. *PLoS ONE, 3*(5), e2212.

Harrison, A., Cleland, J., & Frohlich, J. (2008). Young people's sexual partnerships in KwaZulu-Natal, South Africa: patterns, contextual influences, and HIV risk. *Stud Fam Plann, 39*(4), 295-308.

Hayes, R., Mosha, F., Nicoll, A., Grosskurth, H., Newell, J., Todd, J., et al. (1995). A community trial of the impact of improved sexually transmitted disease treatment on the HIV epidemic in rural Tanzania: 1. Design. *AIDS, 9*(8), 919-926.

Horton, R., & Das, P. (2008). Putting prevention at the forefront of HIV/AIDS. *Lancet, 372*(9637), 421-422.

Jewkes, R., Dunkle, K., Nduna, M., Levin, J., Jama, N., Khuzwayo, N., et al. (2006). Factors associated with HIV sero-positivity in young, rural South African men. *Int J Epidemiol, 35*(6), 1455-1460.

Johnson, B. T., Scott-Sheldon, L. A., Huedo-Medina, T. B., & Carey, M. P. (2011). Interventions to reduce sexual risk for human immunodeficiency virus in adolescents: a meta-analysis of trials, 1985-2008. *Arch Pediatr Adolesc Med, 165*(1), 77-84.

Joint United Nations Programme on HIV and AIDS and World Health Organization. (2007). Guidance on provider-initiated HIV testing and counselling in health facilities. *ISBN 978 92 4 159556 8 (NLM classification: WC 503.1).*

Joint United Nations Programme on HIV/AIDS (UNAIDS) and World Health Organization (WHO). (2007a). Practical Guidelines for Intensifying HIV Prevention: Towards Universal Access. *ISBN 978 92 9173 557 0 (NLM classification: WC 503.2), Geneva.*

Joint United Nations Programme on HIV/AIDS (UNAIDS) and World Health Organization (WHO). (2007b). WHO AND UNAIDS announce recommendations from expert meeting on male circumcision for HIV prevention *http://data.unaids.org/pub/pressrelease/2007/20070328_pr_mc_recommendations_en.pdf.*

Joint United Nations Programme on HIV/AIDS (UNAIDS) and World Health Organization (WHO). (2008). Report on the global HIV/AIDS epidemic 2008. *http://data.unaids.org/pub/GlobalReport/2008/JC1510_2008GlobalReport_en, Geneva.*

Joint United Nations Programme on HIV/AIDS (UNAIDS) and World Health Organization (WHO). (2010). Global report: UNAIDS report on the global AIDS epidemic 2010. *UNAIDS/10.11E | JC1958E ISBN 978-92-9173-871-7 (NLM classification: WC 503.4) http://www.unaids.org/globalreport/Global_report.htm.*

Kalichman, S. C., Ntseane, D., Nthomang, K., Segwabe, M., Phorano, O., & Simbayi, L. C. (2007). Recent multiple sexual partners and HIV transmission risks among people living with HIV/AIDS in Botswana. *Sex Transm Infect, 83*(5), 371-375.

Kamali, A., Byomire, H., Muwonge, C., Bakobaki, J., Rutterford, C., Okong, P., et al. (2010). A randomised placebo-controlled safety and acceptability trial of PRO 2000 vaginal microbicide gel in sexually active women in Uganda. *Sex Transm Infect, 86*(3), 222-226.

Kamali, A., Kinsman, J., Nalweyiso, N., Mitchell, K., Kanyesigye, E., Kengeya-Kayondo, J. F., et al. (2002). A community randomized controlled trial to investigate impact of improved STD management and behavioural interventions on HIV incidence in rural Masaka, Uganda: trial design, methods and baseline findings. *Trop Med Int Health, 7*(12), 1053-1063.

Kaul, R., Kimani, J., Nagelkerke, N. J., Fonck, K., Ngugi, E. N., Keli, F., et al. (2004). Monthly antibiotic chemoprophylaxis and incidence of sexually transmitted infections and

HIV-1 infection in Kenyan sex workers: a randomized controlled trial. *JAMA, 291*(21), 2555-2562.

Kenyon C, & Badri M. (2009). The role of concurrent sexual relationships in the spread of Sexually Transmitted Infections in young South Africans *The Southern African Journal of HIV Medicine, 10*(1), 29-36.

Khumalo-Sakutukwa, G., Morin, S. F., Fritz, K., Charlebois, E. D., van Rooyen, H., Chingono, A., et al. (2008). Project Accept (HPTN 043): a community-based intervention to reduce HIV incidence in populations at risk for HIV in sub-Saharan Africa and Thailand. *J Acquir Immune Defic Syndr, 49*(4), 422-431.

Kim, H. H., & Goldstein, M. (2009). High complication rates challenge the implementation of male circumcision for HIV prevention in Africa. *Nat Clin Pract Urol, 6*(2), 64-65.

Lagarde, E., Taljaard, D., Puren, A., & Auvert, B. (2009). High rate of adverse events following circumcision of young male adults with the Tara KLamp technique: a randomised trial in South Africa. *S Afr Med J, 99*(3), 163-169.

Leclerc-Madlala, S. (2008). Age-disparate and intergenerational sex in southern Africa: the dynamics of hypervulnerability. *AIDS, 22 Suppl 4*, S17-25.

Lissouba, P., Taljaard, D., Rech, D., Doyle, S., Shabangu, D., Nhlapo, C., et al. (2010). A model for the roll-out of comprehensive adult male circumcision services in African low-income settings of high HIV incidence: the ANRS 12126 Bophelo Pele Project. *PLoS Med, 7*(7), e1000309.

Lurie, M., Williams, B. G., & Gouws, E. (1997). Circular Migration and Sexual Networking in rural KwaZulu/Natal: Implications for the Spread of HIV and other Sexually Transmitted Diseases *Health Transition review, 7*, 15-24.

Moyo, W., Levandowski, B. A., MacPhail, C., Rees, H., & Pettifor, A. (2008). Consistent condom use in South African youth's most recent sexual relationships. *AIDS Behav, 12*(3), 431-440.

National Institute of Allergy and Infectious Diseases. (2011). QUESTIONS AND ANSWERS: The HPTN 052 Study: Preventing Sexual Transmission of HIV with Anti-HIV Drugs. http://www.niaid.nih.gov

Peterson, L., Nanda, K., Opoku, B. K., Ampofo, W. K., Owusu-Amoako, M., Boakye, A. Y., et al. (2007). SAVVY (C31G) gel for prevention of HIV infection in women: a Phase 3, double-blind, randomized, placebo-controlled trial in Ghana. *PLoS One, 2*(12), e1312.

Pettifor, A., Macphail, C., Rees, H., & Cohen, M. (2008). HIV and sexual behavior among young people: the South African paradox. *Sex Transm Dis, 35*(10), 843-844.

Pettifor, A. E., van der Straten, A., Dunbar, M. S., Shiboski, S. C., & Padian, N. S. (2004). Early age of first sex: a risk factor for HIV infection among women in Zimbabwe. *AIDS, 18*(10), 1435-1442.

Pilcher, C. D., Joaki, G., Hoffman, I. F., Martinson, F. E., Mapanje, C., Stewart, P. W., et al. (2007). Amplified transmission of HIV-1: comparison of HIV-1 concentrations in semen and blood during acute and chronic infection. *AIDS, 21*(13), 1723-1730.

Pilcher, C. D., Tien, H. C., Eron, J. J., Jr., Vernazza, P. L., Leu, S. Y., Stewart, P. W., et al. (2004). Brief but efficient: acute HIV infection and the sexual transmission of HIV. *J Infect Dis, 189*(10), 1785-1792.

Quinn, T. C., Wawer, M. J., Sewankambo, N., Serwadda, D., Li, C., Wabwire-Mangen, F., et al. (2000). Viral load and heterosexual transmission of human immunodeficiency virus type 1. Rakai Project Study Group. *N Engl J Med, 342*(13), 921-929.

Rottingen, J. A., Cameron, D. W., & Garnett, G. P. (2001). A systematic review of the epidemiologic interactions between classic sexually transmitted diseases and HIV: how much really is known? *Sex Transm Dis, 28*(10), 579-597.

Salomon, J. A., Hogan, D. R., Stover, J., Stanecki, K. A., Walker, N., Ghys, P. D., et al. (2005). Integrating HIV prevention and treatment: from slogans to impact. *PLoS Med, 2*(1), e16.

Schackman, B. R. (2010). Implementation science for the prevention and treatment of HIV/AIDS. *J Acquir Immune Defic Syndr, 55 Suppl 1*, S27-31.

Siegfried, N., Muller, M., Deeks, J. J., & Volmink, J. (2009). Male circumcision for prevention of heterosexual acquisition of HIV in men. *Cochrane Database Syst Rev*(2), CD003362.

Sikweyiya, Y., & Jewkes, R. (2009). Force and temptation: contrasting South African men's accounts of coercion into sex by men and women. *Cult Health Sex, 11*(5), 529-541.

Skoler-Karpoff, S., Ramjee, G., Ahmed, K., Altini, L., Plagianos, M. G., Friedland, B., et al. (2008). Efficacy of Carraguard for prevention of HIV infection in women in South Africa: a randomised, double-blind, placebo-controlled trial. *Lancet, 372*(9654), 1977-1987.

The Voluntary HIV-1 Counseling and Testing Efficacy Study Group. (2000). Efficacy of voluntary HIV-1 counselling and testing in individuals and couples in Kenya, Tanzania, and Trinidad: a randomised trial. *The Lancet, 356*(9224), 103-112.

Tobian, A. A., & Quinn, T. C. (2009). Herpes simplex virus type 2 and syphilis infections with HIV: an evolving synergy in transmission and prevention. *Curr Opin HIV AIDS, 4*(4), 294-299.

Tsai, C. C., Emau, P., Sun, J. C., Beck, T. W., Tran, C. A., Follis, K. E., et al. (2000). Post-exposure chemoprophylaxis (PECP) against SIV infection of macaques as a model for protection from HIV infection. *J Med Primatol, 29*(3-4), 248-258.

United Nations General Assembly. (2001). Declaration of Commitment on HIV/AIDS. New York, United Nations. . *http://www.unaids.org/en/AboutUNAIDS/Goals/UNGASS*.

United Nations Millineum Development Goals. (2000). New York, United Nations. *http://www.un.org/millenniumgoals/aids.shtml*, .

Van Damme, L., Govinden, R., Mirembe, F. M., Guedou, F., Solomon, S., Becker, M. L., et al. (2008). Lack of effectiveness of cellulose sulfate gel for the prevention of vaginal HIV transmission. *N Engl J Med, 359*(5), 463-472.

Van Damme, L., Ramjee, G., Alary, M., Vuylsteke, B., Chandeying, V., Rees, H., et al. (2002). Effectiveness of COL-1492, a nonoxynol-9 vaginal gel, on HIV-1 transmission in female sex workers: a randomised controlled trial. *Lancet, 360*(9338), 971-977.

Van Rompay, K. K. (2010). Evaluation of antiretrovirals in animal models of HIV infection. *Antiviral Res, 85*(1), 159-175.

Van Rompay, K. K., Singh, R. P., Brignolo, L. L., Lawson, J. R., Schmidt, K. A., Pahar, B., et al. (2004). The clinical benefits of tenofovir for simian immunodeficiency virus-infected macaques are larger than predicted by its effects on standard viral and immunologic parameters. *J Acquir Immune Defic Syndr, 36*(4), 900-914.

Van Tieua, H., & Koblina, B. (2009). HIV, alcohol, and noninjection drug use. *Current Opinion in HIV and AIDS 4*, 314-318.

Wald, A., & Link, K. (2002). Risk of human immunodeficiency virus infection in herpes simplex virus type 2-seropositive persons: a meta-analysis. *J Infect Dis, 185*(1), 45-52.

Watson-Jones, D., Weiss, H. A., Rusizoka, M., Changalucha, J., Baisley, K., Mugeye, K., et al. (2008). Effect of herpes simplex suppression on incidence of HIV among women in Tanzania. *N Engl J Med, 358*(15), 1560-1571.

Wawer, M. J., Gray, R. H., Sewankambo, N. K., Serwadda, D., Paxton, L., Berkley, S., et al. (1998). A randomized, community trial of intensive sexually transmitted disease control for AIDS prevention, Rakai, Uganda. *AIDS, 12*(10), 1211-1225.

Weiss, H. A., Dickson, K. E., Agot, K., & Hankins, C. A. (2010). Male circumcision for HIV prevention: current research and programmatic issues. *AIDS, 24 Suppl 4*, S61-69.

Williams, B. G., Lloyd-Smith, J. O., Gouws, E., Hankins, C., Getz, W. M., Hargrove, J., et al. (2006). The potential impact of male circumcision on HIV in Sub-Saharan Africa. *PLoS Med, 3*(7), e262.

Wilson, D., & Halperin, D. T. (2008). "Know your epidemic, know your response": a useful approach, if we get it right. *Lancet, 372*(9637), 423-426.

World Health Organization. (2009). Rapid advice: antiretroviral therapy for HIV infection in adults and adolescents -November 2009. *ISBN 978 92 4 159895 8*, http://www.who.int/hiv/pub/arv/rapid_advice_art.pdf.

Zablotska, I. B., Gray, R. H., Koenig, M. A., Serwadda, D., Nalugoda, F., Kigozi, G., et al. (2009). Alcohol use, intimate partner violence, sexual coercion and HIV among women aged 15-24 in Rakai, Uganda. *AIDS Behav, 13*(2), 225-233.

2

The State of the Science: A 5 - Year Review on the Computer - Aided Design for Global Anti - AIDS Drug Development

Jian Jun Tan[1], Chang Liu[1], Yao Wang[1],
Li Ming Hu[1], Cun Xin Wang[1]* and Xing Jie Liang[2]*
[1]*College of Life Science and Bio-engineering, Beijing University of Technology, Beijing*
[2]*CAS Key Laboratory for Biomedical Effects of Nanomaterials and Nanosafety, National Center for Nanoscience and Technology of China, Beijing*
China

1. Introduction

Since acquired immune deficiency syndrome (AIDS) was recognized by the U.S. centers for disease control and prevention in 1981 (Gallo, 2006), a large number of patients have died due to human immunodeficiency virus (HIV) related causes. In 2009, there were an estimated 33.3 million (31.4 million-35.3 million) persons living with HIV, 2.6 million (2.3 million-2.8 million) persons newly infected by HIV, and 1.8 million (1.6 million-2.1 million) dying due to AIDS. Research on vaccines is one of several strategies to reduce the worldwide harm from AIDS, however, these are early results, and have either not been developed to the point of human testing, or not been fully peer reviewed and replicated by other teams (Girard et al., 2006). Thus, the AIDS patient's treatment continues to focus on seeking the chemical anti-HIV agents. The current anti-HIV drugs approved by Food and Drug Administration (FDA) belong to nucleoside/nucleotide reverse transcriptase inhibitors (NRTIs), non-nucleoside reverse transcriptase inhibitors (NNRTIs), protease inhibitors (PIs), integrase inhibitors (INIs), fusion inhibitors (FIs) and entry inhibitors. The highly active antiretroviral therapy (HAART), which combines over three drugs, has dramatically improved the quality of patients' life (Barbaro et al., 2005; Gulick et al., 2003; Hammer et al., 1996). Three drugs are used together in order to reduce the likelihood of resistance. However, the therapeutic effect is confined by the side effects and toxicity due to long-term use, and the emergence of drug-resistant (Louie & Markowitz, 2002). The multiple steps of HIV replication cycle present novel therapeutic targets other than reverse transcriptase (RT) and protease (PT) for drug development (Greene, 2004; Tan et al., 2010) (Fig. 1). Continued efforts have been made on discovering new inhibitors that target not only RT, PT, IN and the transmembrane glycoprotein gp41, but also other viral targets, achievements on which have been reviewed comprehensively in literatures (Citterio &

Rusconi, 2007; Hazuda et al., 2009; Mastrolorenzo et al., 2007; Qian et al., 2009; Ravichandran et al., 2008; Stanic & Grana, 2009; Tan et al., 2010).

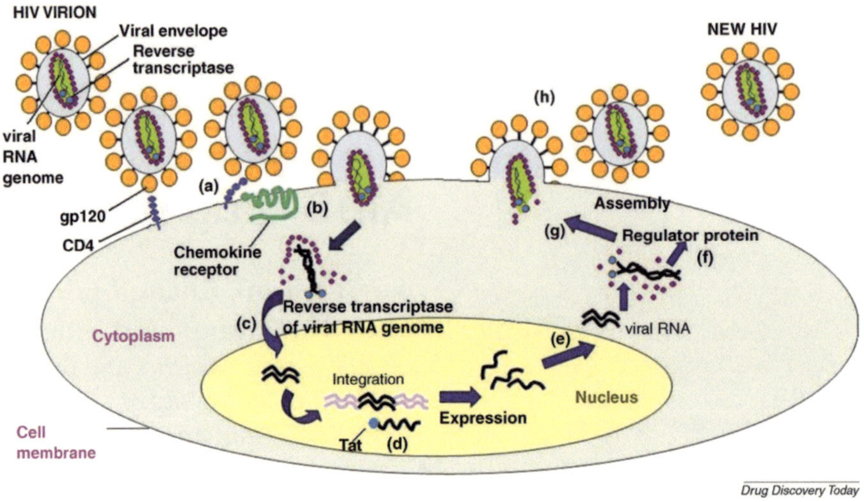

Fig. 1. The reproductive cycle of HIV. (a) Attachment. HIV attaches to CD4 and a chemokine receptor on the surface of a T cell. (b) Fusion. The virus fuses with the cell membrane and releases the virion core into the host cell. (c) Reverse transcription. The HIV enzyme called reverse transcriptase converts the single-stranded viral RNA to double-stranded viral DNA. (d) Integration. The viral DNA is integrated into cellular DNA by the HIV enzyme integrase. (e) Transcription. The virus uses the host enzyme RNA polymerase to create copies of the HIV genomic material and messenger RNA (mRNA). The mRNA is then used to produce long chains of viral proteins. (f) Regulator proteins. These are essential for the HIV viral cycle because they dramatically increase HIV gene expression. (g) Assembly. The HIV enzyme PT hydrolyzes the long chains of viral proteins into functional small proteins. New virions are then assembled with the small viral proteins and RNA. (h) Budding. The newly assembled virions use the cellular envelope as cover and bud off from the host cell.

Computer-aided drug design (CADD) is a rapidly evolving field to provide novel approaches for satisfying the needs of drug discovery (Durrant & McCammon, 2010; Sangma et al., 2010). By employing CADD or a combination of experiments and computational methods, a lot of novel inhibitors have been discovered that can inhibit HIV replication by interacting with the specific target(s). The use of CADD approaches can promote more efficient leads discovery and optimization as well as provide insights into target-ligand interactions. As the broad set of CADD approaches continues to develop, with innovative methods continually appearing, the impacts of CADD on drug discovery will undoubtedly continue to expand. In this chapter, we will take a look at the novel anti-HIV inhibitors discovered by CADD approaches in the past five years.

2. New developments of anti-HIV inhibitors

2.1 HIV fusion/entry inhibitors

The fusion of the viral membrane with host cell, cluster of differentiation 4 (CD4) cell, undergoes the following steps: (1) The N-terminal of the cell surface receptor CD4 binds to

the active cavity of envelope glycoprotein gp120, an essential envelope glycoprotein of HIV mediating the recognition between HIV and CD4; (2) The binding process induces an interacting area exposing to the host cell chemokine, such as C-X-C chemokine receptor type 4 (CXCR4) or C-C chemokine receptor type 5 (CCR5), which are the co-receptors for viral-cell interaction; (3) gp41, another envelope glycoprotein of HIV binding with gp120, is triggered by foregoing events to undergo a great conformational change, thereby allowing the viral-cell membrane fusion and viral genomic materials entry.
Accordingly, the fusion/entry inhibitors are designed to block three main targets, the CD4-gp120, gp120-CCR5/CXCR4 and CD4-gp41 interactions.

2.1.1 The entry inhibitors targeting CD4-gp120

HIV-1 gp120 consists of five conserved (C1-C5) and five variable (V1-V5) protein domains (Horuk, 2009), among which the conserved domains form the core domain of gp120, while the variable domains contribute to the surface of gp120. On the other hand, gp120 is also divided into three functional regions, an inner domain involved in interactions with gp41 and the formation of trimer that is the bioactive conformation of gp120, an outer domain exposed to the molecule surface and is highly glycosylated, and a bridging sheet resulted by the great conformational change following the binding of CD4 and gp120 (Teixeira et al., 2011).
Multi-target HIV-1 entry inhibitors hexa-arginine-neomycin-conjugate (NeoR6) and nona-D-arginine-neomycin-conjugate (Neo-r9) are mimics of V3 loop of gp120 which is involved in the interaction between HIV-1 and CXCR4, exhibiting high antiviral potent and low cytotoxicity. While, Berchanski et al. assumed that both NeoR6 and Neo-r9 may inhibit HIV-1 entry by interfering with the CD4-gp120 binding (Berchanski & Lapidot, 2007). A homology model of unliganded HIV-1 IIIB gp120 was constructed for subsequent docking with NeoR6/Neo-r9. Full geometric-electrostatic docking and flexible docking were performed respectively. It was found that these two multi-target inhibitors were apt to bind to gp120 at the CD4 binding site and mutations in the CD4 binding region greatly attenuate the energetic favor of NeoR6/Neo-r9-gp120 complexes. Simultaneously, another mechanism of anti-HIV-1 activity of NeoR6/Neo-r9 was described as the interference of gp120-CXCR4 interaction. This means that NeoR6/Neo-r9 inhibits HIV-1 in a multi-approach.
The CD4-binding site on gp120, which is a hydrophobic pocket occupied by CD4 Phe43, could be suggested as an ideal target for molecules that interfere with gp120-CD4 interaction. Caporuscio et al. performed a computational analysis containing molecular dynamics (MD) simulation, pharmacophore modeling, virtual screening and molecular docking to identify small molecules targeting the CD4 binding cavity and thereby blocking gp120-CD4 interactions (Caporuscio et al., 2009). Finally, two compounds, **2** and **4** (Fig. 2), with micromolar activity (EC_{50} = 22 and 9 μM, respectively), low toxicity and, more importantly, novel scaffolds were identified from a database containing more than 200,000 available compounds.
BMS-378806 was discovered recently as a small molecule inhibitor targeting the binding of host-cell CD4 with viral gp120 protein and showed potent anti-HIV activity at a nanomolar range (Ho et al., 2006). Docking calculations and the Comparative Molecular Field Analysis (CoMFA) model on BMS-378806 and its analogs revealed that the azaindole ring and methyl groups seem to play an essential role on binding with the CD4 cavity of gp120 through hydrogen bond or hydrophobic interactions. This is consistent with the previous theoretical

studies and facilitated the novel drug design based on scaffolds of BMS-378806 and its analogs (Kong et al., 2006; Teixeira et al., 2009).

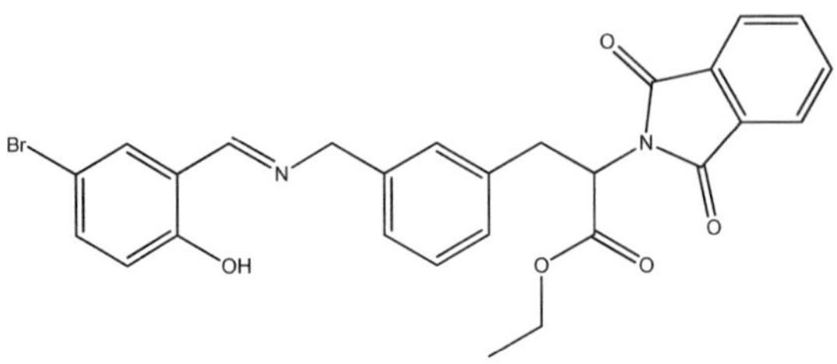

2

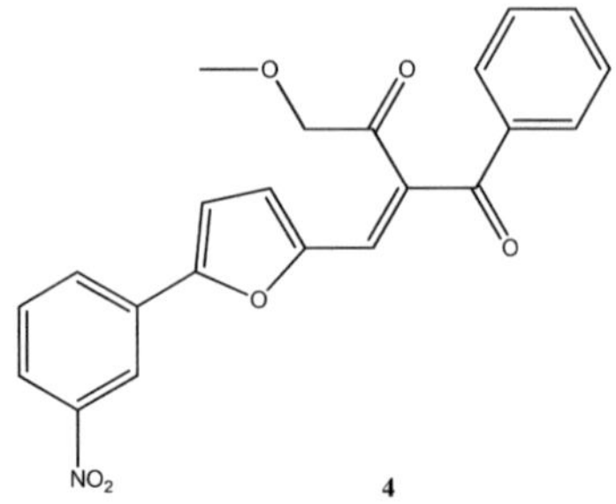

4

Fig. 2. The structure of entry inhibitors

Compound NBD-556 discovered by high-throughput screening few years ago was shown to mimic CD4-induced conformational changes in gp120 and accordingly compete CD4 binding with gp120 (Haim et al., 2009). Starting with the structures of NBD, Lalonde et al. defined the chemotype of NBD with three functional regions and performed two orthogonal screening methods, GOLD docking and ROCS shape-based similarity searching based on these three different regions (Lalonde et al., 2011).

2.1.2 The fusion inhibitors targeting gp41

HIV-1 gp41 is a complex polypeptide, consisting of seven domains, a transmembrane region (TM) which anchors gp41 on the virus surface, a membrane proximal region (MPER) locating near the viral membrane as its name implies, C-terminal helical heptad repead (CHR) and N-terminal helical heptad repeat (NHR) linked by a flexible loop region, a fusion peptide proximal region (FPPR), and a fusion peptide region (FP) which is responsible for binding to host cell membrane. Among which, the CHR and NHR regions are the core structure of gp41 where most peptide inhibitors are derived from (Naider & Anglister, 2009). In fact, gp41 shows bioactivity in a trimeric form as gp120, and contains a critical inhibitory target site—a hydrophobic cavity in the NHR trimer structure for the binding of CHR trimer followed by gp41 6-Helix formation (Strockbine & Rizzo, 2007). However, the total 3D structure of gp41 is still unknown. Thus, this limits the development of HIV-1 FIs targeting gp41.

N-substituted pyrrole derivatives, such as NB-2 and NB-64, were recently identified by Jiang et al. as the novel HIV-1 entry inhibitors which inhibit HIV-1 fusion and entry in low concentration by occupying the gp41 cavity and interfering with the gp41 six-helix bundle (6-HB) formation (Jiang et al., 2004). Molecular docking and mutational analysis revealed that N-substituted pyrrole binds to gp41 cavity through hydrophobic and ionic interactions and conserved residue Lys574 in the cavity is one of the key factors for 6-HB formation and HIV infection. When docking NB-2 into the gp41 hydrophobic pocket, docking results indicated that the carboxyl group of the molecule prefers to bind with Lys574 forming a salt-bridge (He et al., 2007). Also in the molecular docking analysis, a 3D-Quantitative structure-activity relationship (QSAR) CoMFA model was generated based on 23 pyrrole derivatives (He et al., 2007). The obtained model showed a satisfied correlative predictive capacity with statistical results of R^2 = 0.984 and r^2 = 0.463. The descriptors selected for modeling were related to the shape and electron reactivity for C atoms. This indicates that substitution of electron-rich groups on the phenyl ring of pyrrole derivatives may result in improving biological activity. Based on above conclusions, a series of structure-modified N-phenyl-2,5-dimethylpyrrole derivatives with m-COOH on the benzene ring were designed and synthesised with a more effective inhibitory activity than N-phenylpyrrole anologys (Liu et al., 2008). These results suggested that nonpolar interactions are the main interactions of binding, while polar interactions adjust the orientation of the molecules binding into the target site. This guided authors to design and synthesize a series of 2-aryl-5-(4-oxo-3-phenethyl-2-thioxothiazolidinylidene-methyl)furans 3a-o with better inhibitory activity than NB-2 and NB-64 (Jiang et al., 2011). Compounds **12l** and **12m** (Fig. 3) showed high potency against infection by laboratory-adapted and primary HIV-1 IIIB strains with EC_{50} at a low nanomolar level (18 and 14 nM, respectively) and inhibited HIV-1-mediated cell-cell fusion and the gp41 six-helix bundle formation.

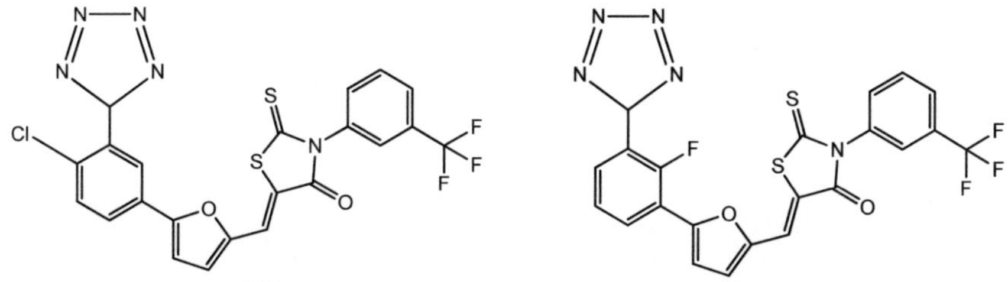

Fig. 3. The molecular structures of designed inhibitors by Jiang et al.

The additional analyses with molecular mechanics Poisson Boltzmann surface area (MM-PBSA)/ molecular mechanics Generalized Born surface area (MM-GBSA) were carried out to predict the binding mode of NB-2/NB-64 and gp41 (Cong et al., 2010). Based on above studies, Tan et al. obtained six new derivatives of NB2 using *de novo* design and screened out a series of molecules with novel structures using the Leapfrog and Autodock programs. They obtained a potent fusion inhibitor (IC_{50} = 41.1 μg/mL) by the structure-based modification. Unfortunately, the inhibitive activity of these compounds isn't greater than that of NB2 (Tan et al., 2011).

2.1.3 The entry inhibitors targeting co-receptor CCR5/CXCR4

A 3D-pharmacophore model was developed based on a great number of pyrrolidine-based and butane-based CCR5 antagonists as HIV-1 entry inhibitors targeting CCR5 (Kong et al., 2008). The most reliable hypotheses consisted of two positive ionizable points and three hydrophobic groups, with R^2 of 0.924. The 74 external compounds were predicted with this model, yielding a correlation coefficient of 0.703. This potent model may be applied to the design and screening of the novel compounds.

Zhuo et al. took a series of 1,3,4-trisubstituted pyrrolidine-based CCR5 receptor inhibitors into account for CoMFA and CoMSIA (Comparative Molecular Similarity Indices) analysis (Zhuo et al., 2008). Compared with CoMSIA model (r^2 = 0.958, q^2 = 0.677), the CoMFA model was more predictive and reliable with better statistical data of r^2 = 0.952 and q^2 = 0.637. Further contour mapping showed that introduction of the electron-rich fluorine atoms into the molecule may promote the antiviral potent in some extent.

To compare the differences between ligand-based and receptor-based approaches, Perez-Nueno et al. performed virtual screenings applied on identifying highly active CXCR4 and CCR5 antagonists, using ligand shape-matching and ligand-receptor docking approaches (Perez-Nueno et al., 2008). For ligand-apporoach virtual screening, the shape-based and the property-based approaches were carried out in a library consisting of 248 and 354 known CXCR4 and CCR5 inhibitors, respectively, and some 4700 similar presumed inactive molecules. For the receptor-based approaches, the models of CXCR4 and CCR5 were built derived from bovine rhodopsin. Then, two highly active molecules, AMD3100 and TAK779, were docked against CXCR4 and CCR5, respectively, followed by a docking-based virtual screening by using the docked AMD3100 and TAK779 conformations as templates. Compared with property-matching and docking-based tools, the ligand-based shape-matching approach provided better performance. Moreover, the enrichments for CXCR4 was better than those for CCR5. Based on above results, Perez-Nueno et al. continued to perform a prospective vitual screening combining docking-based, pharmacophore modeling, QSAR analysis and shape-matching techniques, and five highly activive compounds were finally identified using above computational tools, with the best activity values of 22 nM (molecule **10**, Fig. 4) (Perez-Nueno et al., 2009).

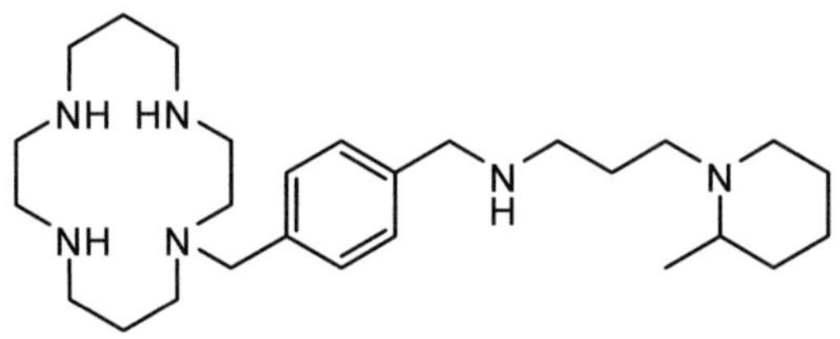

Molecule 10

Fig. 4. The structure of entry inhibitor targeting co-receptor CCR5/CXCR4

2.2 HIV reverse transcriptase inhibitors

2.2.1 The structure of HIV-1 reverse transcriptase

HIV-1 RT transforms a single-stranded viral genomic RNA into a double-stranded DNA that is lately integrated into the genome of the host cell (Himmel et al., 2009). HIV-1 RT is a dimer made up of two subdomains (Fig. 5). One subdomain, a 66-kD subunit (p66), consists of 560 amino acid residues, and the other subdomain, a 51kD subunit (p51), consists of 440 residues and is close to p66. The sequences of the first 440 residues for both p66 and p51 are same. The larger subunit of the RT heterodimer, p66, includes two domains: the N-terminal polymerase domain and the C-terminal Ribonuclease H (RNH) domain. They are responsible for the two catalytic activities of RT (Sarafianos et al., 2009). The N-terminal polymerase domain is made up of four subdomains: fingers (residues 1-85 and 118-155), palm (residues 86-117 and 156-236), thumb (237-318), and connection (319-426) (Jacobomolina et al., 1993). The structures of the individual subdomains in p51 and p66 are same, but the arrangement of subdomains in order is different. The nucleic-acid binding cleft is constructed chiefly by five subdomains (fingers, palm, thumb, connection, and RNH) coming from p66 subunit. The connection and thumb subdomains in p51 subunit construct the floor of the binding cleft. In the presence of nucleic acids, the p66 subunit assumes an "open" conformation, in which the thumb rotates away from the fingers forming a large cleft that affords a space for double-stranded nucleic acid substrates. On the other hand, in the absence of nucleic acid, the p66 subunit presumes a "closed" conformation, in which the thumb rotates toward the fingers to cram this cleft. The binding cleft is formed so that the nucleic acid contacts with both the polymerase and the RNH subdomains; these are placed about 17 or 18 base pairs apart on the nucleic acid substrate.

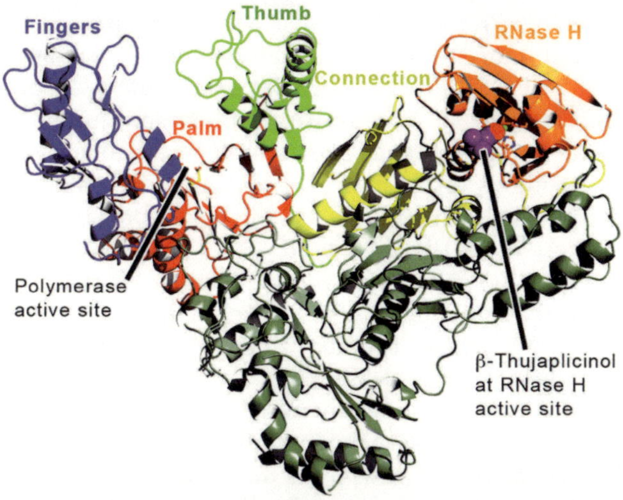

Fig. 5. Overview of RT Structure (Himmel et al., 2009).An RT ribbon diagram of the RT/β-thujaplicinol structure is shown. The subdomains of the p66 subunit (including the RNase H domain) are colored as follows: fingers, blue; palm, red; thumb, green; connection, yellow; RNH, orange; and the p51 subunit, gray. β-thujaplicinol is shown spacefilled in magenta and red.

2.2.2 The quantitative structure activity relationship-based drug design

Pawar et al. studied the correlation of the chemical structure of Isatin analogues and their anti-HIV activity using Multiple Linear Regression Analysis (MLRA) and k Nearest Neighbor Molecular Field Analysis (kNN MFA), respectively (Pawar et al., 2010). New chemical entities were designed according to the results obtained from QSAR studies. The most promising compounds were chosen from molecular modeling studies. Finally, they found that compound **N21** (Fig. 6) showed significant RT inhibitory activity and was comparable with standard Navirapine.

Using isosteric replacement in the central B-ring of diarylpyrimidine compounds, Qin et al. designed a series of diarylaniline and 1,5-diarylbenzene-1,2- diamine derivatives (Qin et al., 2010). The most promising compound **37** (Fig. 6) showed significant anti-HIV activity (EC_{50} values are 0.003 μM against HIV-1 wild-type strains and 0.005 μM against several drug-resistant strains, respectively). Their results demonstrated an important structure-activity relationship (SAR) for diarylanilines that an NH_2 group on the central benzene ring ortho to the anilinemoiety is crucial for interaction with K101 of the NNRTI binding site in HIV-1 RT, likely by forming H-bonds with K101.

Hu et al. studied a series of HIV-1 RT inhibitors (2-amino-6-arylsulfonylbenzonitriles and their thio and sulfinyl congeners) using QSAR. Topological and geometrical descriptors, as well as quantum mechanical energy-related and charge distribution-related descriptors generated from CODESSA, were applied to depict the molecules (Hu et al., 2009). Using Principal component analysis (PCA) distinguishes training set. Six approachs: multiple linear regression (MLR), multivariate adaptive regression splines (MARS), radial basis function neural networks (RBFNN), general regression neural networks (GRNN), projection pursuit regression (PPR) and support vector machine (SVM) were utilized to generate QSAR models between anti-HIV-1 activity and HIV-1 RT binding affinity. The results showed that the capacities of prediction of PPR and SVM models were dominant.

The most common resistant mutation by clinical observation is the substitution of lysine to asparagines at codon 103 of RT (K103N) (Bacheler et al., 2001). In order to obtain the necessary structural information for receptor-based inhibitors design, molecular docking combined with 3D-QSAR was applied to a series of structurally diversed HIV-RT inhibitors (Juan, 2008). Using two methods established 3D-QSAR models. The first method was the flexibility-based molecular alignment (FMA), similar to receptor-based alignment, which sampled the biological space of K103N mutant HIV-RT. FMA was finished by docking the inhibitors to four mutant HIV-RT structures with PDB codes: 1SV5, 2IC3, 1FKP and 1FKO. The best superposition of the inhibitors advised novel inhibition of nevirapine-resistance. The second method was the dataset division which utilized the principal component analysis (PCA) to classify the dataset into training and test sets. Predictive statistical models were obtained using the FMA method for the molecular alignment of compounds based on known structures of HIV-RT complexes. Similarly, employing the most descriptive compounds (MDC) method displayed fitness for the division of dataset compounds. The result showed the relevance of hydrophobic and flexible properties of the inhibitors to favor binding interactions at the active site of mutant HIV-RT.

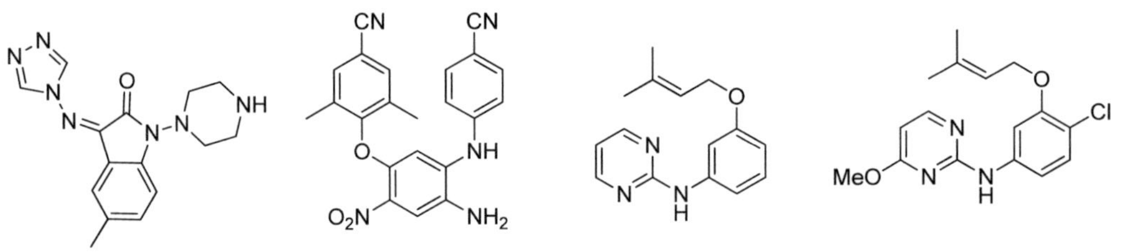

N21 **37** **2a** **2m**

Fig. 6. Structure of reverse transcriptase inhibitors

2.2.3 The fragment-based drug design

Geitmann, M. et al. identified a novel scaffold inhibiting wild type and drug resistant variants of HIV-1 RT in a library consisting of 1040 fragments using screening strategy (Geitmann et al., 2011). The fragments were remarkably different from already known NNRTIs, as demonstrated by a Tversky similarity analysis. A screening project involving surface plasmon resonance (SPR) biosensor-based interaction analysis and enzyme inhibition was used. Ten hits were chosen, and then hits' affinities and resistance profiles were evaluated using wild type and three drug resistant enzyme variants (K103N, Y181C, and L100I). One fragment with EC_{50} at a low μM level against all four tested enzyme variants was chosen.

Employing the BOMB program yielded NNRTI leads (Jorgensen et al., 2006). BOMB generated compounds into an active site by adding user-selected substituents to a core. The core can stuff four substituents and/or linked together. The BOMB libraries include more than 100 cores and 600 substituents, which are general fragments in drugs. A screening search was executed for each compound, each conformer was the best location by all kinds of optimally positioned, and the lowest-energy one was chosen. The output from BOMB contained its predicted activities value, receptor-ligand binding energetic and structural informations, and predicted properties including solubility and cell permeabilities using QikProp program (Jorgensen & Duffy, 2002).

Based on the above design considerations, virtual libraries were formed using two motifs, U-Het-NH-Ph and Het-NH-Ph-U, where U is an unsaturated, hydrophobic group and Het is an aromatic heterocycle. The first motif had been more commonly employed, so initial attention was directed at the latter one. Using NH3 as the core built the ligands, positioned to hydrogen bond with the K101 carbonyl group. Het includes 61 five- and six-membered heterocycles, and 47 alternatives for U. Using above approach obtained 100 lead compounds. In order to narrow the possibilities for the compounds, Monte Carlo simulations using free-energy perturbation simulations were carried out. The present computational strategy had been effective in identifying a 30 μM lead compound **2a** (Fig. 6) that could be rapidly progressed to a 10 nM **2m** (Fig. 6) NNRTI (Jorgensen et al., 2006).

2.3 HIV integrase inhibitors

2.3.1 The structure of HIV-1 integrase

HIV-1 integrase (IN) is a 288-residue enzyme with molecular weight of 32-KD, which is encoded by the pol gene. IN consists of three functional domains as follows: the N-terminal domain (NTD, residues 1-49) with a non-conventional HHCC zinc-finger motif, promoting protein multimerization; the catalytic core domain (CCD, residues 50-212) containing a canonical DDE motif and involved in DNA substrate recognition; the C-terminal domain (CTD, residues 213-288) binding DNA non-specifically and helping to stabilize the IN-DNA complexes (Fig. 7). At present, the structures of IN three respective domains and conjunctional structures of CCD with CTD/NTD have been solved through X-ray and NMR

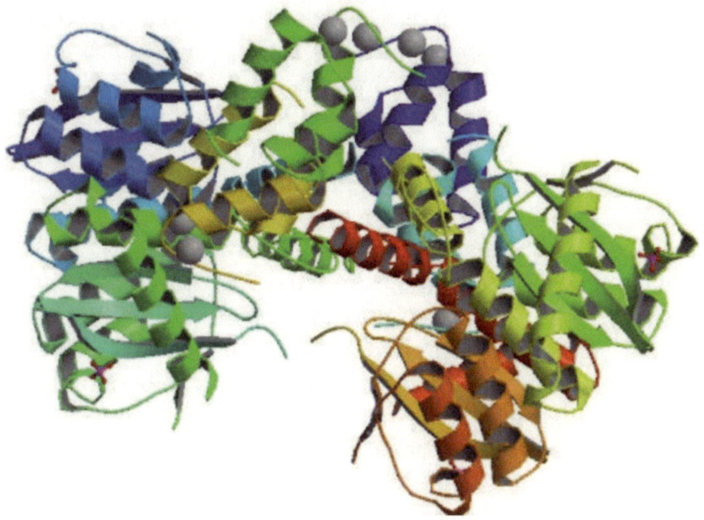

Fig. 7. The structure of HIV integrase (Wang et al., 2001)

spectroscopy (Li et al., 2011). Unfortunately, the full-length structure of IN is still unknown, which thus limit the development of HIV-1 IN inhibitor design. But, the complete structure of the Primate foamy virus (PFV) IN complexed with the substrate DNA and IN inhibitors raltegravir or elvitegravir has recently been obtained (Hare et al., 2010).

IN mediates the integration of viral DNA into host genome in two steps. Firstly, two nucleotides are removed from each 3′-end of each strand of viral DNA to produce new hydroxyl ends (CA-3′OH), which is termed as 3′-processing. Secondly, the recessed 3′-ends of viral DNA are covalently joined to the host genome, which named DNA strand transfer. The DNA strand transfer occurs in nucleus. During the integration procedure, divalent metal ions, such as Mg^{2+} or Mn^{2+}, are necessary.

2.3.2 The Quantitative structure activity relationship-based drug design

QSAR analysis is the most common method for investigates into the relationship of structure and bioactivity, and, more importantly, may provide beneficial suggestion for subsequent novel anti-HIV drug design.

Nunthaboot et al generated a single 3D-QSAR models for 89 HIV-1 IN inhibitors of a whole variety of 11 structurally different classes using CoMFA and CoMSIA (Nunthaboot et al., 2006). The best CoMFA model yielded the $q^2 = 0.698$ and the $r^2 = 0.947$. Contour mapping of CoMFA emphasized steric interactions and electrostatic interactions as the important files contributing to the activities of inhibitors. The best CoMSIA model gave $q^2 = 0.724$ and $r^2 = 0.864$. CoMSIA contour revealed the significance of hydrogen bond between Glu152, Lys156 and Lys159 residues and the side chains of inhibitors. Saiz-Urra *et al* obtained another QSAR model with a r^2 of 0.669 based on 172 compounds that belong to 11 different classes using GETAWAY descriptors, Atom-Weights, Geometry and Topology (Saiz-Urra et al., 2007) .

It's not difficult to see that descriptors applied in QSAR analysis are essential to the predict ability of QSAR model. While, not only descriptors, but also analysis technique, statistic method and other parameters show great influence on reliability and accuracy of predict model. Leonard *et al.* performed 3D-QSAR analysis by molecular shape analysis (MSA) technique based on 36 styrylquinoline derivatives (Leonard & Roy, 2008). Unlike common QSAR, the so-called Jurs descriptors, which are total polar surface area (TPSA), relative polar surface area (RPSA), relative hydrophobic surface area (RASA) and relative positive charge (RPCG), were applied, along with five statistical methods including stepwise regression, genetic function approximation (GFA), multiple linear regression with factor analysis (FA-MLR), partial least squares regression with factor analysis (FA-PLS) and genetic partial least squares (G/PLS). According to results, the best validation statistics were obtained with stepwise regression and GFA derived model with r^2_{pred} and r^2_{test} being 0.611 and 0.664, respectively. More importantly, compared with previous analysis with the same object through CoMFA and docking studies (Ma et al., 2004), the introduction of Jurs descriptors into MSA significantly improved the predictability of QSAR model. Similar research carried out on carboxylic acid derivatives recently (Cheng et al., 2010b) indicated that the combination of the replacement method (RM) method which were used to select descriptors with the support vector machine (SVM) by which mathematical models were obtained, along with 3D-MoRSE (3D-Molecular Representation of Structure based on Electron diffraction) descriptors were the best regression approaches to build QSAR models with the satisfied r^2 of 0.852.

De melo et al. applied multivariate QSAR method to 4,5-dihydroxypyrimidine carboxamides HIV-1 IN inhibitors with four descriptors containing the energy of the highest occupied molecular orbital, the component vector to the overall polarizability in the Y plane, the total energy, and the sum of the bond electrotopological values of carbon-carbon aromatic bonds in which the carbons are not substituted and got a reasonable model with $q^2 = 0.58$, $r^2 = 0.87$ (de Melo & Ferreira, 2009). Interestingly, all of the four descriptors chosen to predict the inhibitory activity of investigated compounds were relate to the electronic distribution, which indicates a requisite relation between the HIV-1 IN inhibition and the electronic distribution of the investigated inhibitors.

Theoretically, QSAR study belongs to ligand-based drug design approach, but the information of receptor is also useful sometimes to QSAR modeling. Dhaked et al. developed a receptor-based 3D-QSAR method—comparative residue interaction analysis (CoRIA) on 81 molecules belonging to 13 structurally different classes of IN inhibitors (Dhaked et al., 2009). This receptor-based model revealed that Asp64, Thr66, Val77, Asp116, Glu152 and Lys159 are key residues influencing the binding of ligands with IN. According to suggestions of the CoRIA models, a **known molecule** (Fig. 8) of data set was modified to a **new molecule** (Fig. 8) with higher anti-HIV activity by intensifying the van der Waals interaction with residues Asp64 and Asp116 and the Columbic interaction of residue Thr66, and while reducing the Columbic interaction with Val77. The activity value (pIC_{50}) was improved from 4.92 to the best 5.22

Ravichandran et al.. obtained a QSAR model with R^2_{CVext} of 0.630 and R^2_{Pred} of 0.688 using 1,3,4-oxadiazole substituted naphthyridine derivatives (Ravichandran et al., 2010). The descriptors valence connectivity index order, lowest unoccupied molecular orbital and dielectric energy exhibited significant affect on the inhibition of HIV-1 IN activity by 1,3,4-oxadiazole substituted naphthyridine derivatives. Coefficient of these descriptors indicated that highly branched, unsaturated and long chain groups as well as high electro negativity are favorable for HIV-1 IN inhibitory activity; in contrary, the increased dielectric constant of the compounds is unfavorable. The selected descriptors could serve as a novel guideline for the design of novel and potent antagonists targeting HIV-1 IN.

Chalcones are discovered as a novel class of HIV IN inhibitors with satisfied antiviral activity. But, unfortunately, many chalcones are non-specific inhibitors and possess cytotoxicity. Based on two chalcones previously reported (Deng et al., 2006), Deng et al subsequently developed five six-feature pharmacophores and two four-feature pharmacophores aiming to discover non-chalcone-based compounds with low cytoxicity . The best pharmacophore model was applied as a query to search a small molecule database, 44 compounds were chosen and showed high inhibitory potency at IC_{50} values <100 μM. Among these molecules, compound **62** (Fig.8) stood out finally as the most active molecule with IC_{50} value of 1.9 μM and 0.6 μM for 3-processing and strand transfer process, respectively (Deng et al., 2006).

Sharma et al. generated a pharmacophore model based on a series of 3-keto salicylic acid chalcones and related amides as novel HIV-1 IN inhibitors (Sharma et al., 2011). A set of pharmacophoric sites were obtained, including H-bond acceptor (A), H-bond donor (D), hydrophobic group (H), negatively charged group (N) and aromatic ring (R). To identify a common pharmacophore hypothesis, the top twenty pharmacophore hypotheses were selected to undergo further analysis by partial least square (PLS) regression-based 3D-QSAR. The best hypothesis exhibited the highest predicted ability of $q^2 = 0.57$ and $r^2 = 0.74$, consisting of six features, two H-bond acceptors, two hydrophobic groups, a negative group and one aromatic ring. Subsequently, CoMFA and CoMSIA 3D-QSAR model were built based on pharmacophore mapping. The combinational application of pharmacophore model with QSAR analysis afforded the best model with q^2 and r^2 values of 0.54 and 0.94, respectively, which would guide the rational design of more potent novel 3-keto salicylic acid IN inhibitors.

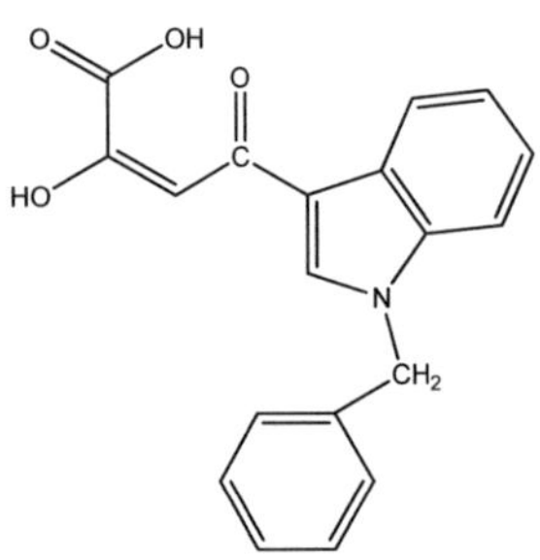

Known molecule

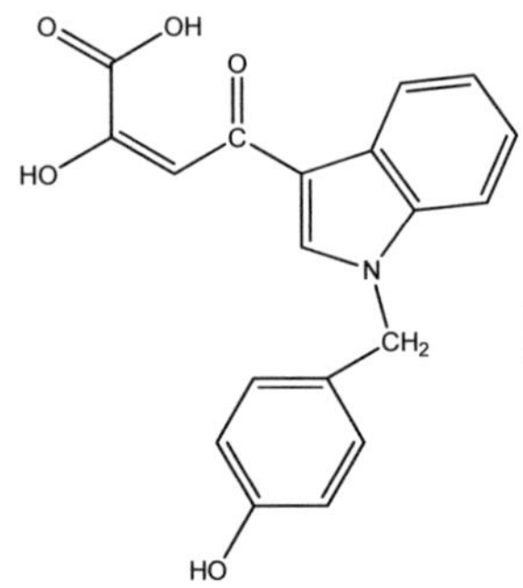

New molecule

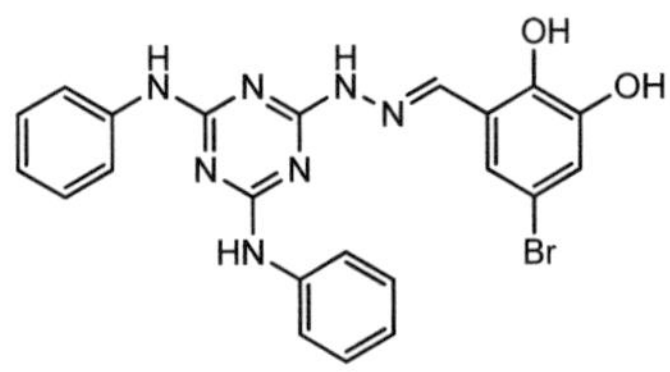

62

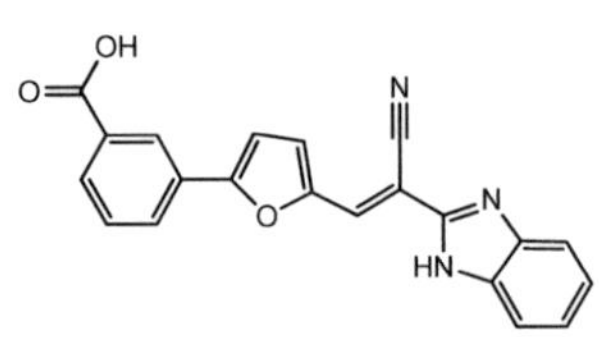

BAS-0314191

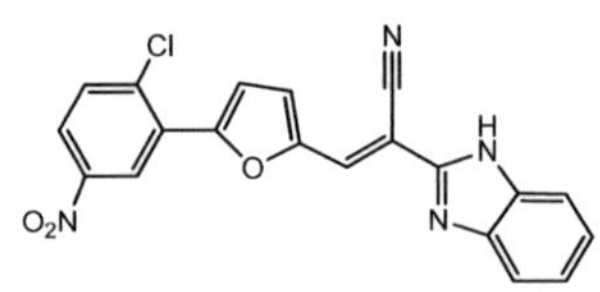

BAS-0717929

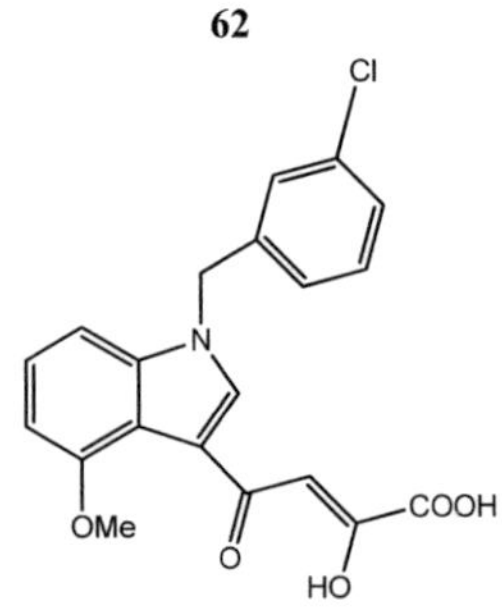

34

Fig. 8. The structure of integrase inhibitors

2.3.3 Combined the receptor-based and ligand-based drug design approach

As QSAR analysis, the pharmacophore model is built based on the structural information of ligands. While, only ligand-based or receptor-based research is not enough perfectly sometimes (Dayam et al., 2008) because the inhibition of inhibitors against IN is implemented through a integral processing with anticipation of both the IN enzyme and inhibitor molecules. Accordingly, it's becoming increasingly popular to combine the receptor-based drug design (RBDD) and ligand-based drug design (LBDD) approach so that both the small molecules and receptor can be taken into account and the result would be more rational and valid.

Tintori et al employed an innovative virtual screening approach consisting of the electron-ion interaction potential technique, druglike property calculation, pharmacophoric model generation, and docking studies, with which both the long- and short- range interactions between molecules could be calculated (Tintori et al., 2007). As result, 12 compounds were eventually screened out from a database containing over 200,000 molecules to in vitro assay and one of them **BAS-0314191** (Fig. 8) displayed a comparative satisfied activity with IC_{50} value. Subsequent substructure codification identified a better molecule **BAS-0717929** (Fig.

8) with a higher IC_{50} value from 69 to 10 μM. Using the same approach as Tintori, other hit compounds as IN binding inhibitors with corresponding IC_{50} values with **BAS-0717929** (Fig. 8) were discovered from a 200,000 molecule-contained database (Mugnaini et al., 2007).

Tintori et al. applied a novel multistep computational protocol for the development of structure-based pharmacophores which combined pharmacophore generation with conformational analysis, docking studies and MD simulation (Tintori et al., 2008). A conformational search was initially performed from the flexible loop region of IN to cluster the conformations with low enough energy. Then, three pharmacophore models were generated containing hydrogen bond acceptors, hydrogen bond donors and hydrophobic features based on the best conformation found in the most populated cluster and followed by a database screening using these three hypotheses alternately. As result, one hit compound was identified finally and showed satisfied EC_{50} value of 30 μM and IC_{50} values of 25 μM and 3 μM toward 3-processing and strand transfer, respectively.

Zhang et al. have recently developed a 3-D pharmacophore model from two diketoacids (DKAs) inhibitors, MK-0518 and S-1360 (Zhang et al., 2009). For the strong anti-HIV potency and reliable drug-like properties, they mapped inhibitor conformations into the pharmacophore model and superimposed it in their docking model with IN core domain. Thus, the corresponding positions between the pharmacophore model and IN residues were identified, according which the pharmacophore was improved further. Finally, a better pharmacophore model including one hydrophobic feature, three hydrogen pair features and one hydrogen-bond donor feature was generated and displayed a higher retrieval capability and universality than previous studies (De Luca et al., 2008).

Ferro et al. combined SBDD with LBDD approach to investigate the binding mechanism of HIV IN inhibitors and then obtained a set of structurally attractive lead compounds (Ferro et al., 2009). Employing combination of ligand-based pharmacophore and receptor-based docking approach, a series of 4-[1-(4-fluorobenzyl)-1H-indol-3-yl]-2-hydroxy -4-oxobut-2-enoic acids which have the 1H-benzylindole skeleton (Barreca et al., 2005; Ferro et al., 2007) were discovered as potent anti HIV-1 IN agents selectively inhibiting strand transfer step of IN. Moreover, docking result revealed that there is a large hydrophobic cavity defined by nonpolar residues L68, I73, V75, L158 and I162 in IN core domain, which is probably occupied by the 4-fluorophenyl ring of the inhibitor. Based on above results, Ferro et al. subsequently designed a series of new chloro-fluoro-benzylindoles analogues (Ferro et al., 2010) from the leading compound named CHI-1043 characterized by the presence of a methoxy group at C-4 of the indole system and bearing a fluorine atom on the para position of the benzyl moiety which was identified previously (De Luca et al., 2008). The best molecule, derivative **34** (Fig. 8), displayed a good antiviral activity (IC_{50} = 30 nM, inhibit the in vitro strand-transfer step) and selectivity index, and, more important, higher efficiency and lower cytotoxicity than CHI-1043 (Ferro et al., 2010).

2.4 HIV protease inhibitors

2.4.1 The structure of HIV protease

HIV PT can process the viral into mature and infectious virus particle. Many studies reveal that it cause mature infectious virus particles through cleavage of the viral Gag and GagPol precursor proteins. HIV-1 PT is a homodimer with 99 residues per subunit (Fig. 9), and each subunit is composed of nine β-strands and one α-helix (Noel et al., 2009). β-Strands 2 to 8 are involved in the formation of a jelly-rollβ-barrel topology within each subunit. The dimeric interface contains an antiparallel β-sheet formed by the interdigitation of the N- and C-terminal β-strands in each subunit and by an interlocking and balanced pair of threonines, Thr26, in the active site (Noel et al., 2009). The active site-needing proteolysis is embed in the flap tips and crossing the subunit interface. At the subunit interface and the base of the active-site flap tips, Trp6 and Trp42 providing intrinsic fluorescence (FL) probes of the folding reaction. The result of NMR studies revealed that the mutations of HIV-1 PT variants at or near the interface always break the balance of monomer-dimer.

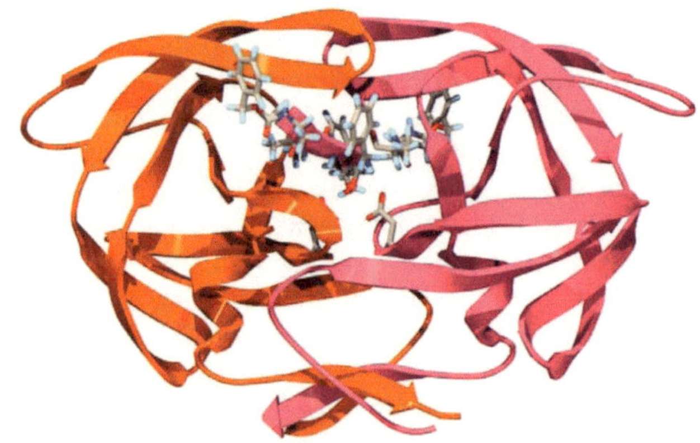

Fig. 9. Structure of HIV PR complexed with TL-3 (PDB: 3TLH) (Brik & Wong, 2003).

2.4.2 Development of HIV protease inhibitors by CADD

Nelfinavir is a potent, non-peptidic inhibitor of HIV-1 PT, which turns out to be successful in the treatment of AIDS. But the potency of Nelfinavir ever-reduced along with HIV develops drug-resistance. Perez et al reported three new variants of Nelfinavir in their studies (Perez et al., 2007). They used minimization and MD simulations methods to optimize and modify original Nelfinavir. Three new inhibitors were designed employing binding free energies calculation and structure modification. The new inhibitors showed greater affinity for HIV-1 PT than Nelfinavir.

Nanoparticles as a new technology have been extensively used in many research fields. Yuan Cheng et al reported the design of carbon nanotubes as HIV-1 PIs (Cheng et al., 2010a). Using docking and MD simulation methods, they designed carbon nanotubes and explored the binding mode between carbon nanotubes and HIV-1 PT. They designed an atomistic model to investigate free energy and interaction between receptor and ligand. In addition, in order to investigate the behaviors of the PT in MD experiment, they used a coarse-grained model based on the atomistic model. The result of dynamics showed that the carbon nanotubes can preferable bind the active site of the HIV PR. It can stop the active flaps in turn to blocking the function of the PT. At the same time, they found that the simulation track is strongly influenced by the size of the carbon nanotube.

Jha et al. established effective prediction model of QSAR on some N-aryl-oxazolidinone-5-carboxamides for higher anti-HIV PT activities (Jha & Halder, 2010). Stepwise regression developed significant models showing importance of atom based descriptors like refractotopological state atom indices, Wang-Ford charges and different whole molecular descriptors. The high prediction ability of these QSAR models was confirmed by challenging these against an external dataset.

HIV-1 PT can specifically recognize their peptide substrates in extended conformations. General approaches for designing HIV-1 PIs often consist of peptidomimetics that feature this conformation. Arora et al evaluated the potential of triazole linked β-strand mimetics as inhibitors of HIV-1 PT activity employing the combination of computational and experimental approaches (Arora et al., 2009). Their studies suggested that nonpeptidic β-strand mimetics, termed triazolamers, offer attractive starting points for the rational design of PIs.

3. Perspectives

This chapter gives a brief review of recent achievements in discovering anti-HIV inhibotorss by using CADD method. Readers are suggested to peruse the original articles for more detailed information. In addition to NRTIs, NtRTIs, NNRTIs, PIs, INIs, FIs and entry inhibitors provide great potential for the treatment patients of HIV infections. Studies on the viral proteins Tat, Rev, Vif and Nef may further afford new drug targets. Latest technological advances (Fischer & Hubbard, 2009) (e.g., protein crystallography, X-ray crystallography, computer resource, cheminformatics & bioinformatics), the growing number of chemical and biological databases, and an explosion in programs and software are providing an ever betterment tools for the design of anti-HIV inhibitors.

4. Acknowledgment

This work was supported by International S&T Cooperation Program of China (No. 2010DFA31710) and National Key Basic Research Program of China (2009CB930200).

5. References

Arora, P. S.; Jochim, A. L.; Miller, S. E., & Angelo, N. G. (2009). Evaluation of triazolamers as active site inhibitors of HIV-1 protease. *Bioorganic & Medicinal Chemistry Letters,* Vol. 19, No. 21, pp. 6023-6026, ISSN 0960-894X

Bacheler, L.; Jeffrey, S.; Hanna, G.; D'Aquila, R.; Wallace, L.; Logue, K.; Cordova, B.; Hertogs, K.; Larder, B.; Buckery, R.; Baker, D.; Gallagher, K.; Scarnati, H.; Tritch, R., & Rizzo, C. (2001). Genotypic correlates of phenotypic resistance to efavirenz in virus isolates from patients failing nonnucleoside reverse transcriptase inhibitor therapy. *Journal of Virology,* Vol. 75, No. 11, pp. 4999-5008, ISSN 0022-538X

Barbaro, G.; Scozzafava, A.; Mastrolorenzo, A., & Supuran, C. T. (2005). Highly active antiretroviral therapy: Current state of the art, new agents and their pharmacological interactions useful for improving therapeutic outcome. *Current Pharmaceutical Design,* Vol. 11, No. 14, pp. 1805-1843, ISSN 1381-6128

Barreca, M. L.; Ferro, S.; Rao, A.; De Luca, L.; Zappala, M.; Monforte, A. M.; Debyser, Z.; Witvrouw, M., & Chimirri, A. (2005). Pharmacophore-based design of HIV-1 integrase strand-transfer inhibitors. *Journal of Medicinal Chemistry,* Vol. 48, No. 22, pp. 7084-7088, ISSN 0022-2623

Berchanski, A., & Lapidot, A. (2007). Prediction of HIV-1 entry inhibitors neomycin-arginine conjugates interaction with the CD4-gp120 binding site by molecular modeling and multistep docking procedure. *Biochimica et Biophysica Acta,* Vol. 1768, No. 9, pp. 2107-2119, ISSN 0006-3002 (Print) 0006-3002 (Linking)

Brik, A., & Wong, C. H. (2003). HIV-1 protease: mechanism and drug discovery. *Organic & Biomolecular Chemistry,* Vol. 1, No. 1, pp. 5-14, ISSN 1477-0520

Caporuscio, F.; Tafi, A.; Gonzalez, E.; Manetti, F.; Este, J. A., & Botta, M. (2009). A dynamic target-based pharmacophoric model mapping the CD4 binding site on HIV-1 gp120 to identify new inhibitors of gp120-CD4 protein-protein interactions. *Bioorganic & Medicinal Chemistry Letters,* Vol. 19, No. 21, pp. 6087-6091, ISSN 1464-3405 (Electronic) 0960-894X (Linking)

Cheng, Y.; Li, D.; Ji, B.; Shi, X., & Gao, H. (2010a). Structure-based design of carbon nanotubes as HIV-1 protease inhibitors: atomistic and coarse-grained simulations. *Journal of Molecular Graphics & Modelling,* Vol. 29, No. 2, pp. 171-177, ISSN 1873-4243 (Electronic) 1093-3263 (Linking)

Cheng, Z.; Zhang, Y., & Fu, W. (2010b). QSAR study of carboxylic acid derivatives as HIV-1 Integrase inhibitors. *European Journal of Medicinal Chemistry,* Vol. 45, No. 9, pp. 3970-3980, ISSN 1768-3254 (Electronic) 0223-5234 (Linking)

Citterio, P., & Rusconi, S. (2007). Novel inhibitors of the early steps of the HIV-1 life cycle. *Expert Opinion on Investigational Drugs,* Vol. 16, No. 1, pp. 11-23, ISSN 1354-3784

Cong, X. J.; Tan, J. J.; Liu, M.; Chen, W. Z., & Wang, C. X. (2010). Computational Study of Binding Mode for N-substituted Pyrrole Derivatives to HIV-1 gp41. *Progress in Biochemistry and Biophysics,* Vol. 37, No. 8, pp. 904-915, ISSN 1000-3282

Dayam, R.; Al-Mawsawi, L. Q.; Zawahir, Z.; Witvrouw, M.; Debyser, Z., & Neamati, N. (2008). Quinolone 3-carboxylic acid pharmacophore: Design of second generation HIV-1 integrase inhibitors. *Journal of Medicinal Chemistry,* Vol. 51, No. 5, pp. 1136-1144, ISSN 0022-2623

De Luca, L.; Barreca, M. L.; Ferro, S.; Iraci, N.; Michiels, M.; Christ, F.; Debyser, Z.; Witvrouw, M., & Chimirri, A. (2008). A refined pharmacophore model for HIV-1 integrase inhibitors: Optimization of potency in the 1H-benzylindole series. *Bioorganic & Medicinal Chemistry Letters,* Vol. 18, No. 9, pp. 2891-2895, ISSN 0960-894X

de Melo, E. B., & Ferreira, M. M. C. (2009). Multivariate QSAR study of 4,5-dihydroxypyrimidine carboxamides as HIV-1 integrase inhibitors. *European Journal of Medicinal Chemistry,* Vol. 44, No. 9, pp. 3577-3583, ISSN 0223-5234

Deng, J. X.; Kelley, J. A.; Barchi, J. J.; Sanchez, T.; Dayam, R.; Pommier, Y., & Neamati, N. (2006). Mining the NCI antiviral compounds for HIV-1 integrase inhibitors. *Bioorganic & Medicinal Chemistry,* Vol. 14, No. 11, pp. 3785-3792, ISSN 0968-0896

Dhaked, D. K.; Verma, J.; Saran, A., & Coutinho, E. C. (2009). Exploring the binding of HIV-1 integrase inhibitors by comparative residue interaction analysis (CoRIA). *Journal of Molecular Modeling,* Vol. 15, No. 3, pp. 233-245, ISSN 1610-2940

Durrant, J. D., & McCammon, J. A. (2010). Computer-aided drug-discovery techniques that account for receptor flexibility. *Current Opinion in Pharmacology,* Vol. 10, No. 6, pp. 770-774, ISSN 1471-4892

Ferro, S.; Barreca, M. L.; De Luca, L.; Rao, A.; Monforte, A. M.; Debyser, Z.; Witvrouw, M., & Chimirri, A. (2007). New 4-[(1-benzyl-1H-indol-3-yl)carbonyl]-3-hydroxyfuran-

2(5H)-ones, beta-diketo acid analogs as HIV-1 integrase inhibitors. *Archiv der Pharmazie,* Vol. 340, No. 6, pp. 292-298, ISSN 0365-6233

Ferro, S.; De Luca, L.; Barreca, M. L.; De Grazia, S.; Christ, F.; Debyser, Z., & Chimirri, A. (2010). New chloro,fluorobenzylindole derivatives as integrase strand-transfer inhibitors (INSTIs) and their mode of action. *Bioorganic & Medicinal Chemistry,* Vol. 18, No. 15, pp. 5510-5518, ISSN 1464-3391 (Electronic) 0968-0896 (Linking)

Ferro, S.; De Luca, L.; Barreca, M. L.; Iraci, N.; De Grazia, S.; Christ, F.; Witvrouw, M.; Debyser, Z., & Chimirri, A. (2009). Docking Studies on a New Human Immodeficiency Virus Integrase-Mg-DNA Complex: Phenyl Ring Exploration and Synthesis of 1H-Benzylindole Derivatives through Fluorine Substitutions. *Journal of Medicinal Chemistry,* Vol. 52, No. 2, pp. 569-573, ISSN 0022-2623

Fischer, M., & Hubbard, R. E. (2009). fragment-based ligand discovery. *Molecular Interventions,* Vol. 9, No. 1, pp. 22-30, ISSN 1534-0384

Gallo, R. C. (2006). A reflection on HIV/AIDS research after 25 years. *Retrovirology,* Vol. 3, No., pp. -, ISSN 1742-4690

Geitmann, M.; Elinder, M.; Seeger, C.; Brandt, P.; de Esch, I. J. P., & Danielson, U. H. (2011). Identification of a Novel Scaffold for Allosteric Inhibition of Wild Type and Drug Resistant HIV-1 Reverse Transcriptase by Fragment Library Screening. *Journal of Medicinal Chemistry,* Vol. 54, No. 3, pp. 699-708, ISSN 0022-2623

Girard, M. P.; Osmanov, S. K., & Kieny, M. P. (2006). A review of vaccine research and development: The human immunodeficiency virus (HIV). *Vaccine,* Vol. 24, No. 19, pp. 4062-4081, ISSN 0264-410X

Greene, W. (2004). The brightening future of HIV therapeutics. *Nature Immunology,* Vol. 5, No. 9, pp. 867-871, ISSN 1529-2908

Gulick, R. M.; Meibohm, A.; Havlir, D.; Eron, J. J.; Mosley, A.; Chodakewitz, J. A.; Isaacs, R.; Gonzalez, C.; McMahon, D.; Richman, D. D.; Robertson, M., & Mellors, J. W. (2003). Six-year follow-up of HIV-1-infected adults in a clinical trial of antiretroviral therapy with indinavir, zidovudine, and lamivudine. *Aids,* Vol. 17, No. 16, pp. 2345-2349, ISSN 0269-9370

Haim, H.; Si, Z.; Madani, N.; Wang, L.; Courter, J. R.; Princiotto, A.; Kassa, A.; DeGrace, M.; McGee-Estrada, K.; Mefford, M.; Gabuzda, D.; Smith, A. B., 3rd, & Sodroski, J. (2009). Soluble CD4 and CD4-mimetic compounds inhibit HIV-1 infection by induction of a short-lived activated state. *PLoS Pathogens,* Vol. 5, No. 4, pp. e1000360, ISSN 1553-7374 (Electronic) 1553-7366 (Linking)

Hammer, S. M.; Katzenstein, D. A.; Hughes, M. D.; Gundacker, H.; Schooley, R. T.; Haubrich, R. H.; Henry, W. K.; Lederman, M. M.; Phair, J. P.; Niu, M.; Hirsch, M. S.; Merigan, T. C.; Blaschke, T. F.; Simpson, D.; McLaren, C.; Rooney, J., & Salgo, M. (1996). A trial comparing nucleoside monotherapy with combination therapy in HIV-infected adults with CD4 cell counts from 200 to 500 per cubic millimeter. *New England Journal of Medicine,* Vol. 335, No. 15, pp. 1081-1090, ISSN 0028-4793

Hare, S.; Gupta, S. S.; Valkov, E.; Engelman, A., & Cherepanov, P. (2010). Retroviral intasome assembly and inhibition of DNA strand transfer. *Nature,* Vol. 464, No. 7286, pp. 232-236, ISSN 1476-4687 (Electronic) 0028-0836 (Linking)

Hazuda, D.; Iwamoto, M., & Wenning, L. (2009). Emerging Pharmacology: Inhibitors of Human Immunodeficiency Virus Integration. *Annual Review of Pharmacology and Toxicology,* Vol. 49, No., pp. 377-394, ISSN 0362-1642

He, Y.; Liu, S.; Jing, W.; Lu, H.; Cai, D.; Chin, D. J.; Debnath, A. K.; Kirchhoff, F., & Jiang, S. (2007). Conserved residue Lys574 in the cavity of HIV-1 Gp41 coiled-coil domain is critical for six-helix bundle stability and virus entry. *Journal of Biological Chemistry,* Vol. 282, No. 35, pp. 25631-25639, ISSN 0021-9258 (Print) 0021-9258 (Linking)

Himmel, D. M.; Maegley, K. A.; Pauly, T. A.; Bauman, J. D.; Das, K.; Dharia, C.; Clark, A. D.; Ryan, K.; Hickey, M. J.; Love, R. A.; Hughes, S. H.; Bergqvist, S., & Arnold, E. (2009). Structure of HIV-1 Reverse Transcriptase with the Inhibitor beta-Thujaplicinol Bound at the RNase H Active Site. *Structure,* Vol. 17, No. 12, pp. 1625-1635, ISSN 0969-2126

Ho, H. T.; Fan, L.; Nowicka-Sans, B.; McAuliffe, B.; Li, C. B.; Yamanaka, G.; Zhou, N.; Fang, H.; Dicker, I.; Dalterio, R.; Gong, Y. F.; Wang, T.; Yin, Z.; Ueda, Y.; Matiskella, J.; Kadow, J.; Clapham, P.; Robinson, J.; Colonno, R., & Lin, P. F. (2006). Envelope conformational changes induced by human immunodeficiency virus type 1 attachment inhibitors prevent CD4 binding and downstream entry events. *Journal of Virology,* Vol. 80, No. 8, pp. 4017-4025, ISSN 0022-538X (Print) 0022-538X (Linking)

Horuk, R. (2009). Chemokine receptor antagonists: overcoming developmental hurdles. *Nature Reviews Drug Discovery,* Vol. 8, No. 1, pp. 23-33, ISSN 1474-1784 (Electronic) 1474-1776 (Linking)

Hu, R. J.; Doucet, J. P.; Delamar, M., & Zhang, R. S. (2009). QSAR models for 2-amino-6-arylsulfonylbenzonitriles and congeners HIV-1 reverse transcriptase inhibitors based on linear and nonlinear regression methods. *European Journal of Medicinal Chemistry,* Vol. 44, No. 5, pp. 2158-2171, ISSN 0223-5234

Jacobomolina, A.; Ding, J. P.; Nanni, R. G.; Clark, A. D.; Lu, X. D.; Tantillo, C.; Williams, R. L.; Kamer, G.; Ferris, A. L.; Clark, P.; Hizi, A.; Hughes, S. H., & Arnold, E. (1993). Crystal-structure of human-immunodeficiency-virus type-1 reverse-transcriptase complexed with double-stranded dna at 3.0 angstrom resolution shows bent DNA. *Proceedings of the National Academy of Sciences of the United States of America,* Vol. 90, No. 13, pp. 6320-6324, ISSN 0027-8424

Jha, T., & Halder, A. K. (2010). Validated predictive QSAR modeling of N-aryl-oxazolidinone-5-carboxamides for anti-HIV protease activity. *Bioorganic & Medicinal Chemistry Letters,* Vol. 20, No. 20, pp. 6082-6087, ISSN 0960-894X

Jiang, S.; Lu, H.; Liu, S.; Zhao, Q.; He, Y., & Debnath, A. K. (2004). N-substituted pyrrole derivatives as novel human immunodeficiency virus type 1 entry inhibitors that interfere with the gp41 six-helix bundle formation and block virus fusion. *Antimicrobial Agents and Chemotherapy,* Vol. 48, No., pp. 4349-4359, ISSN

Jiang, S.; Tala, S. R.; Lu, H.; Abo-Dya, N. E.; Avan, I.; Gyanda, K.; Lu, L.; Katritzky, A. R., & Debnath, A. K. (2011). Design, synthesis, and biological activity of novel 5-((arylfuran/1H-pyrrol-2-yl)methylene)-2-thioxo-3-(3-(trifluoromethyl)phe nyl)thiazolidin-4-ones as HIV-1 fusion inhibitors targeting gp41. *Journal of Medicinal Chemistry,* Vol. 54, No. 2, pp. 572-579, ISSN 1520-4804 (Electronic) 0022-2623 (Linking)

Jorgensen, W. L., & Duffy, E. M. (2002). Prediction of drug solubility from structure. *Advanced Drug Delivery Reviews,* Vol. 54, No. 3, pp. 355-366, ISSN 0169-409X

Jorgensen, W. L.; Ruiz-Caro, J.; Tirado-Rives, J.; Basavapathruni, A.; Anderson, K. S., & Hamilton, A. D. (2006). Computer-aided design of non-nucleoside inhibitors of HIV-1 reverse transcriptase. *Bioorganic & Medicinal Chemistry Letters,* Vol. 16, No. 3, pp. 663-667, ISSN 0960-894X

Juan, A. A. S. (2008). 3D-QSAR models on clinically relevant K103N mutant HIV-1 reverse transcriptase obtained from two strategic considerations. *Bioorganic & Medicinal Chemistry Letters,* Vol. 18, No. 3, pp. 1181-1194, ISSN 0960-894X

Kong, R.; Tan, J. J.; Ma, X. H.; Chen, W. Z., & Wang, C. X. (2006). Prediction of the binding mode between BMS-378806 and HIV-1 gp120 by docking and molecular dynamics simulation. *Biochimica et Biophysica Acta,* Vol. 1764, No. 4, pp. 766-772, ISSN 0006-3002 (Print) 0006-3002 (Linking)

Kong, R.; Xu, X. M.; Chen, W. Z.; Wang, C. X., & Hu, L. M. (2008). Pharmacophore Model Generation Based on Pyrrolidine- and Butane-derived CCR5 Antagonists. *Acta Physico-Chimica Sinica,* Vol. 23, No. 9, pp. 1325-1331, ISSN 1000-6818

Lalonde, J. M.; Elban, M. A.; Courter, J. R.; Sugawara, A.; Soeta, T.; Madani, N.; Princiotto, A. M.; Kwon, Y. D.; Kwong, P. D.; Schon, A.; Freire, E.; Sodroski, J., & Smith, A. B., 3rd. (2011). Design, synthesis and biological evaluation of small molecule inhibitors of CD4-gp120 binding based on virtual screening. *Bioorganic & Medicinal Chemistry,* Vol. 19, No. 1, pp. 91-101, ISSN 1464-3391 (Electronic) 0968-0896 (Linking)

Leonard, J. T., & Roy, K. (2008). Exploring molecular shape analysis of styrylquinoline derivatives as HIV-1 integrase inhibitors. *European Journal of Medicinal Chemistry,* Vol. 43, No. 1, pp. 81-92, ISSN 0223-5234

Li, X.; Krishnan, L.; Cherepanov, P., & Engelman, A. (2011). Structural biology of retroviral DNA integration. *Virology,* Vol. 411, No. 2, pp. 194-205, ISSN 1096-0341 (Electronic) 0042-6822 (Linking)

Liu, K.; Lu, H.; Hou, L.; Qi, Z.; Teixeira, C.; Barbault, F.; Fan, B. T.; Liu, S.; Jiang, S., & Xie, L. (2008). Design, synthesis, and biological evaluation of N-carboxyphenylpyrrole derivatives as potent HIV fusion inhibitors targeting gp41. *Journal of Medicinal Chemistry,* Vol. 51, No. 24, pp. 7843-7854, ISSN 1520-4804 (Electronic) 0022-2623 (Linking)

Louie, M., & Markowitz, M. (2002). Goals and milestones during treatment of HIV-1 infection with antiretroviral therapy: a pathogenesis-based perspective. *Antiviral Research,* Vol. 55, No. 1, pp. 15-25, ISSN 0166-3542

Ma, X. H.; Zhang, X. Y.; Tan, J. J.; Chen, W. Z., & Wang, C. X. (2004). Exploring binding mode for styrylquinoline HIV-1 integrase inhibitors using comparative molecular field analysis and docking studies. *Acta Pharmacologica Sinica,* Vol. 25, No. 7, pp. 950-958, ISSN 1671-4083 (Print) 1671-4083 (Linking)

Mastrolorenzo, A.; Rusconi, S.; Scozzafava, A.; Barbaro, G., & Supuran, C. T. (2007). Inhibitors of HIV-1 protease: Current state of the art 10 years after their introduction. from Antiretroviral drugs to antifungal, antibacterial and antitumor agents based on aspartic protease inhibitors. *Current Medicinal Chemistry,* Vol. 14, No. 26, pp. 2734-2748, ISSN 0929-8673

Mugnaini, C.; Rajamaki, S.; Tintori, C.; Corelli, F.; Massa, S.; Witvrouw, M.; Debyser, Z.; Veljkovic, V., & Botta, M. (2007). Toward novel HIV-1 integrase binding inhibitors: Molecular modeling, synthesis, and biological studies. *Bioorganic & Medicinal Chemistry Letters,* Vol. 17, No. 19, pp. 5370-5373, ISSN 0960-894X

Naider, F., & Anglister, J. (2009). Peptides in the treatment of AIDS. *Current Opinion in Structural Biology,* Vol. 19, No. 4, pp. 473-482, ISSN 1879-033X (Electronic) 0959-440X (Linking)

Noel, A. F.; Bilsel, O.; Kundu, A.; Wu, Y.; Zitzewitz, J. A., & Matthews, C. R. (2009). The folding free-energy surface of HIV-1 protease: insights into the thermodynamic basis for resistance to inhibitors. *Journal of Molecular Biology,* Vol. 387, No. 4, pp. 1002-1016, ISSN 1089-8638 (Electronic) 0022-2836 (Linking)

Nunthaboot, N.; Tonmunphean, S.; Parasuk, V.; Wolschann, P., & Kokpol, S. (2006). Three-dimensional quantitative structure-activity relationship studies on diverse structural classes of HIV-1 integrase inhibitors using CoMFA and CoMSIA. *European Journal of Medicinal Chemistry,* Vol. 41, No. 12, pp. 1359-1372, ISSN 0223-5234

Pawar, V.; Lokwani, D.; Bhandari, S.; Mitra, D.; Sabde, S.; Bothara, K., & Madgulkar, A. (2010). Design of potential reverse transcriptase inhibitor containing Isatin nucleus using molecular modeling studies. *Bioorganic & Medicinal Chemistry,* Vol. 18, No. 9, pp. 3198-3211, ISSN 0968-0896

Perez-Nueno, V. I.; Pettersson, S.; Ritchie, D. W.; Borrell, J. I., & Teixido, J. (2009). Discovery of novel HIV entry inhibitors for the CXCR4 receptor by prospective virtual screening. *Journal of Chemical Information and Modeling,* Vol. 49, No. 4, pp. 810-823, ISSN 1549-9596 (Print) 1549-9596 (Linking)

Perez-Nueno, V. I.; Ritchie, D. W.; Rabal, O.; Pascual, R.; Borrell, J. I., & Teixido, J. (2008). Comparison of ligand-based and receptor-based virtual screening of HIV entry inhibitors for the CXCR4 and CCR5 receptors using 3D ligand shape matching and ligand-receptor docking. *Journal of Chemical Information and Modeling,* Vol. 48, No. 3, pp. 509-533, ISSN 1549-9596 (Print) 1549-9596 (Linking)

Perez, M. A.; Fernandes, P. A., & Ramos, M. J. (2007). Drug design: new inhibitors for HIV-1 protease based on Nelfinavir as lead. *Journal of Molecular Graphics & Modelling,* Vol. 26, No. 3, pp. 634-642, ISSN 1093-3263 (Print) 1093-3263 (Linking)

Qian, K.; Morris-Natschke, S. L., & Lee, K. H. (2009). HIV Entry Inhibitors and Their Potential in HIV Therapy. *Medicinal Research Reviews,* Vol. 29, No. 2, pp. 369-393, ISSN 0198-6325

Qin, B. J.; Jiang, X. K.; Lu, H.; Tian, X. T.; Barbault, F.; Huang, L.; Qian, K. D.; Chen, C. H.; Huang, R.; Jiang, S. B.; Lee, K. H., & Xie, L. (2010). Diarylaniline Derivatives as a Distinct Class of HIV-1 Non-nucleoside Reverse Transcriptase Inhibitors. *Journal of Medicinal Chemistry,* Vol. 53, No. 13, pp. 4906-4916, ISSN 0022-2623

Ravichandran, S.; Veerasamy, R.; Raman, S.; Krishnan, P. N., & Agrawal, R. K. (2008). An overview on HIV-1 reverse transcriptase inhibitors. *Digest Journal of Nanomaterials and Biostructures,* Vol. 3, No. 4, pp. 171-187, ISSN 1842-3582

Ravichandran, V.; Shalini, S.; Sundram, K., & Sokkalingam, A. D. (2010). QSAR study of substituted 1,3,4-oxadiazole naphthyridines as HIV-1 integrase inhibitors. *European*

Journal of Medicinal Chemistry, Vol. 45, No. 7, pp. 2791-2797, ISSN 1768-3254 Electronic) 0223-5234 (Linking)

Saiz-Urra, L.; Gonzalez, M. P.; Fall, Y., & Gomez, G. (2007). Quantitative structure-activity relationship studies of HIV-1 integrase inhibition. 1. GETAWAY descriptors. *European Journal of Medicinal Chemistry,* Vol. 42, No. 1, pp. 64-70, ISSN 0223-5234

Sangma, C.; Chuakheaw, D.; Jongkon, N., & Gadavanij, S. (2010). Computer Techniques for Drug Development from Thai Traditional Medicine. *Current Pharmaceutical Design,* Vol. 16, No. 15, pp. 1753-1784, ISSN 1381-6128

Sarafianos, S. G.; Marchand, B.; Das, K.; Himmel, D. M.; Parniak, M. A.; Hughes, S. H., & Arnold, E. (2009). Structure and Function of HIV-1 Reverse Transcriptase: Molecular Mechanisms of Polymerization and Inhibition. *Journal of Molecular Biology,* Vol. 385, No. 3, pp. 693-713, ISSN 0022-2836

Sharma, H.; Patil, S.; Sanchez, T. W.; Neamati, N.; Schinazi, R. F., & Buolamwini, J. K. (2011). Synthesis, biological evaluation and 3D-QSAR studies of 3-keto salicylic acid chalcones and related amides as novel HIV-1 integrase inhibitors. *Bioorganic & Medicinal Chemistry,* Vol. 19, No. 6, pp. 2030-2045, ISSN 1464-3391 (Electronic) 0968-0896 (Linking)

Stanic, A., & Grana, J. C. (2009). Review of antiretroviral agents for the treatment of HIV infection. *Formulary,* Vol. 44, No. 2, pp. 47-54, ISSN 1082-801X

Strockbine, B., & Rizzo, R. C. (2007). Binding of antifusion peptides with HIVgp41 from molecular dynamics simulations: quantitative correlation with experiment. *Proteins-Structure Function and Bioinformatics,* Vol. 67, No. 3, pp. 630-642, ISSN 1097-0134 (Electronic) 0887-3585 (Linking)

Tan, J. J.; Cong, X. J.; Hu, L. M.; Wang, C. X.; Jia, L., & Liang, X. J. (2010). Therapeutic strategies underpinning the development of novel techniques for the treatment of HIV infection. *Drug Discovery Today,* Vol. 15, No. 5-6, pp. 186-197, ISSN 1359-6446

Tan, J. J.; Zhang, B.; Cong, X. J.; Yang, L. F.; Liu, B.; Kong, R.; Kui, Z. Y.; Wang, C. X., & Hu, L. M. (2011). Computer-aided Design, Synthesis, and Biological Activity Evaluation of Potent Fusion Inhibitors Targeting HIV-1 gp41. *Medicinal Chemistry,* Vol. 7, No. 4, pp. 309-316, ISSN 1573-4064

Teixeira, C.; Gomes, J. R.; Gomes, P., & Maurel, F. (2011). Viral surface glycoproteins, gp120 and gp41, as potential drug targets against HIV-1: Brief overview one quarter of a century past the approval of zidovudine, the first anti-retroviral drug. *European Journal of Medicinal Chemistry,* Vol. 46, No. 4, pp. 979-992, ISSN 1768-3254 (Electronic) 0223-5234 (Linking)

Teixeira, C.; Serradji, N.; Maurel, F., & Barbault, F. (2009). Docking and 3D-QSAR studies of BMS-806 analogs as HIV-1 gp120 entry inhibitors. *European Journal of Medicinal Chemistry,* Vol. 44, No. 9, pp. 3524-3532, ISSN 1768-3254 (Electronic) 0223-5234 (Linking)

Tintori, C.; Corradi, V.; Magnani, M.; Manetti, F., & Botta, M. (2008). Targets Looking for Drugs: A Multistep Computational Protocol for the Development of Structure-Based Pharmacophores and Their Applications for Hit Discovery. *Journal of Chemical Information and Modeling,* Vol. 48, No. 11, pp. 2166-2179, ISSN 1549-9596

Tintori, C.; Manetti, F.; Veljkovic, N.; Perovic, V.; Vercammen, J.; Hayes, S.; Massa, S.; Witvrouw, M.; Debyser, Z.; Veljkovic, V., & Botta, M. (2007). Novel virtual screening protocol based on the combined use of molecular modeling and electron-ion interaction potential techniques to design HIV-1 integrase inhibitors. *Journal of Chemical Information and Modeling,* Vol. 47, No. 4, pp. 1536-1544, ISSN 1549-9596

Zhang, X. Y.; Liu, B.; He, H. Q.; Yang, D., & Wang, C. X. (2009). Human Immunodeficiency Virus Integrase Pharmacophore Model Derived from Diketoacids Inhibitors. *Acta Physico-Chimica Sinica,* Vol. 25, No. 5, pp. 817-824, ISSN 1000-6818

Zhuo, Y.; Kong, R.; Cong, X. J.; Chen, W. Z., & Wang, C. X. (2008). Three-dimensional QSAR analyses of 1,3,4-trisubstituted pyrrolidine-based CCR5 receptor inhibitors. *European Journal of Medicinal Chemistry,* Vol. 43, No. 12, pp. 2724-2734, ISSN 1768-3254 (Electronic) 0223-5234 (Linking)

3

HIV Prevention Needs Epidemiological Data

Anatole Tounkara et al.*
SEREFO HIV/TB research and Training Center, University of Bamako Mali

1. Introduction

Infection with human immune deficiency virus (HIV) is a challenging problem to public health, because it often involves long term treatment with advanced drugs to prolong survival of patients diagnosed with the infection. As an important public health preventive measure, it is necessary to give an HIV-infected individual antiretroviral therapy (ART). This measure facilitates the reduction of the risk of the infected individual from transmitting the virus to others by reducing the viral load in that person. But often, the drug regimens used are surrounded by such questions as the best timing for initiation of therapy as well as benefits and risks associated with delay or early treatment. As a result health caregivers for HIV need to have a continuous update of their knowledge and skills on HIV care and counseling so that they can manage and support individuals with HIV/AIDS with the best and most effective strategy. One way to develop an effective preventive response against HIV is to understand how the infection spreads and the factors that contribute to new infections.

Data from epidemiological studies indicate that, worldwide the prevalence of HIV increased from 29 million in 2001 to 33.4 million in 2008. Similarly, other opportunistic infections such as tuberculosis, cryptococcal meningitis as well as the drug-resistant forms of these diseases altogether add up to make the management of HIV a complex activity. Whereas the incidence is declining in many parts of the world due to access to effective drug regimens, the trend in developing countries has stabilized or slightly increased. Available data from 11 West African countries indicate that national prevalence of HIV/AIDS had been stable in these countries ranging from <1% in Senegal and Niger, to 6.7% in Guinea Bissau. With the exception of Senegal and Ghana, the prevalence rates of these countries were higher in the urban than in the rural areas. The spread of HIV in this region is of great concern to many organizations and governments because of predictions of its increase, yet data are scarce and not regularly revised to reflect current estimates for the countries in this region. In addition, there is the presence of both HIV-1 and HIV-2 in this region. Though more importance is placed on the former than the latter because it is thought to be more easily transmissible while conflicting reports have been shown for the later regarding its

*Abdulrahman S. Hammond[2], Bassirou Diarra[1], Almoustapha Maiga[1], Yaya Sarro[1], Amadou Kone[1], Samba Diop[1] and Aboubacar Alassane Oumar[1]
[1]*SEREFO HIV/TB research and Training Center, University of Bamako, Mali*
[2]*SAIC Frederick, Maryland, USA*

protection of HIV-1 and a lower progression to disease. There is great enthusiasm by many stakeholders in establishing preventive measures to control increase in HIV-1 in the region, however, not much is done about estimation of transmission dynamics and monitoring of coverage of interventions.

In Mali, estimates from 2006 indicated that the overall prevalence of HIV was 1.3% in the general population, 2.2% among young adults (between the ages of 15 and 30), and 35.3% among sex workers (Samake, 2006). The main factors associated with HIV infection in Mali are limited access to treatment and extreme poverty. However, other factors such as poor health conditions, low literacy levels and certain cultural practices like male dominance of women, low condom use, and a relatively high prevalence of sexually transmitted diseases, all contribute to HIV transmission in Mali. Here, we review some of the preventive methods adopted for the management of HIV in Mali. Our review includes current epidemiological data in the general population and the different forms of circulating HIV strains as well as HIV transmission risk behaviors among patients diagnosed with HIV infection in Mali. We also discuss progress made with effective distribution of drug regimens and throw light on the debates of when to start therapy as well as the benefits and demerits of these measures.

2. Epidemiology

2.1 Overview of HIV infection in Mali

Mali is a landlocked country situated in West Africa with a size of 1,241,248 Km^2 and a population of approximately 14.5 million inhabitants. The country is divided into 8 administrative regions with Bamako as the capital. The north stretches deep into the Sahara and is inhabited mainly by the Tuaregs and the nomadic Fulani tribes. Two major rivers, Niger and Senegal, flow through the southern region. A number of countries share border with Mali and includes Algeria in the north, Niger in the east, Burkina Faso in the south-east, Cote D'Ivoire and Guinea in the south, and Mauritania and Senegal in the west. Distribution of HIV prevalence varies from one region to another. Based on two surveys the highest recorded prevalence is observed to be in the Bamako region, where majority of inhabitants live.

A report of HIV/AIDS was first made in 1985 in Mali. In 2001, the Demographic and Health Survey indicated a prevalence of 1.7% among adults (Pichard, 1988; Ballo, 2001). This survey hinted that the prevalence in the general population could increase three-fold if appropriate preventive measures are not put in place to curtail the spread of the infection. Consequently, with a strong commitment from the government a National AIDS Program (NAP) was formed and by 2006 the rate had decreased to 1.3%. The NAP was again restructured in 2002 by which time rates of HIV infection was higher among young women (mostly pregnant women with prevalence ≤5%) between the ages of 25 to 29 years than young men. Similarly, among the 30-34 years age group, women had 2.2% prevalence against 1% prevalence for men. Table 1 shows the distribution of HIV prevalence in Mali between the regions. Overall, prevalence is higher in the urban areas (1.3%) than in the rural (0.6%). Though there are poor records of transmission and prevalence rates, the survey in 2006 showed that sex workers were the highest risk group with 35.3% rates, followed by young street vendors (5.9%), drivers (2.5%), while casual workers and the unemployed youth shared the same rate (2.2%) (Samake, 2006).

It is worthy of mention that Mali is a poor country with about 70% of the population in extreme poverty. In addition, a similar proportion, mainly women are illiterate. A number of socio-cultural practices such as excision and tattooing are commonly found among the population. The 2006 sentinel study indicated that there was early onset of sexual activity among young women and in addition there is generally low condom use by young males between the ages of 15 and 24 years. These together posed a risk factor for infection among the young population in which 2 out of 3 did not believe in the existence of HIV/AIDS (Samake, 2006).

ADMINISTRATIVE MAP OF MALI

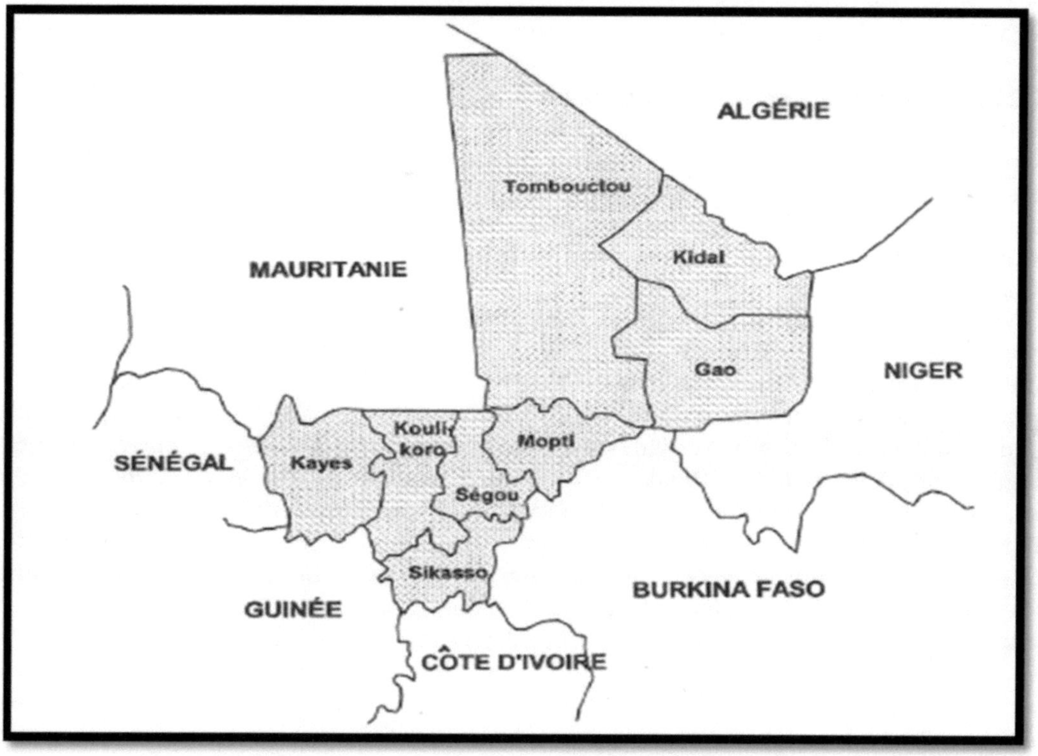

Fig. 1. Map of Mali showing the 8 administrative regions (Samake, 2006).

Regions of Mali	Prevalences	
	2001	2006
Kayes	1.9	0.7
Koulikoro	1.9	1.2
Sikasso	1	0.6
Segou	1.9	1.3
Mopti	1.4	1.4
Gao	0.7	1.1
Tombouctou	0.7	0.5
Kidal	0.7	0.6
Bamako	2.5	1.9

Note: This table shows the differences between the two national surveys of HIV prevalence in the different regions of Mali. As can be seen HIV prevalence decreased in the period 2001 to 2006.

Table 1. HIV prevalence in 2001 and 2006 from different administrative regions of Mali.

In 2001, the Malian initiative of access to antiretroviral therapy (IMAARV) was created. This initiative organizes, implements and follows up antiretroviral therapy in patients infected with HIV. The most important effort of the Malian government was to make free the distribution of antiretroviral drugs for all patients including diagnosis and follow up. This measure allowed the acquisition of regular data from different groups working in HIV field.
Thus, the data presented in this chapter represents those from different groups working in Mali, and includes epidemiological data from the Malian health system and research reports.

2.2 HIV prevalence among the educated & non-educated folk

Although HIV epidemic is related to certain behaviors that exposes an individual to the virus and subsequently increases the risk of the individual to infection, unsafe behaviors are the main contributing factors to transmission of HIV in Mali. For instance, condom use among young males between the ages of 15 and 25 is around 30% and 14% for young women. Similarly, condom use is low among military personnel, truck drivers and vendors of all kinds.
Given that knowledge about HIV is important in identifying and better understanding populations most at risk for HIV infection, the national control program embarked upon different strategies and campaigns to assess knowledge and behavior of students about HIV regarding the different routes of transmission. In the study that also assessed the prevalence and predictors of HIV infection among 950 high school and University students in three regions of Mali, namely, Bamako, Sikasso and Koulikoro, it was observed that the prevalence rate was respectively 3.6, 1.8, and 3.4%. Overall prevalence of HIV was 3.1% and both HIV-1 and 2 were circulating in the schools, although there was more HIV-1 (93.1%) than HIV-2. The study however, did not observe any association between HIV status and the following predictors: age, sex, marital status, religion, education level, ever had intercourse, current sexual partner, condom use at last sexual intercourse, casual sex and study site. By regression coefficient (1.25; $p < 0.01$) the study showed that the main significant predictor of HIV infection was knowledge of route of infection (White, 2009). Thus it demonstrated that the most feasible strategy for slowing down the HIV/AIDS epidemic is education towards risk reduction and prevention of infection. It is not known yet whether there have been follow up studies to understand why the students who had knowledge of the route of transmission of HIV infection were more at risk so that better and more effective strategies can be designed to prevent future occurrence.

2.3 HIV Infection in jail

Few studies were conducted in the Malian prisons. This is particularly due to the strict government regulations that protect the occupants of these prisons. The prisoners are known to be at high risk for HIV infection because of unsafe behaviors in these places (Pichard, 1988). Thus knowledge of prevalence in this group has relevant impact on designing strategies for prevention in these areas. To this end, some studies have looked at attitude, risk behaviors and knowledge of HIV within jail population, and noted that most inmates of a jail had limited knowledge of the definition of HIV/AIDS. Only 2.7% knew that AIDS is an Acquired Immunodeficiency Syndrome and can be transmitted through body fluids and by sex. The study also showed limited knowledge of routes of transmission for both HIV and Sexually Transmitted Diseases (STDs), and only 7.5% of the study population knew their HIV status (TCHOUZOU, 2008).

Recommendations from this study led the national program against HIV/AIDS to initiate large campaigns in 2006, regarding the routes of transmission of HIV in order to educate people in different communities including prisoners. Topics covered in these campaigns included sexual transmission, intravenous drug use, mother-to-child transmission of HIV, risks from blood products and transfusion, organ donor or tissue transplantation as well as risks of occupational exposures to the virus. Similarly, there is a need to conduct follow-up studies to determine the prevalence of HIV so that improved recommendations can be made for implementation, particularly in the jails.

2.4 HIV prevalence among blood donors

Whereas HIV overall prevalence in Mali is currently 1.3%, prevalence among blood donors is 2.6% (Diarra, 2009). Estimates from the National Center of Blood Transfusion (Centre National de Transfusion Sanguine [CNTS], Bamako, Mali) indicate that this rate had risen from 3% in 1999 to 4.5% in 2009 (Tounkara, 2004; Tounkara, 2009) and decrease to 2.6% in 2007 (Diarra, 2009). Young adults (between 18 and 25 years) accounted for 41% of overall blood donors. It is important to note that, 1.13% of the blood donors with HIV were also co-infected with Hepatitis B virus (HBV) (Table 2). Of these, 88.5% are men (over 25 years of age), while young adults make up 43%. About 80% of the blood donors from the cohort at CNTS were recruited from family members of patients who need blood transfusion. From this cohort some studies have shown that majority of the HIV seropositive individuals had thrombocytopenia, with a platelet count lower than 150 x $10^3/mm^3$ (Tounkara, 2004). Compared to HIV seronegative individuals, the HIV infected had longer bleeding time, a diminution of the rate of prothrombin, and an elevated partial time for thromboplastin. Taken together, these data suggest a modification of hemostasis over the course of HIV infection (Tounkara A, 2004). Also, a proportion of blood donors were found to have human cytomegalovirus (HCMV). Among these, 89% were AIDS patients, 71% were HIV-infected and 58% were uninfected with HIV. About 40% of the blood donors co-infected with HIV and HCMV also had pneumonia compared to those infected with only HIV (Maiga, 2003; Tounkara, 2004).

	HBV Status		
HIV Status	Positive, n (%)	Negative, n (%)	Total, n (%)
Positive	131 (1.13)	387 (3.34)	518 (4.47)
Negative	1591 (13.73)	9483 (81.80)	11 074 (95.53)
Total	1722 (14.86)	9870 (85.14)	11 592 (100)

Abbreviations: HBV, hepatitis B virus; HIV, human immunodeficiency virus; n, number of donors; %, percentage of the specific cell based on the total number of donors (11 592).
Note: This table represents HIV and HBV infection alone as well as the prevalence of co-infection among Malian Blood donors.

Table 2. HIV/HBV Coinfection Frequency among Blood Donors in Mali

Studying HIV prevalence among blood donors will help to refine strategies used in recruiting blood donors, and significantly reduce HIV transmission in the general population.

2.5 Circulating recombinants forms of HIV in Mali

A lot of interest has been generated by the scientific community in seeking to understand the range of variability of HIV so that the spread of an epidemic can be tracked between different population and places, as well as develop strategies to control the virus. Firstly, HIV is thought to be the most variable virus, and its clinical characteristics alone are not sufficient to explain the outcomes of infection. In addition, it has subtypes with distinct geographic distribution and recombination can occur between and within subtypes (Korber, 2003). Thus creating a further increase in the genetic diversity in many parts of the world and thereby a complex challenge to control. As a result, the role of genetic variability in HIV infection has received extensive consideration both for understanding of the natural history of the disease and for developing strategies for control of the virus. Currently 9 subtypes have been identified worldwide in the HIV-1 group M (A, B, C, D, F, G, H, J and K). Viruses E and I in the envelope are recombinant strains (Peeters, 1999). In 2009 estimates showed that approximately 2.6 million [2.3 - 2.8 million] new infections were due to HIV-1 subtype non-B, and these were predominantly among infected individuals in the Americas, Western Europe, and in Australia (Report 2010 of UNAIDS). More than 50% of HIV infections worldwide are associated with the HIV-1 subtype C, with South Africa having the highest majority, while subtypes A and D are commonly found in East Africa. The prevalence of recombinant forms of HIV has been increasing, and in Europe it rose from 17% during the period 1996-1999 to 28% in the period 2000-2003 and again to 35% in 2006-2009. The most common recombinant strain in circulation in some regions of Africa and West Asia is the HIV-1 Circulating Recombinant Form (HIV-1 CRF).

A number of studies have characterized subtypes in Mali and other West African states, and have noted that the recombinant CRF02_AG is the main HIV-1 infecting strain in this region. Sequencing analysis has revealed that early failures to Triomune ® (d4T/3TC/NVP) in adults occurred because the viruses in circulation were recombinant CRF02_AG (Marcelin, 2007). Recent primary drug resistance studies conducted in Mali (in Bamako and Segou) on 198 samples obtained from ARV-naive patients showed CRF02_AG to be the most prevalent strain, with respectively 70.5 and 72% occurring in 2005 and 2006 (Derache, 2008). A second recombinant strain was CRF06_cpx with 19.5% and 11% infections respectively occurring in the same period. Other subtypes and recombinants in circulation were also found, but with a lower prevalence in these two years. Overall, there was a greater genetic diversity in the year 2006 compared to 2005. Indeed, in 2005, two pure subtypes (C and G) and a recombinant (CRF01_AE) were found, while in 2006, three pure subtypes (A, F2 and G) and 3 recombinants (CRF01_AE, CRF09_cpx and CRF18_cpx) were identified (Derache, 2007). The prevalence of CRF02_AG appeared to be stable, while that of CRF06_cpx decreased, giving way to other subtypes, including CRF09_cpx and CRF18_cpx which are new strains in Mali. The recombinant CRF09_cpx, is a mosaic virus from different subtypes (A, F and G), and although it was first described in 2004, in West Africa, it is now the most predominant recombinant strain in the region. This recombinant appears to have structural similarities as well as important genetic distances like the first CRF02_AG isolated (McCutchan, 2004). As for the recombinant CRF18_cpx, this was first identified in 2005 in Cuba, but now, seems native to Central Africa. Indeed, it consists of various segments from the CRF13_cpx, CRF04_cpx and 36 other viruses, is predominantly found in Central Africa (Thomson, 2005). Similarly, a recent study in Mali found a subtype namely, CRF05_DF (Maiga, 2010). This subtype, CRF05_DF, was first described in Belgium in 2000 from a patient linked to the Democratic Republic of Congo (DRC) (Laukkanen, 2000). Thereafter, Casado and colleagues identified another strain in 2003 in the DRC (Casado, 2003).

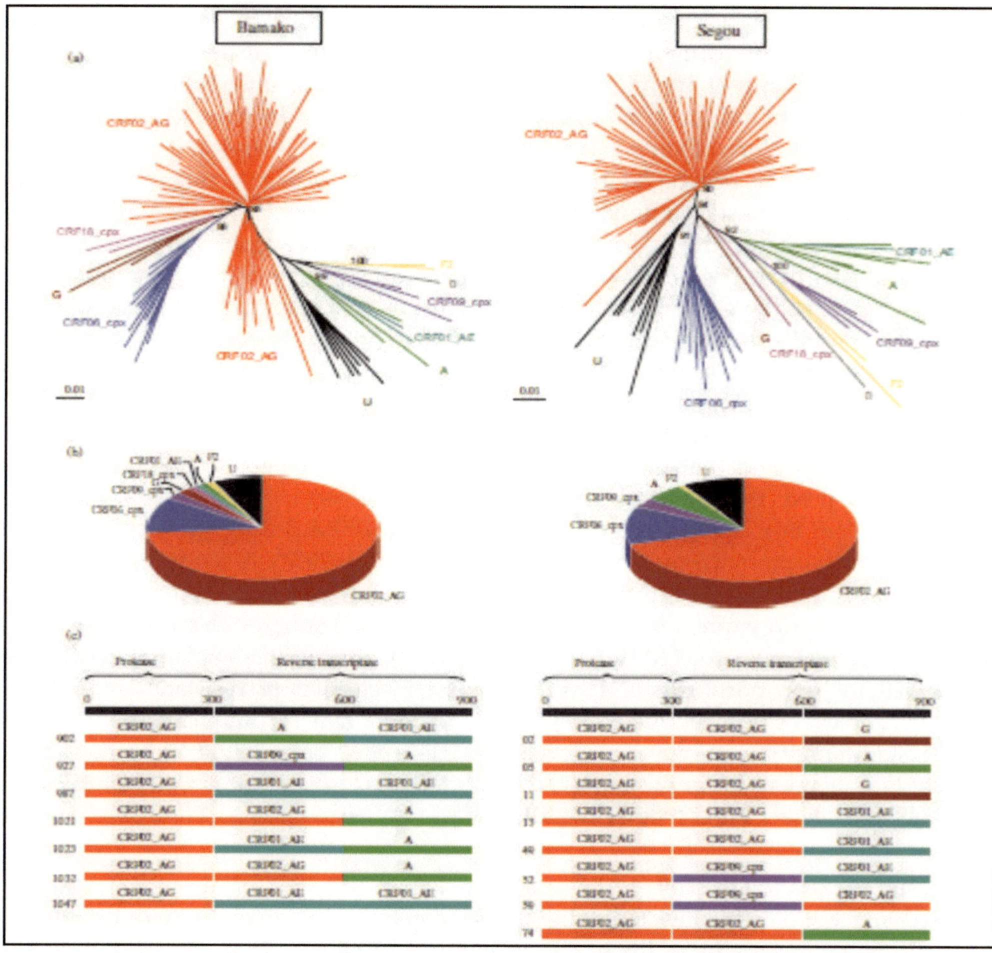

Fig. 2. Phylogenetic analysis from different subtypes in Mali. Results are presented for Bamako on the left and for Segou on the right. (a) Unrooted phylogenetic trees of pol nucleotides sequences. Sequences from references strains appear in bold. Each colour corresponds to a subtype or CRF. (b) Graphic representation of subtypes repartition. (c) pol gene mosaic viruses ('unknown U' viruses), with recombination points and subtypes involved. (Derache, 2008)

As seen from the phylogenetic data above (Fig. 1), Mali has a large genetic diversity of HIV-1 viral strains and the potential to generate new recombinants. While evaluating antiretroviral resistance of HIV strains in Mali a recent study conducted among 746 ARV treatment-naive HIV-1 patients showed that the majority carried the CRF02_AG subtype CRF06_cpx (Maiga, 2010). Indeed, many of the viruses sequenced in this study were either recombinant intersubtypes or had unique recombinant forms (URF). A large proportion 72%% of these were the recombinant CRF02_AG. It is therefore important to monitor the emergence and spread of new recombinants because the appearance of a particular polymorphism within a new recombinant could lead to resistance mutation profiles in individuals or a different response to antiretroviral therapy. For now, the CRF02_AG is believed to be the most prevalent (72%) in Mali and overall it appears to have similar characteristics to the subtype B.

The genetic variability of HIV viral strains involves genes encoding the viral enzymes, which are targets of therapeutic drugs. This variability occurs because of errors in viral reverse transcriptase. Knowledge of the genetic subtype as well as the inter-subtype recombinant nature of HIV-1 strains might be of crucial importance for the development of future HIV vaccine. Some substitutions of amino acids are found at high frequencies at positions involved in resistance to ARVs in subtype B. Thus, over 50% of non-B virus infecting in naive patients carry at least three PI resistance mutations, while it concerns only 8% of the virus subtype B (Holguin, 2002). To assess the impact of this polymorphism on resistance to ARVs, many phenotypic studies have been conducted on the gene for PR gene with many mutations of minor resistance in subtype non-B. Although many results conclude that patients infected with HIV-1 subtype non-B also respond well to treatment than patients infected by subtype B, some studies show a decreased sensitivity to certain subtypes IP. For example, the recombinant CRF02_AG, naturally bearing mutations K20I and M36I, replicates better in the presence of IP, thus reducing its sensitivity to these molecules, including NFV (Kinomoto, 2005). In addition, Perno et al demonstrated that the minor mutation M36I of PR gene, polymorphic in non-subtype B was predictive of virological failure after 24 weeks of antiretroviral therapy containing a PI, in fact, appearance of major mutations L90M during virologic failure was associated with the presence of the mutation M36I (Perno, 2004). A study in Uganda also showed that mutations associated with resistance to NVP was detected more frequently 6-8 weeks after delivery in women infected with subtype D than subtype A after taking a single dose of NVP in the context of PMTCT (Kiwanuka, 2008). The authors explain this result by a potential natural polymorphism of IT to push faster selection of resistance mutations to Nevirapine. A recent study conducted in Japan identified a new recombinant strain of HIV-2, CRF01_AB. Although no recombinant forms of HIV-2 have been found in Mali, there is a possibility that this new strain may soon be identified here, given that it was identified from samples obtained from Cote d'Ivoire (Ibe, 2010).

2.6 HIV drug resistance in Mali

The management of patients infected with HIV is complex and follows a long duration. It will therefore improve the quality of life of people living with HIV, if drug resistance is avoided. Several research studies on resistance mutations were performed in Mali. In 2007, Derache and colleagues evaluated the presence of resistance mutations in 98 naive patients receiving antiretroviral therapy, and showed the presence of K103N in two individuals. This mutation resulting in NNRTI resistance, render NVP or EFV inefficient (Derache, 2007). Similarly, another study estimated the presence of resistance mutations in 109 patients treated in Segou by Triomune ® (d4T +3 TC + NVP) in a median time of 8 months, and showed 11 cases of resistance to the presence of different mutations as follows: 2 cases of M184V alone, 1 case of Y181C alone, 8 cases including 5 associations Y181C + M184V, K103N + M184V + 2 and 1 association G190A + M184V K101E + G190A (Marcelin, 2007). These data demonstrates the need for the management of early failures to drug treatments and shows the importance of using other NRTIs in second-line treatments. Based on the 2007 version of an algorithm of interpretation by International AIDS Society (IAS) Derache and colleagues showed an overall prevalence for primary resistance of 11.5% (made up of 1.5% for NRTIs (K219Q), 9% to NNRTIs (Y181C, K101E, V90I, A98G and V106I and V108I) and 1% for PI (L33F and M46L)) (Derache, 2008). These identified mutations corresponded to the treatments used except for the mutations V90I, A98G and V106I which were associated with resistance to TMC 125 or Etravirine according to the IAS algorithm. No significant difference between 2005 and 2006 in

the prevalence of primary resistance of different classes of antiretroviral drugs has been observed. A similar study of treatment-naive patients recently showed a higher prevalence of primary resistance (9.9%) than was previously reported by Derache and colleagues (Haidara, 2010; Derache, 2008). So also have other studies reported late failures to drug treatment in Mali and in Burkina Faso with median treatment duration lasting 18 months (Sylla, 2008). Recently, two studies looked at resistance mutations among treatment-naïve patients in Mali. In the first study, 10% of patients failing second-line drug treatments were found to have failed therapy to all available drug molecules used in the country (Maiga, 2010). In the same study, resistance associated to ETR was found in ARV-naïve patients with HIV-1 subtype B. Previously, the genetic barriers to integrase inhibitors for HIV-1 subtype B had been compared to those of CRF02_AG and although they both have similar barriers, the CRF02_AG carried a higher genetic barrier at positions 140 and 151 of the integrase (Maiga, 2009). Thus, the finding in which ETR was implicated is important because it will facilitate the establishment of second and third line ARV treatments in a developing country such as Mali (Maiga, 2010). In the second study, of 57 HIV-2 treatment-naïve patients, 3 of 36 had a PR and RT-resistance mutation, implying that either resistant virus to these class strategy are circulating in Mali or the patients were taking ART without medical supervision. Of the remaining 21 patients, 1 had resistance mutations to both RT and PR, while a second had resistance to RT only. The presence of these mutations in both of these treatment-naïve patients indicates inadequate compliance to treatment (Oumar, 2010).
Although there is the risk that resistant viruses are spread throughout the country, and thereby pose an additional public health challenge, currently there is not enough data at the national level on the transmission of resistant virus. Despite this, the data shown from the studies mentioned above indicate the magnitude of the problem which may limit therapeutic choices in a resource-limited country such as Mali. And because, resistance is a major concern for long-term treatment in this place, it is necessary to improve adherence to treatment as well as routine monitoring to avoid an escalation of the evolution of primary resistance. One approach to resolving this is to broaden genotypic testing for treatment failures, and have a wider range of antiretroviral drug regimen to cover cases involving resistant strains. Although individual classes of antiretroviral are low, overall primary resistance in Mali is high. Exceptions are the NNRTIs which are relatively high (9%) probably due to their frequent use. In the past at least, a single-dose of NVP was used for the prevention of mother to child transmission and needs monitoring.

3. Conclusions/recommendations

Considerable efforts have been made towards HIV prevention and treatment in Mali. Lessons learnt from some epidemiological data showed that the efforts must be sustained in order to make significant changes to the behavior of young adults regarding HIV infection in Mali. As shown the prevalence of HIV alone is variable between social groups. Surprisingly, the prevalence among those co-infected with HIV and HBV was so high that this particular group must be targeted for further education and counseling. Despite this, it must be remembered that the biggest challenge is the rising numbers in circulating recombinant forms of HIV due to the occurrence of several mutations resistant to antiretroviral drugs. Therefore in Mali, there is an urgent need to increase access to antiretroviral drugs. In addition, newer approaches must be developed to improve compliance as well as follow up monitoring of viral load levels of the patients. Also, it will be more useful if knowledge about HIV and the level and frequency of risk behaviors related to the transmission of HIV is stepped up as part of a national educational campaign, with the hope to change unsafe behaviors towards a better one.

4. Acknowledgements

We are grateful to the Malian Ministry of Health, Malian National HIV program and their partners particularly the ESTHER group, for giving us access to data on different national surveys, and to the University of Bamako for their support of this work. Funding was obtained from DCR/NIAID/NIH for this chapter.

5. References

Auerbach DM, Darrow WM, Jaffe HW,& Curran JW. 1984. Cluster of cases of the acquired immune Deficiency syndrome: patients linked by sexual contact. *Am J Med* 76: 487-492

Asamoah-Odei E, Garcia-Callga JM, & Boerma T. 2004. HIV prevalence and trends in sub-Sahara Africa: no decline and large subregional differences. *Lancet* 364: 35-40

Ballo MB, Traore SM, Niambele I, Ba S, Ayad M,& N'diaye S, 2001. Troisième Enquête Démographique et de Santé du Mali 2001 (EDSM-IV), *CPS/MS*, 332 pages.

Brun-Vezinet F, Katlama C, Roulot D, Lenoble L, Alizon M, Madjar JJ, Rey MA, Girard PM, Yeni P, Clavel F, Gadelle S, & Harzic M. 1987. "Lymphadenopathy-associated virus type 2 in AIDS and AIDS-related complex. Clinical and virological features in four patients." *Lancet* 1(8525): 128-32 Casado G,Thomson MM, Delgado E, Sierra M, Vazquez-De Parga E, Perez-Alvarez L, Ocampo A,& Najera R. 2003. Near full-length genome characterization of an HIV type 1 CRF05_DF virus from Spain. *AIDS Res Hum Retroviruses* 19:719-25.

Chamberland ME, Castro KG, Haverkos HW, Miller BI, Thomas PA, Reiss R, Walker J, Spira TJ, Jaffe HW,& Curran JW.1984.Acquired immunodeficiency syndrome in the United States: an analysis of cases outside high-incidence groups. *Ann Intern Med.* Nov;101(5):617-23.

Clavel F. (1987). "HIV-2, the West African AIDS virus." *AIDS* 1(3): 135-40.

Clavel F, Mansinho K, Chamaret S, Guetard D, Favier V, Nina J, Santos-Ferreira MO, Champalimaud JL, & Montagnier L. 1987. Human immunodeficiency virus type 2 infection associated with AIDS in West Africa. *N Engl J Med* 316:1180-5.

Derache A, Maiga AI, Traore O, Akonde A, Cisse M, Jarrousse B, Koita V, Diarra B, Carcelain G, Barin F, Pizzocolo C, Pizarro L, Katlama C, Calvez V,& Marcelin AG. 2008. Evolution of genetic diversity and drug resistance mutations in HIV-1 among untreated patients from Mali between 2005 and 2006. *J Antimicrob Chemother* 62:456-63.

Derache A, Traore O, Koita V, Sylla A, Tubiana R, Simon A, Canestri A, Carcelain G, Katlama C, Calvez V, Cisse M,& Marcelin AG. 2007. Genetic diversity and drug resistance mutations in HIV type 1 from untreated patients in Bamako, Mali. *Antivir Ther* 12:123-9.

Diarra A, Kouriba B, Baby M, Murphy E, Lefrere JJ, 2009. HIV, HCV, HBV and syphilis rate of positive donations among blood donations in Mali: lower rates among volunteer blood donors. *Transfus Clin Biol.*16(5-6):444-7.

Haidara A, Chamberland A, Sylla M, Aboubacrine SA, Cissé M, Traore HA, Maiga MY, Tounkara A, Nguyen VK,& Tremblay C; Appuyer le Traitement Anti Rétroviral en Afrique de l'Ouest (ATARAO) Group 1. 2010. High level of primary drug resistance in Mali. *HIV Med.* 1;11(6):404-11.

Holguin, A, Alvarez A, & Soriano V. 2002. High prevalence of HIV-1 subtype G and natural polymorphisms at the protease gene among HIV-infected immigrants in Madrid. *AIDS* 16:1163-70.

Korber A, Dissemond J, Hillen U, Goos M,& Esser S. 2003. [HIV-positive patient with multiple ulcers. Lues maligna]. *Hautarzt* 54:1098-102.

Korber B, Muldoon M, Theiler J, Gao F, Gupta R, Lapedes A, Hahn BH, Wolinsky S, & Bhattacharya T. 2000. Timing the ancestor of the HIV-1 pandemic strains. *Science* 288:1789-1796.

Kinomoto M, Appiah-Opong R, Brandful JA, Yokoyama M, Nii-Trebi N, Ugly-Kwame E, Sato H, Ofori-Adjei D, Kurata T,Barre-Sinoussi F, Sata T, & Tokunaga K. 2005. HIV-1 proteases from drug-naive West African patients are differentially less susceptible to protease inhibitors. *Clin Infect Dis* 41:243-51.

Kiwanuka N, Laeyendecker O, Robb M, Kigozi G, Arroyo M, McCutchan F, Eller LA, Eller M, Makumbi F, Birx D, Wabwire-Mangen F, Serwadda D, Sewankambo NK, Quinn TC, Wawer M,& Gray R. 2008. Effect of human immunodeficiency virus Type 1 (HIV-1) subtype on disease progression in persons from Rakai, Uganda, with incident HIV-1 infection. *J Infect Dis* 197:707-13.

Laukkanen T, Carr JK, Janssens W, Liitsola K, Gotte D, McCutchan FE, Op de Coul E, Cornelissen M, Heyndrickx L, van der Groen G, & Salminen MO. 2000. Virtually full-length subtype F and F/D recombinant HIV-1 from Africa and South America. *Virology* 269:95-104.

Maiga A, Fofana DF, AIT-ARKHOUB Z, Cissé, M, Diallo F, Haidara M, Traoré HA, Coulibaly H, Akonde A, Pizarro L, Brucker G, Murphy R, Katlama C, Tounkara A, Marcelin AG,& Calvez V. 2010. "Echec Virologique aux traitements Antirétroviraux de seconde ligne et Profil des Mutations de Résistance chez des Patients infectés par le VIH-1 à Bamako au Mali." *5ème Conférence francophone Casablanca Maroc* 28 - 31 Mars.résumé N° 333

Maiga AI, Descamps D, Morand-Joubert L, Malet I, Derache A, Cisse M, Koita V, Akonde A, Diarra B, Wirden M, Tounkara A, Verlinden Y, Katlama C, Costagliola D, Masquelier B, Calvez V,& Marcelin AG. 2010. Resistance-associated mutations to etravirine (TMC-125) in antiretroviral-naive patients infected with non-B HIV-1 subtypes. *Antimicrob Agents Chemother* 54:728-33

Maïga AI, Malet I, Soulie C, Derache A, Koita V, Amellal B, Tchertanov L, Delelis O, Morand-Joubert L, Mouscadet JF, Murphy R, Cissé M, Katlama C, Calvez V,& Marcelin AG. 2009. Genetic barriers for integrase inhibitor drug resistance in HIV type-1 B and CRF02_AG subtypes. *Antivir Ther.*;14(1):123-9.

Maïga I, Le Faou A, Muller CP, & Venard V.2005. Unexpected high prevalence of hepatitis B and HIV infections in Malian medical students. *Eur J Clin Microbiol Infect Dis.* Jul;24(7):501-2.

Marcelin AG, Jarrousse B, Derache A, Ba M, Dakouo ML, Doumbia A, Haidara I, Maiga A, Carcelain G, Peytavin G, Katlama C,& Calvez V. 2007. HIV drug resistance after the use of generic fixed-dose combination stavudine/lamivudine/nevirapine as standard first-line regimen. *AIDS* 21:2341-3.

McCutchan F E, Sankale JL., M'Boup S, Kim B, Tovanabutra S, Hamel DJ, Brodine SK, Kanki PJ,& Birx DL. 2004. HIV type 1 circulating recombinant form CRF09_cpx from west Africa combines subtypes A, F, G, and may share ancestors with CRF02_AG and Z321. *AIDS Res Hum Retroviruses* 20:819-26.

Oumar AA, Dao S, Lambert C, Traoré S, Katile D, Sidibé Y, Tulkens PM, Goubau P, & Ruelle J.2010. Traitement du VIH-2 au Mali et Profil de résistance aux antirétroviraux. 5ème *Conférence Francophone VIH/Sida, Casablanca* Maroc du 28-31 Mars 2010. Abstract N°170/33A

Peeters M, & Delaporte, E. 1999. Genetic diversity of HIV infection worldwide and its consequences. *Med Trop* (Mars). 1999;59(4 Pt 2):449-55.

Perno C F, Cozzi-Lepri A, Forbici F, Bertoli A, Violin M, Stella Mura M, Cadeo G, Orani A, Chirianni A, De Stefano C, Balotta C,& d'Arminio Monforte A. 2004. Minor mutations in HIV protease at baseline and appearance of primary mutation 90M in patients for whom their first protease-inhibitor antiretroviral regimens failed. *J Infect Dis* 189:1983-7.

Pichard E, Guindo A, GrossetteG, Fofana Y, Maiga Y I, Koumare B, Traore S, Maiga M, Brun-Vezinet F, & Rosenheim M, 1988. L'infection par le virus de l'Immunodéficience humaine (VIH) au Mali. *Med Trop* 48 (4) ; 345-349

Samake S, Traore SM, Ba S, Dembele E, Diop M, Mariko S,& Libite PR. 2006. Quatrième Enquête Démographique et de Santé du Mali 2006 (EDSMIV), CPS/MS, 410 pages

Selik RM, Harverkos HH, Curran JW. 1978. Acquired immune deficiency syndrome (AIDS) trends in the United States, 1978-1982. *Am J Med.* 76: 493-500

Sidibe T, Sangho H, Traore MS, Cissé MB, Diallo B, Keîta MM,& Gendrel D. 2006. Knowledge, attitudes, and practices of adolescents in an urban school environment in Bamako, Mali, around family planning, sexually transmitted infections, and AIDS]. *Mali Med.*;21(1):39-42.

Sylla M, Chamberland A, Boileau C, Traoré HA, Ag-Aboubacrine S, Cissé M, Koala S, Drabo J, Diallo I, Niamba P, Tremblay-Sher D, Machouf N, Rashed S, Nickle DC, Nguyen VK, & Tremblay CL; ATARAO Group. 2008. Characterization of drug resistance in antiretroviral-treated patients infected with HIV-1 CRF02_AG and AGK subtypes in Mali and Burkina Faso. *Antivir Ther.* ;13(1):141-8.

TCHOUZOU Tabeth Hilaire, 2008. Evaluation des connaissances, comportements et attitudes a risk de l'infection VIH /SIDA dans la population carcérale de la maison d'arrêt de Bamako.*These de Medecine, Universite de Bamako, Mali*

Thomson MM, Casado G, Posada D, Sierra M,& Najera R. 2005. Identification of a novel HIV-1 complex circulating recombinant form (CRF18_cpx) of Central African origin in Cuba. *AIDS* 19:1155-63.

UNIAID/WHO. AIDS epidemic update, December, 2005. UNIAID/WHO; Genevor, Switszerland

UNAIDS/WHO. AIDS epidemic update. December 2010. www.unaids.org

White HL, Kristensen S, Coulibaly DM, Sarro YS, Chamot E,& Tounkara A. 2009. Prevalence and predictors of HIV infection amongst Malian students. *AIDS Care.* Jun;21(6):701-7.

WHO, UNAIDS, UNICEF. Towards universal access. Scaling up priority HIV/AIDS interventions in the health sector. Progress report 2009. Geneva:WHO press; 2009.pp.1-162.

World Health Organisation. Rapid advice. Antiretroviral therapy for HIV infection in adults and adolescents. Geneva:WHO press;2009.pp.1-25. www.who.int/hiv/pub/arv/rapid_advice_art.pdf

Part 2

Clinical Evidence of Secondary Manifestations of Both the Disease and the Treatment

4

Facial Lipoatrophy and AIDS

Flávia Machado Gonçalves Soares
and Izelda Maria Carvalho Costa
[1]*Physician at the Secretariat of Health of the Federal District*
[2]*Professor at the University of Brasilia*
Brasil

1. Introduction

Since AIDS has become a chronic and manageable disease, it is essential to recognize and treat the conditions associated with the infection itself and with the adverse effects of antiretroviral drugs. Facial lipoatrophy associated with HIV / AIDS has become epidemic. Therefore, all of those involved in assisting this group of patients should recognize the signs of lipodystrophy syndrome as well as the recommended treatment options, which should always be incorporated into the therapeutic arsenal for patients with HIV/AIDS.

2. Lipodystrophy associated with HIV/AIDS

2.1 Background

From 1996, a series of new anatomical and metabolic changes began to be described in patients with HIV/AIDS, especially in those undergoing highly active antiretroviral therapy. The patients presented peripheral fat atrophy as well as central fat accumulation. At the same time, it was observed that redistribution of body fat was accompanied by insulin resistance and several abnormalities in serum lipids. These changes were later described in general terms as HIV-associated lipodystrophy and/or HIV lipodystrophy syndrome (HLS).

The HLS was officially described by the Food and Drug Administration (FDA), the United States agency regulating the release and use of drugs, in 1997.

The first morphological signs of HLS were described about two years after the introduction of protease inhibitors (PI). However, the introduction of PI coincides with the inclusion of a second nucleoside analog reverse transcriptase inhibitor called stavudine.

Initially, HLS was called Crixbelly, since the first cases of redistribution of body fat were observed after the use of Crixivan® (Indinavir), a drug belonging to the PI class. The association between the use of Indinavir and the redistribution of body fat was described in 1998, with the use of computed tomography showing the increase in visceral fat in these individuals. With the emergence of new PI, it was concluded that the redistribution of body fat was not an exclusive effect of Indinavir, and the name was abandoned.

After observing clinical similarities between patients with Cushing's syndrome and patients with HLS, Miller at al. (1998) began to call it "pseudo-Cushing's syndrome". However,

subsequent studies showed no changes in the hypothalamic-pituitary-adrenal axis of HIV-seropositive patients, and this nomenclature was also abandoned.
Currently, several synonyms are used for HLS, such as body fat redistribution syndrome, metabolic syndrome associated with antiretroviral therapy or, more recently, HIV/ART-associated dyslipidemia.

2.2 Clinical aspects

The first body changes to be noticed were accumulation of fat in the abdominal region and on the back of the neck, the so-called buffalo hump.
Other anatomical changes include lipoatrophy of the face, arms and legs and prominence of superficial veins, associated or not with accumulation of fat in the abdomen, neck and breast. The metabolic changes include lipid changes and abnormalities in glucose homeostasis. Metabolic changes may be associated or not with anatomical changes.
Lipid changes found in HLS are an increase in serum triglycerides (TG) and/or total cholesterol levels at the expense of low-density lipoproteins (LDL), with a tendency to decreased levels of high-density lipoproteins (HDL).
Hypertriglyceridemia is mainly due to elevated levels of *de novo* lipogenesis and to delayed clearance of TG in the postprandial period. Studies have also revealed that a significantly higher proportion of patients receiving PI presented increased fasting serum levels of apolipoproteins B and E, possibly due to their increased synthesis, which could be related to the manifestation of hyperlipidemia. Moreover, the so-called metabolic syndrome, in which abdominal obesity - a component of HLS - correlates with changes in lipid metabolism, was present in 18% of the patients undergoing ART, especially in patients using PI.
Glucose abnormalities may manifest as glucose intolerance, peripheral insulin resistance or diabetes mellitus (DM).
The mechanisms of action through which ARV such as protease inhibitors cause insulin resistance are a reduction in glucose uptake mediated by insulin in skeletal muscle and adipocytes, interfering with glucose transmembrane transporters GLUT-4, and their effect on the transcription factor sterol regulatory element binding protein-1c (SREBP-1), affecting the metabolism of glucose as they produce imperfect expressions of the gamma receptor activated by peroxisome proliferator (PPAR-gamma).
The lactic acidosis that occurs in the syndrome is mainly caused by nucleoside analog reverse transcriptase inhibitors. It is secondary to the mitochondrial dysfunction caused due to inhibition of mitochondrial deoxyribonucleic acid (DNA) polymerase by this class of drugs. The establishment of lactic acidosis is slow and the symptoms are not specific.
It is unclear whether the loss of bone mineral density is a component of the same syndrome. Avascular necrosis has been considered a complication of HLS, since hyperlipidemia and the HIV infection itself are known risk factors for osteonecrosis of the femoral head.
Metabolic changes are associated with increased risk of cardiovascular events.
Hyperinsulinemia associated with insulin resistance is a risk factor recognized in patients not infected with HIV and may contribute to increased risk of acute myocardial infarction in patients using ARV.
Thus, HIV-positive patients, with significantly higher prevalence of elevated fasting glucose and triglyceride levels and low levels of HDL cholesterol are at increased risk of

atherosclerosis, coronary heart disease and diabetes mellitus. The risk of developing diabetes is 6 to 10% in these patients, and is further increased in obese patients coinfected with hepatitis C or with a family history of DM . There are reports of an increase of 16% in the incidence of myocardial infarction per year of antiretroviral treatment.

Among the fat redistribution anatomical changes, three groups are identified: lipoatrophy, lipohypertrophy and mixed forms.

Lipoatrophy and lipohypertrophy may occur independently or may occur together in the same patient.

There is central or localized accumulation of fat in lipohypertrophy. Accumulation of fat may occur in the abdomen, neck, back, breast and other sites in a localized form. The abdomen acquires a global aspect and fat tissue is commonly deposited intra-abdominally, in viscera or between them. Increased intra-abdominal pressure may predispose to abdominal hernias that may eventually require surgical correction.

Accumulation of fat in the upper trunk surrounding the chest and extending up to the armpits was observed in male patients, as well as accumulation of fat in the anterior cervical region and in the suprapubic region in men and women.

An increase in the breasts of female patients mostly occurs due to a fat component and is not necessarily associated with glandular hypertrophy. In male patients, gynecomastia can occur (glandular hypertrophy) or pseudo-gynecomastia (fat accumulation).

Lipohypertrophy is more associated with older patients who are initiating treatment, using protease inhibitors, and who have more elevated body mass.

Loss of peripheral subcutaneous tissue is observed in lipoatrophy. In addition to that, upper and lower limbs get thinner, the skin gets thinner and allows almost anatomical visualization of muscle groups and superficial blood vessels. This condition may give the patient a pseudo-athletic aspect. Evidence of blood vessels is also often confused with venous insufficiency (pseudo varicose veins).

For some authors, the heterogeneity of the findings concerning HIV-associated lipodystrophy may reflect the existence of more than one syndrome.

2.3 Diagnosis

There is still no universally accepted definition for HLS, which explains the difficulty in determining a case as wells as its prevalence, etiology and treatment.

The most commonly used method to determine a case of lipodystrophy includes the subjective description of changes in body fat. Two multicenter studies were conducted in an attempt to define a case of lipodystrophy. The Lipodystrophy Case Definition Study compared patients with and without clinical evidence of lipodystrophy, in agreement between patients and physicians. Laboratory, anthropometry and radiology data, such as dual X-ray absorptiometry (DEXA) and computed tomography (CT), were compared between the two groups of patients. The definition of lipodystrophy generated had sensitivity and specificity of 80%, but has proved to be too complex to be used in clinical practice. The Fat Redistribution and Metabolic Changes in HIV Infection Study compared laboratory testings and anthropometry and radiology data on distribution of body fat among HIV-infected and non-infected patients. The study showed that the only change in body fat associated with HIV infection was generalized lipoatrophy. The results do not explain the high prevalence of intra-abdominal obesity in HIV-positive patients, but is in accordance with other studies, which claim that lipoatrophy is the hallmark of body changes in HIV-infected individuals.

Some diagnostic criteria were proposed in the First International Workshop on Lipodystrophy and Adverse Reactions to Drugs, held in June 1999 in San Diego. The clinical criteria described were sunken face, depressed temples, sunken eyes, prominent zygomatic arch, emaciated appearance, prominent non-varicose veins in the arms and legs, loss of skin folds, loss of the contours and fat from the gluteal region. Accumulation of fat was categorized into 5 areas: increased abdominal girth, breast enlargement, dorsocervical fat accumulation, facial fat accumulation (although possibly rarer than facial lipoatrophy), and the presence of lipomas. Methods for evaluation and monitoring of fat deposition include patient's report, clinical evaluations, anthropometric measurements and imaging studies.

Objective criteria for diagnosis of lipodystrophy have not been established yet. The absence of standardized values in relation to fat in the general population and the heterogeneity of clinical manifestations of lipodystrophy make the diagnosis even more difficult. A gold standard technique for measuring body fat is not available yet. However, some methods such as anthropometry, bioelectrical impedance analysis (BIA), DEXA, computed tomography, magnetic resonance imaging (MRI) and ultrasound have been used.

Anthropometry and impedance analysis cannot measure localized fat. CT and MRI methods are costly, which restricts their use. The use of US is promising because it is simple, noninvasive, available and low-cost, although it is more operator-dependent than the other techniques. The fact that measurement of absolute values of localized fat does not elucidate the occurrence of body-fat changes is also a limiting factor.

High-resolution MRI allowed the identification of a clear disruption in the adipose tissue of HIV patients, and changes in the tissue architecture seem to appear earlier than changes detected by DEXA or by clinical examination.

The US showed moderate agreement between its findings and the lipoatrophy reported by the physician or patient in clinical evaluation. According to the authors, the anatomy of the face, the patient's age and quality of the skin affect how subcutaneous fat is perceived externally. Even so, they see the US as a potentially useful tool in evaluating patients due to its low-cost, accessibility and absence of radiation.

Considering all of these limitations, describing the loss or accumulation of fat in specific areas and determining the degree of intensity through clinical evaluation and in a way that doctors and patients agree continue to be the best way to define the problem individually.

Most studies on lipodystrophy syndrome are based on the presence of symptoms subjectively reported by patients, clinical signs found in the physical examination carried out by a doctor or on a combination of both. These observations may or may not be confirmed by diagnostic methods.

Objective measurement of facial fat is more difficult to obtain than measurement of body fat. A questionnaire of the FRAM study (2006) asked patients to assess any change in fat in the region of the cheeks, near the nose and mouth, and give it a score from 1 to 6. A similar score system varying from 1 to 7 was used by health professionals to assess fat in the region of the cheeks of the participants. A longitudinal ratio of the data obtained from patients and healthcare professionals can be used, as well as monitoring based on serial photographs, if the patient consents.

The diagnosis of lipoatrophy is still often based on the patient's perception and on clinical evaluation, which have shown a good correlation.

2.4 Epidemiology

It is very difficult to evaluate the prevalence of HLS, since there is no clear definition of the disease, with well-defined criteria for characterizing a case. Also, there are no accurate diagnostic methods for detection of fat redistribution or quantification of loss or gain of body fat.

As the condition is characterized by several changes in body composition, whether atrophy, hypotrophy or hypertrophy, which may be present together or separately, it becomes more difficult to fit the patients into well-defined groups.

The prevalence of lipodystrophy reported in the literature varies widely, with articles that describe rates of 7 to 84% among patients with HIV/AIDS using antiretrovirals or not. Such variations are possibly due to the diagnostic criteria used, despite the lack of standardization for these criteria.

Generally speaking, the prevalence of at least one body change is approximately 50%.

A study conducted by Cabrero et al. (2010) with 965 patients in 98 different health facilities showed that the patients noticed some kind of body change in 55.1% of the cases. Concerning the physicians' perception in relation to body changes, this ratio changes to 55.2% of the cases. The most commonly reported change was lipoatrophy, which was mentioned by 46.8% of the patients and 49.4% of the physicians, followed by lipohypertrophy. There was no gender difference in terms of perception of body changes. The concordance between patients and physicians in terms of the changes detected was 83%.

Hendrickson et al. (2009) also agree that lipoatrophy is one of the most common manifestations associated with the use of ARV and cite a frequency range of 13 to 63%.

Viskovic et al. (2009) believe that lipoatrophy is the most common and disfiguring of the body changes of the syndrome. They evaluated 151 patients with HIV, of whom about 39% reported lipoatrophy in some place, while about 45% of the physicians noticed fat loss in the clinical examination. Among the patients, 11% reported facial lipoatrophy, while the doctors noticed clinically detectable facial lipoatrophy in 15% of the patients.

2.5 Physiopathogenesis

The exact mechanism that leads to the development of anatomical and metabolic changes is still unclear. Several hypotheses have been suggested and, separately, none of them explain all aspects of these changes, which are probably multifactorial in origin. Some hypothesis are: mitochondrial toxicity related to the use of NRTIs; dysregulation of the tumor necrosis factor α (TNFα); inhibition of cytochrome P 450, related to protease inhibitors; hypercorticolism (pseudo Cushing's syndrome); local effects of HIV on production of cortisol and changes in other steroid hormones, among others.

When HLS arose, it was initially associated with the use of PI, a frequent component of ART. Studies have suggested that PI mediated lipoatrophy by changing the regulatory element of steroids and binding to protein 1, which is involved in the differentiation of adipocytes.

Ledru et al. (2000) have also showed that PIs have an effect on cellular proteases, which contributes to the accumulation of T cells, which produce TNFα. This seems to favor lipodystrophy as it contributes to changes in lipid metabolism. Other authors have also shown that TNFα levels and its receptors seem to be associated with the development of lipodystrophy in patients undergoing ART.

More recently, NRTI, another frequent component of ART, has been implicated as a cause of lipodystrophy.

Among the NRTIs, lipoatrophy is more associated with the use of stavudine and zidovudine. Lipoatrophy occurs in 30% of the patients after 2 years of use of stavudine, while it occurs in only 6% of the patients using tenofovir.

NRTIs deplete the deoxyribonucleic acid (DNA) of mitochondria, inhibiting mitochondrial DNA polymerase, which may result in apoptosis of adipocytes. It has been suggested that thymidine analogue NRTIs (stavudine, zidovudine) are more toxic to the mitochondrial DNA than the new non-thymidine analogue NRTI, such as abacavir; although all of the drugs belonging to this class can cause depletion of mitochondrial DNA.

Lipohypertrophy is more associated with the use of PIs; although efavirenz, an NNRTI, is involved in the appearance of pseudo-gynecomastia. Even though lipoatrophy is more associated with NRTI, efavirenz is also implicated in the progression of lipoatrophy.

Pacenti et al. (2006) identified genes modulated by PI and NRTI in early adipogenesis and suggest that the regulation of transcription factors and modulation of the Wnt gene are the route through which PIs lead to inhibition of adipocyte differentiation and negative regulation of the expression of specific markers for adipocytes such as leptin, MRAP, Cd36/FAT and S100A8. The effect of NRTIs on adipocyte differentiation and on gene expression profiling was milder than that of PI, although NRTI have shown modulation in the expression of tissue inhibitors of metalloproteinases and of transcription factors, such as Aebp1, which can act on the determination of the phenotype of adipocytes. The authors conclude that abnormal expression of these genes may underlie lipodystrophy associated with ART.

Genetic predisposition is another important factor in the pathogenesis of lipodystrophy. Ranade et al. (2008) identified a subgroup of patients who were especially vulnerable to the metabolic side effects of ART. After genetic analysis, they identified the resistin gene as being implicated in susceptibility to HIV-associated lipodystrophy.

Mitochondrial DNA haplogroup H was also identified as having strong association with the presence of atrophy in patients treated with nucleoside analog reverse transcriptase inhibitors. On the other hand, haplogroup T has shown borderline significance as a protective factor in the development of lipoatrophy in the same group of patients.

Some studies suggest that fat redistribution and metabolic abnormalities associated with HIV infection are related to changes in the endocrine function of adipose tissue. The adipose tissue, besides its function of storing fat, is an active endocrine tissue and the major determinant of insulin sensitivity, modulating the metabolism of glucose and lipids through the secretion of adipocytokines.

Verkauskiene et al. (2006) have shown that HIV-infected children with signs of redistribution of body fat have lower levels of adiponectin, associated with insulin resistance and dyslipidemia. In this study, leptin concentration showed no significant effect on the redistribution of body fat.

Lipoatrophy may occur in the absence of PI or NRTI therapy, with studies suggesting that antiretroviral drugs are not the only causal factor. In the HIV Outpatient Study (2001), 1,077 patients were evaluated in relation to changes in body fat distribution. Lipoatrophy was associated with the use of indinavir, a PI, for more than two years and with the use of stavudine, an INTR. However, independently, risk factors unrelated to drug use were strongly associated with lipoatrophy, including advanced age (> 40 years), white race, CD4 count <100 cells/mm3, decreased body mass index, and higher duration and severity of the HIV disease itself. The number of non-pharmacological risk factors increased the likelihood of developing lipoatrophy. The results suggest that the cause of lipoatrophy is multifactorial and that it may be a result of HIV infection of long duration. The expression of tumor necrosis factor α (TNF) by subcutaneous adipocytes *in vitro* is higher among patients with lipoatrophy, and this suggests that sustained activation of inflammatory cytokines in HIV infection may mediate lipoatrophy.

Interleukin 6 (IL-6) is a multifunctional cytokine that acts as an inflammatory, immune and metabolic mediator. Thus, its involvement in various events related to HIV infection is questioned. Increased production of IL-6 in patients infected with HIV and undergoing antiretroviral therapy is known. Saumoy et al. (2008) evaluated the influence of the IL-6-174G>C genotype on the risk of developing fat redistribution syndrome in HIV-infected patients undergoing combined antiretroviral therapy, but no significant difference was found.

Beyond the risk factors for HIV facial lipodystrophy which have already been identified, as the use of protease inhibitors, age, low CD4, high viral load, duration of ARV, white race and being female, other influences which have not yet been identified may also be associated with the development of HLS.

Whatever the etiology of HLS, be it caused by drug therapy, genetic predisposition, immune reconstitution, activation of cytokines, direct action of HIV infection, hormonal influences or other unidentified influences, the fact is that fat loss is apparently irreversible.

3. Facial lipoatrophy

3.1 Definition

Among the areas affected by lipoatrophy, one of the most common components of the syndrome, the face is the region where fat loss is more evident and impressive.

Facial lipoatrophy consists of a progressive loss of facial fat, mainly due to decreased malar fat (Bichat's fat pad) and temporal fat. Facial lipoatrophy stimulates the appearance of new skin furrows, the intensity of facial expression lines, in addition to intensifying areas of depression and visualization of the skull. All of this leads to wrinkling of the face, which precociously ages the individual; in women, loss of facial fat leads to a loss of femininity of the face. Moreover, the aspect of an emaciated and haggard face started to be seen once again as a 'facies of the disease', bringing back the old stigma of the "face of AIDS", in addition to the fear of involuntary disclosure of the diagnosis.

3.2 Classification

The lack of criteria for diagnosing and assessing fat loss in facial lipoatrophy (HIV facial wasting) is also a complicating factor in the establishment of a classification of disease severity.

The Facial Lipoatrophy Severity Index (FLSI) was developed by Brazilian physicians based on the parameters used for the classification of psoriasis severity. This tool aims at objectively measuring the degree of atrophy and improvement with treatment.

The FLSI evaluates three regions of the face. The malar region corresponds to the zygomatic and buccal areas, limited by the infraorbital border and lower edge of the mandible. Other anatomical structures considered are the zygomatic bone, the body of mandible projection, the zygomaticus major muscle, the canine fossa and maxilla.

The temporal region corresponds to the anterior temporal fossa, limited by the temporal line of the frontal bone and zygomatic arch (zygomatic process of the temporal bone and temporal process of the zygomatic bone).

The pre-auricular region corresponds to the masseter, between the zygomatic arch and the angle and lower edge of the mandible.

The depth and extent of the affected area in the malar, temporal, and preauricular regions are individually assessed. The depth of the atrophic areas is scored from 0 to 4, with 0 being absence of atrophy, 1, mild atrophy, 2, moderate atrophy, 3, severe atrophy, and 4, very severe atrophy. The extent of the affected area is scored from 0 to 5, with 0 being absence of involvement, 1, involvement of less than 20% of the region assessed, 2, from 21 to 50%, 3, from 51 to 70%, 4, from 71 to 90%, and 5, from 91 to 100%.

A partial number is calculated for each area assessed by multiplying the score relative to depth by the one relative to the affected area and by a correction factor.

The correction factor was determined for each region of the face and corresponds to the degree of importance of each one of them in facial lipoatrophy. Correction factors are 0.7 for the malar region, 0.2 for the temporal region and 0.1 for the preauricular region.

Since fat loss is not symmetrical, the most affected side is considered in the assessment.

The partial scores of the three regions are then added, yielding a final score.

The Brazilian Ministry of Health classifies facial lipoatrophy into grades I through IV, based on the application of the FLSI.

Grade I, or mild facial lipoatrophy, corresponds to an FLSI from zero to 5.9. In such cases there is a slight depression, but there is no evidence of anatomical structures in the region nor loss of facial contour. The skin is normal to digital pressure.

Grade II or moderate facial lipoatrophy corresponds to an FLSI from 6.0 to 10. Depression is more visible with early visualization of anatomical structures, especially the zygomatic arch and increase of nasolabial folds. There is no loss of facial contour or projection of the maxilla. Upon digital pressure, the skin is normally depressed but return to the resting state is delayed.

Grade III or severe FL corresponds to an FLSI from 10.1 to 15. Structures in the malar region are well observed, such as the zygomatic bone, visualization of the canine fossa, partial visualization of the zygomaticus major muscle and mild or moderate depression of the lower edge of the mandible. Loss of facial contour and projection of the maxilla may occur. Upon digital pressure, the skin depresses slightly and is very slow to return to the resting state.

Grade IV, or very severe FL, corresponds to an FLSI from 15.1 to 20. There is almost complete visualization of the anatomical contours, revealing the bone and muscles of the face. There is loss of facial contour, with visualization of the upper and lower surfaces of the zygomatic arch in the temporal and preauricular regions. Upon digital pressure, the skin hardly depresses.

The FLSI can vary from 0 to 20, and the Brazilian Ministry of Health recommends treatment for patients with a score equal to or greater than 6.

Other classifications are adopted in the international literature, all of them with a degree of subjectivity for being evaluator-dependent.

3.3 Psychological impact

Changes in body image can be extremely disruptive in terms of psychosocial well-being, increasing the stigma of the disease. Although it is also visible in the arms, legs and buttocks, lipodystrophy is most apparent on the face.

With the progression of the symptoms, patients begin to show facies that are typical of lipodystrophy syndrome. This brought back the stigma of AIDS and the need for specialists working with HIV/AIDS patients to identify these changes and seek treatment options.

Patients have described facial lipodystrophy as a visible marker to identify HIV carriers, perceived as the "face of AIDS," or the "Kaposi's sarcoma of the 21st century." Moreover, it causes problems in social and family relationships, which in some cases trigger disturbances in social relations, leading to the isolation of patients. One of the major consequences of lipodystrophy is treatment dropout due to the psychosocial effects of body fat redistribution.

Given the prevalence of changes caused by fat redistribution, it is clear that HIV-associated facial lipoatrophy is becoming epidemic. It stigmatizes those affected causing a major impact on their quality of life. Usually, these patients have good disease control and good health, but their facial features suggest otherwise and the psychological effects are often devastating.

Patients with facial lipoatrophy are exposed and cannot afford to keep their condition a secret. This may result in discrimination at work, affect relationships and sexual function and even adherence to treatment. This influences the patients' sense of well-being, as well as their body image and self-esteem. In some cases, patients become socially isolated.

It is a fact that facial lipoatrophy causes a major psychological impact and can reduce patient compliance with treatment.

3.4 Treatment

Since the causes of HIV-associated lipodystrophy are not well known and it is not yet clear how the syndrome develops, it is difficult to delineate treatment attempts. So far, some treatments are available for facial lipodystrophy, either conservative or interventional, pharmacological or surgical, with varying results and side effects.

3.4.1 Conservative treatments

Among the conservative treatments of FL, the possibility of adjustment of antiretroviral therapy has been considered, allocating drugs that are less associated with the development of HIV facial wasting. Change of antiretroviral therapy in response to lipoatrophy should be cautious due to the risk of viral rebound or adverse reactions to the drugs introduced.

Some studies have shown that the exchange of a thymidine analogue nucleoside reverse transcriptase inhibitor for a non-thymidine analogue results in a slight increase in peripheral fat after 24 weeks, measured by DEXA and CT, although the effect has not been shown to be clinically evident. The replacement of stavudine with abacavir or tenofovir showed maintenance of the immunological pattern, with the advantage of stabilization of anatomical changes, and even their slight improvement. A prolonged interruption to treatment (greater than 6 months), however, does not yield a clinically evident improvement in lipoatrophy in some studies.

Nonetheless, physicians should consider the sensitivity of the virus to the drugs and disease severity, as well as the potential risks of drug therapy when changing treatment regimens.

One of the possible interventions in drug therapy is the use of antidiabetic agents.

Thiazolidinediones (rosiglitazone, pioglitazone) are antidiabetic agents that improve insulin resistance in type 2 diabetes mellitus. They can lead to fat gain in some patients and may increase fat mass in some familial forms of lipoatrophy. Some studies show conflicting results about the increase of subcutaneous fat tissue with the use of rosiglitazone. Large-scale studies are needed.

Studies with metformin are not consensual and most have a short follow-up. Some data suggest reduction of subcutaneous fat with its use, including visceral and limb fat, being more useful in patients with glucose disorders.

Anabolic actions are among the most important effects of the growth hormone (GH). The therapeutic use of human GH began 49 years ago. Recombinant GH has been used since 1985, which enabled pituitary hormone replacement therapy with less risk to patients. The most common indications for the use of GH are deficient growth, either idiopathic or secondary, adults with GH deficiency or insufficiency, and weight loss due to AIDS. The

FDA has approved a type of growth hormone to treat muscle wasting in HIV-positive patients when they present with hormonal suppression. The use of this treatment in public health programs is limited by high cost, about $ 36,000 per year. The international literature reports that short-term treatment increases total body weight and lean body mass, with consequent improvement of physical capacity and quality of life. The regimen to be employed among HIV/AIDS patients and the duration of treatment are not well established.

Although commonly used to fight body mass loss, anabolic steroids may actually reduce subcutaneous fat and worsen HIV-associated lipoatrophy. Although human GH has been widely used in HIV-associated fat accumulation, particularly in the abdominal (visceral) region, its use to treat facial lipoatrophy is controversial. Honda et al. (2007) evaluated the use of subcutaneous GH in HIV-1 patients who had moderate to severe facial lipoatrophy. The authors concluded that GH is effective and relatively safe for the treatment of moderate to severe facial lipoatrophy and that the cost-effectiveness of its use should be further discussed.

The use of GH is also limited by the fact that the benefits obtained with its use do not persist for more than 12 weeks after its interruption and by a decreased sensitivity to insulin, already impaired in the syndrome.

Some new drug treatments have been suggested for HIVLS, but more scientific studies to gauge their true clinical applicability are needed.

Leptin is an amino acid which is a product of the human leptin gene. It regulates the energy, neuroendocrine and functional homeostases of the body. Recombinant human leptin is an emerging possibility to treat lipoatrophy caused by its genetic deficiency and may have some application in lipoatrophy associated with HIV/AIDS.

As one of the causes of lipoatrophy is mitochondrial toxicity caused by ARVs, antioxidants and mitochondrial cofactors could also be of value in its prevention or treatment.

Nutritional counseling and physical exercises are adjuvant therapies for metabolic and body alterations in HIVLS. Aerobic exercises reduce the levels of TGC and cholesterol, especially LDL and, through the burning of fat, they help to reverse some bodily changes related to the central accumulation of fat. Resistance exercises help with muscle mass gain, improving the appearance of the chest, arms and legs, in addition to being useful to treat osteopenia. A diet rich in fiber and adequate in energy and protein can prevent the development of body fat deposits. However, these measures have no impact on facial subcutaneous fat that has already been lost.

3.4.2 Surgical treatments

Disorders of body fat distribution associated with antiretroviral therapy are currently considered irreversible. Several studies have explored therapeutic strategies, but none of these strategies allow for sufficient recovery of adipose tissue to a consistent clinical perception.

To the HIV/AIDS Treatment and Training Foundation in Spain, surgery is the only option to reverse the manifestations of lipodystrophy, which can be atrophy, hypertrophy, or a combination of both.

One promising technique to treat facial lipoatrophy is subcutaneous filling – the cutaneous fillers.

The use of dermal fillers was introduced in 1981, when bovine collagen began to be implanted into the skin to smooth away the appearance of facial wrinkles. Since then, new materials have been developed to improve effectiveness and safety parameters.

The ideal filler should be a nontoxic material that does not induce hypersensitivity or foreign body reactions, which does not degenerate over time or induce calcification, and which is chemically inert and easily implanted. These substances must be biocompatible, must not cause allergic reactions, and must be easily managed and stable over time. Moreover, the cost of treatment should be accessible to patients.

3.4.2.1 Dermal fillers

Injectable fillers are currently important tools in the non-invasive arsenal of rejuvenation procedures, in the correction of congenital or acquired facial defects and, more recently, in the treatment of facial lipoatrophy associated with HIV/AIDS.

According to their availability, chemical composition and degradation, fillers can be classified as temporary or permanent, organic or inorganic, and autologous or heterologous.

With regard to durability, some studies rely on a third sub-group, which would be that of semi-permanent fillers. Some authors define semi-permanent products as those with durability between one and two years. Permanent fillers would then last over 2 years and temporary fillers, less than one year.

Some fillers, when implanted, increase facial volume by direct filling and expansion of receptor sites. This is the case of silicone, collagen, and certain polyacrylamides. Others also create volume directly, but promote a foreign body reaction for a given period of time, stimulating progressive and long-lasting collagen deposition. PMMA, polylactic acid and calcium hydroxyapatite are examples of this second category.

Hoping to find a filler with greater durability, researchers tested a series of non-resorbable particles in mice, and polymethylmethacrylate (PMMA) molecules were the best tolerated, with the lowest rate of allergic reactions.

Polymethylmethacrylate was synthesized for the first time in 1902. It was patented in 1928 as Plexiglas and it was mainly used as bone cement in the medical field. Initially available in the form of pellets, in 1937 the material could also be found in the form of granules and molding powder.

Neurosurgeons began using PMMA during the Second World War to perform cranioplasty because of the resistance and lightness of the material. PMMA is still used in the reconstruction of cranial defects because of its excellent tissue compatibility, the ease with which it is handled in surgery, its strength and radiolucency, as well as its accessibility, low thermal and electrical conductance and lightness. In 1946, PMMA represented approximately 95% of the prostheses in the market.

Medical research progressed and PMMA also began to be used for the fixation of femural orthopedic prosthesis. The use of PMMA as bone cement was introduced by Charnley and Smith in the 60s. Since then it has been widely used in surgery to fill the spaces between the prosthesis and bone.

The inert chemistry and biocompatibility of polymethylmethacrylate have been accepted since Jude introduced the first hip prosthesis made of this material in 1947.

The first hard PMMA ophthalmic lenses were made by Kevin Tuohey in 1948. Its use in ophthalmology has also brought a lot of knowledge about this material.

So far, PMMA continues to be used as bone cement in orthopedics, as repair material in craniofacial neurosurgery, as a material for intraocular lenses in ophthalmology and as dental cement in dentistry.

The PMMA molecule appears to be chemically inert, so conducting prior allergy testing is not necessary when the product is used in isolation. Animal experiments have shown that the keys to skin biocompatibility are the spherical shape of particles, their smooth and regular surface and the size of polymethylmethacrylate microspheres. The size of the molecules is important because very small particles can be easily phagocytosed and the largest ones do not pass easily through a No. 26 needle. Repeated rinsing of the microspheres reduces impurities and increases tolerance to the product by reducing the number of foreign body giant cells around the injected particles of PMMA.

Since PMMA microspheres are not biodegradable and are too large to migrate or be phagocytosed by macrophages, a permanent tissue increase is expected, consisting of 80% of the volume of autologous connective tissue. Lemperle et al. (1991) suggested that PMMA particles are resistant to phagocytosis and degradation and are not carcinogenic. This study attributes resistance to phagocytosis to the smooth surface of the particles and reports that, after four months, a delicate fibrous capsule is formed around each particle, which prevents displacement of the implant.

The PMMA implant has immediate and long term results, considering it is a biocompatible and inert filler, which give it characteristics of a permanent implant.

The injected microspheres cause a stimulus in the tissue that ultimately induces formation of new collagen fibers.

The tissue stimulation induced by PMMA microspheres is caused by a mild inflammation produced by monocytes, histiocytes and fibroblasts at the site of application, which can subsequently produce collagen fibers. Allen et al. (1992), in a longitudinal study, noticed the cellular reactions after the injection of inert implants. Such reactions were followed by a series of events of variable magnitude. In the first 24 hours, neutrophils and small round cells predominate; within 48 hours, there is a predominance of monocytes and, in 7 days, there is formation of foreign body giant cells. In two weeks, the cellular response is already moderate; in 4 weeks, fibroblasts appear; in 6 weeks, foreign body giant cells are noted and deposition of collagen is intensified; in eight weeks, chronic inflammatory cells are scattered along a massive deposition of collagen. Thereafter, the cellular reaction to the foreign body is stabilized and in six months giant cells and a small level of cellular response are present with a reduced amount of dense collagen; there is also conversion of fibroblasts into fibrocytes. From then on there was greater permanence of the implant in place. Collagen compounds mixed with PMMA microspheres then became a source of great expectations for researchers and the medical community.

In presentations made available internationally, PMMA microspheres were first suspended in gelatin. Of the 578 patients who initially received the product, 15 developed granulomas within 6 to 18 months after application. It was concluded, therefore, that impurities stimulated macrophages and were the cause of the formation of granulomas. In addition, some patients had palpable nodules that were attributed to the rapid absorption of the gelatin carrying the microspheres, which allowed them to agglutinate. This vehicle was then replaced by a collagen solution, which is more viscous and more durable in the tissue. After applying the product to the deep dermis, collagen is degraded by the body within 1 to 3 months and is completely replaced by the patient's own collagen within a similar period of time, ensuring increased volume.

The collagen used in foreign formulations is of bovine origin. The antigenicity of bovine collagen is reduced by the action of a pepsin, which removes the more antigenic end portion of the collagen molecule, without destroying the helical nature of the collagen fibers.

Commercial formulations available in most countries are a suspension of 20% purified PMMA microspheres of 30 to 42 micrometers in diameter in a 3.5% bovine collagen solution. It also contains 0.3% lidocaine to reduce discomfort after application. This product has been approved and made available in over 50 countries since 1994, with an estimated 400,000 patients treated so far and a complication rate of 0.01%. It has been marketed under the trade name Artecoll since 1996 in the European Union, 1998 in Canada and in Mexico, since 1999. The product was approved by the FDA in October 2006, and is marketed in the U.S. under the name Artefill, with the same composition as that of Artecoll, but with reduced nanoparticles and more uniform-sized spheres.

Because bovine collagen is a foreign protein, 3% of patients may develop an immune reaction, possibly a type IV allergic reaction, although antibodies to bovine collagen can be seen in the serum of patients. Thus, a prior allergy test is essential. A small amount of pure collagen solution, usually 0.05 to 0.1 ml, is injected intradermally on the surface of the forearm. Reading is done in 72 hours and again after 1 month. Edema and/or erythema make the test positive. About 1.2% of patients with negative test results develop an immune reaction in a subsequent application, so a second test should be performed 30 days after the first. Some authors suggest a new test for treatments after a period of 12 months.

The association of bovine collagen to PMMA substantially increases the cost of the product, which becomes a limiting factor for situations in which large amounts of the filler are needed, such as in the treatment of facial lipodystrophy, and very impractical for use in public health programs.

Several countries use associated PMMA -Artfill, Artecoll- and the number of patients treated worldwide surpassed 250,000 in 2005. Among these, only 0.01% had granuloma formation.

Most papers published in the international literature on PMMA implants are about collagen-associated products (Artecoll or Artfill).

The Brazilian Sanitary Surveillance Agency (ANVISA), similar to the FDA in the United States, has approved the use of PMMA without association with collagen for the treatment of HIV-associated facial lipodystrophy. However, this product has also been used to treat nasolabial folds, to correct the atrophy of bone eminences, especially malar and mental, to treat Parry-Romberg syndrome (progressive hemifacial atrophy), and to correct the nasal dorsum, scars and atrophic ear lobe.

The injectable product used in Brazil consists of polymerized microspheres of PMMA ranging from 30 to 50 micrometers in size, coated with magnesium carboxygluconate hydrolactic gel. The ratio microspheres/gel is 3:10. It is available in 10 ml vials or ready-to-use syringes of 1 or 3 ml, stored at room temperature. It was initially introduced in Brazil in 1996. Since there are no animal components in its structure, prior allergy testing is not needed.

The great advantages of the PMMA used in Brazil are the fact that it does not require prior allergy testing and presents no risk of prion disease transmission. Because it is a permanent filler, the results are lasting. In addition, it has a very low cost compared to other fillers on the market. The cost of Metacryll, one of the PMMA-based products sold, is about US$20/ml. Studies have shown safety and efficacy with the use of this product, with a high rate of satisfaction among patients and low incidence of side effects. In fact, an increase in the number of CD4 + cells after treatment of FL with this implant has been described. Improvements in the quality of life, social relationships, and psychological state of the patient are reported after treatment of FL, with improvement of the immune system.

The literature describes the use of many other fillers in the treatment of FL. In the United States and Canada, some forms of injectable liquid silicone have been successfully used to treat HIV-associated facial lipoatrophy. The term silicone was assigned to a family of polymers with one basic element: silicon. These polymers vary in their viscosity from an oil to a jelly. The pure silicone recommended for dermal filling is siloxane, which is a class of chemical compounds with alternating chains of silicon, oxygen and methane. The pure, sterile and filtered form is recommended for use as filler.

The combination of puncture and silicone deposition leads to an inflammatory reaction with polymorphonuclear cell migration, followed by a moderate lymphocytic infiltrate. This infiltrate can be observed for six months. There is a discreet phagocytic activity and a small number of giant cells can be seen, which do not evolve to the formation of granulomas. The low volumes of silicone injected soon settle in the deep dermis and subcutaneous tissue and are surrounded by pseudocapsules of preexisting collagen, which later give rise to a newly-formed thin collagen capsule.

Immediate reactions include erythema, edema, and possibly ecchymosis. Soon after injection, small papules may appear at the site of the injection, but they disappear after a few hours or within 3 weeks. There are reports of dyschromias, but they are infrequent. Excessive elevation may occur due to overcorrection or excess volume injected. Cases of erythema and granuloma formation are associated with impurity of the material, inadequate location or injection of large volumes. Migration of the silicone, which is often the main fear among professionals and patients, only occurs when volumes above 1 ml are used in a single site, which is often necessary in the treatment of FL.

In some studies, injectable liquid silicone appeared to be the most cost-effective treatment in the United States. However, a longer follow-up of treated patients is needed to determine the efficacy, permanency, and long-term safety of liquid silicone injection in the treatment of HIV-associated facial lipoatrophy.

A limiting factor to this procedure is that its use is prohibited in many countries.

Polylactic acid filler was the first to be approved by the FDA for the treatment of facial lipoatrophy associated with the use of ARVs. FDA approval was based on four studies that documented the safety and efficacy of the product in 278 patients with facial lipoatrophy.

Polylactic acid is a synthetic polymer which is biodegradable and immunologically inert. Once injected, the microparticles of polylactic acid may stimulate collagen production, which allows a gradual and progressive increase in the volume of the lipoatrophic area. Polylactic acid belongs to the family of alpha-hydroxyl acids and has been available for over 30 years for various uses in medicine.

Polylactic acid is injected into the deep dermis in order to increase the number of fibroblasts and their activity, resulting in increased collagen synthesis. It has two modes of action. Initially, there is a temporary increase in volume of the treated area and it is essential that patients be well advised not to be disappointed when this initial volume decreases. The initial volume is created by injection of the volume of sterile water used to reconstitute the polylactic acid, which is resorbed in 48 to 72 hours. The second mode of action is the stimulation of collagen formation.

It may take several sessions before the desired effect on the contour of the face is noted. Polylactic acid is completely degraded in nine months.

Carey et al. (2007) conducted a randomized, multicentric study with a follow-up of 24 and 96 weeks, comparing adult patients with facial lipoatrophy induced by ARVs who were injected with polylactic acid in their deep dermis with a control group. These authors showed that treatment of facial lipoatrophy with polylactic acid in adult patients infected with HIV provided only a modest increase in facial thickness, but not in facial volume. In contrast, patients' perception of improved well-being, quality of life and cosmetic benefits was significant. Polylactic acid does not interfere with fat loss from other regions of the body. The authors further point out that other comparative studies are needed to establish the optimal treatment for HIV-associated facial lipoatrophy.

However, because polylactic acid is a biodegradable product, its effects are temporary and retreatment may be eventually necessary. Furthermore, multiple application sessions are necessary for its administration. Still, subcutaneous nodules have been described after injection of this material. There is also the high cost of this procedure. Thus, other alternative options for patients with facial lipoatrophy are important.

Hyaluronic acid is a polysaccharide component of soft tissue and it is identical in all species and types of tissue. There are commercial formulations that have already been approved by the FDA.

Injectable hyaluronic acid is obtained by bacterial fermentation and has a low incidence of adverse reactions. This incidence has fallen further in recent years, from 1/1400 patients in 1999 to 1/1800 patients in 2000. This decrease is explained by the production of more purified forms of hyaluronic acid by the pharmaceutical industry.

Hyaluronic acid has been used successfully to treat HIV-associated facial lipoatrophy. However, as with other temporary fillers, large volumes are often needed to achieve full correction, which tends to decrease after 6 to 12 months. The high cost of large volumes and the need to repeat treatment are major limiting factors.

Calcium hydroxyapatite gel is an injectable filler composed of 30% calcium hydroxyapatite microspheres and 70% of a carrier aqueous gel. Although synthetic, its components are identical to the mineral portion of bones and teeth. It is a biocompatible, non toxic and non-antigenic material.

It was approved by the FDA in 2006 for correction of the signs of facial fat loss in HIV patients. This implant provides an immediate correction. The carrier gel is absorbed in a few weeks, leaving the microspheres that serve as matrix for neocollagenesis and formation of new tissue. The major limiting factors for its use are also its high cost and the fact that it is a new filler about which there are no long term studies.

Polyacrylamide gel is a non-biodegradable polymer, non-allergenic and non toxic, composed of 96% non-pyrogenic water and 4% polyacrylamide. It is the only filler in which a thin layer of collagen capsule develops around the gel, isolating it from the host tissue. As a result of the encapsulation process, the implant can be readily identified and if removal is needed, it can be easily removed by the expression of the capsule, expelling the material from its interior. Therefore, polyacrylamide is considered an injectable prosthesis.

Polyacrylamide gel is nonbiodegradable and it is suggested to be biologically inert. The cosmetic effects of polyacrylamide filling are permanent, avoiding the need for further treatment.

A practical limitation of therapy with facial fillers is the cost associated with these products. The cost of polyacrylamide in 2007 in Canada was about US$ 175.00 per milliliter; patients require about 10 to 25 ml of the product. The total cost of the treatment would therefore range from US$ 1,750.00 to US$ 4,375.00 . In addition to the cost, which makes the use of this filler very impractical, the rate of infection described in the literature is higher than with the use of other fillers.

Cost is really a limiting factor in the choice of fillers, especially considering that in the case of FL the volumes needed are higher than those for other cosmetic indications. In a study of treatment of HIV/AIDS facial lipoatrophy with large particle-size hyaluronic acid, trade name SubQ, the estimated value per patient was 950 Euros, considering that each patient received an average of 6 ml of the product and the cost of 1 ml of the material was 160 Euros. Other formulations of hyaluronic acid have a starting cost of US$ 123 per unit, with a total average cost of US$ 687 for treating an area of the face. Polylactic acid has an approximate cost of US$ 123 per ml, with a total average price of US$ 3,690 per facial area treated. Silicone has a total cost of $ 8,750 for facial area treated, as described in the literature. Hydroxyapatite costs about $ 280 / ml, with an average cost of treatment reported in the literature of $ 7560 for facial area.

Because HIV-associated lipoatrophy is caused by loss of subcutaneous fat of the own patient, it would seem logical that the transfer of autologous fat was the most appropriate therapeutic option. A recent study reported 29 patients with HIV-associated facial lipoatrophy who received autologous fat transplantation by the Coleman's method. The technique was deemed reliable and photographic records done 6 months after treatment showed the permanency of the fat graft. However, the authors noted that most patients with HIV-associated facial lipoatrophy have no suitable fat donor areas, so many are not candidates for this procedure. Jones (2005) performed fat grafts in 10 patients with HIV-associated facial lipoatrophy with the same methods and similar results. Nevertheless, in almost all cases, correction did not last for more than 12 months. Another recent study also suggested that, although the filling with autologous fat is effective for this condition, patients with HIV-associated facial lipoatrophy have minimal fat donor sites and that this treatment requires new filling sessions over time. HIV patients often lose subcutaneous fat in the abdomen and buttocks, which are usually fat donor sites.

Comparative studies with groups treated with different fillers available in the market should be conducted to better establish the cost effectiveness of each product; the high cost of most fillers in the market limits their use in the treatment of FL.

In an attempt to obtain new fillers to be used mainly in treatments for rejuvenation of the face, new products may be developed and made available in the market. The cost of newly launched products, the durability of the materials, and the existence of research to ensure their effectiveness and safety are important factors that should bolster the use of fillers in medical practice, in particular, their use in the treatment of FL.

4. References

[1] Martinez E, Mocroft A, Garcia-Viejo M et al. Risk of Lipodystrophy in HIV-1-infected patients treated with protease inhibitors: a prospective cohort study. Lancet. 2001;357(9256): 592-98.

[2] Carr A, Samaras K, Burton S et al. A syndrome of peripheral lipodystrophy, hyperlipidaemia and insulin resistance in patients receiving HIV protease inhibitors. AIDS. 1998; 12(7):F51-F58.

[3] Collins E, Wagner C, Walmsley S. Psychosocial impact of the lipodystrophy syndrome in HIV infection. AIDS Read. 2000;10(9): 546-51.

[4] Brasil. Ministério da Saúde. Secretaria de Vigilância em Saúde. Departamento de DST, AIDS e Hepatites Virais. Manual de Tratamento da Lipoatrofia Facial: Recomendações para o preenchimento facial com polimetilmetacrilato em portadores de HIV/AIDS. Série A. Normas e Manuais Técnicos. Série Manuais 81. Brasília: Ministério da Saúde, 2009.

[5] Miller K, Yanovski J, Shankar R et al. Visceral abdominal-fat accumulation associated with use of indinavir. *Lancet*. 1998;351(9106):871-5.

[6] Miller KK, Daly PA, Sentochnik D et al. Pseudo-Cushing's syndrome in human immunodeficiency virus-infected patients. Clin Infect Dis. 1998;27(1):68-72.

[7] Valente AMM, Reis AF, Machado DM et al. HIV lipodystrophy syndrome. Arq Bras Endocrinol Metab. 2005; 49(6):871-81.

[8] Behrens GMN, Stoll M, Schimidt RE. Lipodystrophy Syndrome in HIV Infection: What is it, What Causes it and How Can it Be Managed? Drug Saf. 2000; 23(1):57-76.
[9] Gkrania-Klotsas E, Klotsas AE. HIV and HIV treatment: effects on fats, glucose and lipids. Br Med Bull. 2007;84(1):49-68.
[10] Castelo Filho A, Abrão P. Alterações metabólicas do paciente infectado por HIV. Arq Bras Endocrinol Metab. 2007;51(1):93-6.
[11] Finucane KA, Archer CB. Dermatological aspects of medicine: highly active antiretroviral therapy and the treatment of human immunodeficiency virus. Clin Exp Dermatol. 2010;35(1):107-9.
[12] Carr A, Emery S, Law M et al. An objective case definition of lipodystrophy in HIV-infected adults. Lancet. 2003;361(9359):726–735.
[13] Tien PC, Benson C, Zolopa AR et al. The study of fat redistribution and metabolic change in HIV infection (FRAM): methods, design, and sample characteristics. Am J Epidemiol. 2006;163(9): 860-869.
[14] Milinkovic A, Martinez E. Current perspectives on HIV-associated lipodystrophry syndrome. Journal of Antimicrobial Chemotherapy. 2005; 56(1): 6-9.
[15] Josse G, Gensanne D, Aquilina C et al. Human immundeficiency vírus atrophy induces modification of subcutaneous adipose tissue architecture: in vivo visualization by high-resolution magnetic resonance imaging. Br J Dermatol. 2009;160(4):741-6.
[16] Viskovic K, Richman I, Klasnic K et al. Assessment of Ultrasound for Use in Detecting Lipoatrophy in HIV-Infected Patients Taking Combination Antiretroviral Therapy. AIDS Patient Care STDS. 2009;23(2):79-84.
[17] Barli JG, Junod P, LeBlanc R et al. HIV-associated lipodystrophy syndrome: A review of clinical aspects. Can J Infct Dis Med Microbiol. 2005; 16(4): 233-243.
[18] Bacchetti P, Grispshover B, Grunfeld C et al. Fat distribution in men with HIV infection. J Acquire Immune Defic Synd. 2005; 40:121-131.
[19] Cabrero C, Griffa L, Burgos A. Prevalence and Impact of Body Physical Changes in HIV Patients Treated with Highly Active Antiretroviral Therapy: Results from a Study on Patient and Physician Perceptions. AIDS Patient Care STDS. 2010;24(1):5-13.
[20] Chen D, Misra A, Garg A. Clinical review 153: Lipodystrophy in human immunodeficiency virus-infected patients. J Clin Endocrinol Metab. 2002;87(11):4845–4856.
[21] Carter VM, Hoy JF, Bailey M et al. The prevalence of lipodystrophy in an ambulant HIV-infected population: It all depends on the definition. HIV Med. 2001;2(3):174–180.
[22] Lichtenstein KA, Ward DJ. Clinical assessment of HIV-associated lipodystrophy in an ambulatory population. Clinical Science. 2001; 15(11):1389-1398.
[23] Hendrickson SL, Kingsley LA, Ruiz-Pesini E et al. Mitochondrial DNA Halogroups Influence Lipoatrophy After Highly Active Antiretroviral Therapy. J Acquir Immune Defic Syndr. 2009;51(2):111-116.
[24] Bugge H, Negaard A, Skeie L et al. Hyaluronic acid treatment of facial fat atrophy in HIV-positive patients. HIV Med. 2007; 8(8):475-482.
[25] Li HY, Silva ACCM, Santos S. Síndrome Lipodistrófica e HIV/AIDS. J Bras Aids. 2002;3(2): 23-35.
[26] Ledru E, Christeff N, Patey O, Truchis P, Melchior JC, Gougeon ML. Alteration of tumor necrosis factor-α T-cell homeostasis following potent antiretroviral therapy:

contribution to the development of human immunodeficiency virus-associated lipodystrophy syndrome. Blood. 2000; 95(10):3191-3198.
[27] Pacenti M, Barzon L, Favaretto F, Fincati K, Romano S, Milan G et al. Microarray analasys during adipogenesis identifies new genes altered by antiretroviral drugs. AIDS. 2006; 20(13):1691-1705.
[28] Ranade K, Geese WJ, Noor M, Flint O, Tebas P, Mulligan K et al. Genetic analysis implicates resistin in HIV lipodystrophy. AIDS. 2008; 22(13): 1561-1568.
[29] Verkauskiene R, Dollfus C, Levine M, Faye A, Deghmoun S, Houang M et al. Serum Adiponectin and Leptin Concentrations in HIV-Infected Children with Fat Redistribution Syndrome. Pediatric Research. 2006; 60(2):225-230.
[30] Rezai AR, Nakajima K, Beall GN, Mitsuyasu RT, Hirano T, et al. Infection with HIV is associated with elevated IL-6 levels and production. J Immunol. 1990; 144: 480-484.
[31] Saumoy M, Lopez-Dupla M, Veloso S. The IL-6 system in HIV-1 infection and in HAART-related fat redistribution szndromes. Aids. 2008, 22(7): 893-903.
[32] Baril MD, Junod P, LeBlanc R et al. HIV-associated lipodystrophy syndrome: A review of clinical aspects. Infect Dis Med Microbiol. 2005;16(4): 233-43.
[33] Jones D. HIV Facial Lipoatrophy: Causes and Treatment Options. Dermatol Surg. 2005;31(11Pt2):1519-29.
[34] Kavouni A, Catalan J, Brown S et al. The face of HIV and AIDS: can we erase the stigma? AIDS Care. 2008;20(4):485-7.
[35] Paton NI, Earnest A, Ng YM, Karim F, Aboulhab J. Lipodystrophy in a cohort of human immunodeficiency virus-infected asian patients: prevalence, associated factors, and psychological impact. Clinical Infectious Disease. 2002; 35(5): 1244-9.
[36] Pujol RM, Domingo P, Francia E, Sanbeat MA, Alomar A, Vasquez G, et al. HIV-1 protease inhibitor associated partial lipodystrophy: clinicopathologic review of 14 cases. J Am Acad Dermatol. 2000; 42 (2Pt1): 193-8.
[37] Narins RS. Minimizing Adverse Events Associated with Poly-L-latic Acid Injection. Dermatol Surg. 2008;34(Supp1):S100-S104.
[38] Wohl DA, Brown TT. Management of Morphologic Changes Associated with Antiretroviral Use in HIV-Infected Patients. J Acquir Immune Defic Syndr. 2008; 49(Supply 2): S93-S100.
[39] Wannmacher L. Hormônio de crescimento: uma panacéia? ISNN. 2006; 3(8): 1810-19.
[40] Yin MT, Glesby MJ. Recombinant human growth hormone therapy in HIV-associated wasting and visceral adiposity. Expert Rev Anti Infect Ther 2005; 3(5):727-738.
[41] Honda M, Yogi A, Ishizuka N. Effectiveness of Subcutaneous Growth Hormona in HIV-1 Patients with Moderate to Severe Facial Lipoatrophy. Intern Med 2007;46:359-62.
[42] Spinola-Castro AM, Siviero-Miachon AA, Silva MTN, Guerra-Junior G. O papel do hormônio de crescimento no tratamento dos distúrbios endócrino-metabólicos do paciente com a síndrome da imunodeficiência adquirida (Aids). Arq Brás Endocrinol Metab. 2008; 52(5):818-32.
[43] Kelesidis T, Kelesidis I, Chou S et al. Narrative Review: The Role of Leptin in Human Physiology: Emerging Clinical Applications. Annals of Internal Medicine. 2010; 152(2): 93-101.
[44] Fundación para la Formación e Información sobre Tratamiento en el VIH/sida(FIT). Documento de Consenso. Tratamiento quirurgico de la lipodistrofia asociada a la

infección por VIH. Conclusiones de uma Reunión Multidisciplinar. Enferm Infecc Microbiol Clin. 2007;25(5): 324-8.
[45] Wolfram D, Tzankov A, Pisa-Katzer H. Surgery for Foreign Body Reactions due to Injectable Fillers. Dermatology. 2006;213(4):300-4.
[46] Sturm LP, Cooter RD, Mutimer KL et al. A Systematic Review of Permanent and Semipermanent Dermal Fillers for HIV-Associated Facial Lipoatrophy. AIDS Patient Care STDS. 2009;23(9): 699-714.
[47] Lemperle G, Ott H, Charrier U, Hecker J, Lemperle M. PMMA microspheres for intradermal implantation. I. Animal Research. Ann Plast Surg. 1991; 26(1):57-63.
[48] Frazer RQ, Byron RT, Osborne PB et al. PMMA: An Essential Material in Medicine and Dentistry. J Long Term Eff Med Implants. 2005;15(6):629-39.
[49] Alster TS, West TB. Human-derived and new synthetic injectable materials for soft-tissue augmentation: Current status and role in cosmetic surgery. Plast Reconstr Surg. 2000; 105 (7): 2515-25.
[50] Lemperle G, Gauthier-Hazan N, Lemperle M. PMMA microspheres (Artecoll) for long-lasting correction of wrinkles: Refinements and statistical results. Aesthetic Plast Surg. 1998; 22(5): 356-65.
[51] Judet, J. Protheses en resins acrylic. Mem Acad Chir. 1947; 73:561 apud Cohen SRMD, Holmer REMD. A long-lasting injectable wrinkle filler material: report of a controlled, randomized, multicenter clinical trial of 251 subjects. Plast Reconstr Surg. 2004; 114(4): 964-76.
[52] Reichnberger MA, Stoff AF, Ritcher D. Polymethilmethacrylate for managing frontal bone deformities. Aesth Plast Surg. 2007; 31(9): 397-400.
[53] Costa IMC, P Salaro CP, Costa MC. Polymethylmethacrylate facial implant: a successful personal experience in Brazil for more than 9 years. Dermatol Surg. 2009;35(8):1221-7.
[54] Lemperle F, Morhenn V, Charrier U. Human histology and persistence of various injectable filler substances for soft tissue augmentation. Aesthetic Plast Surg. 2003; 27(5): 354-66.
[55] Odo MEY, Chichierchio AL. Práticas em Cosmiatria e Medicina Estética - Evolução dos Implantes e Toxina Botulínica.1a. ed. São Paulo: Tecnopress; 2000.
[56] Allen O. Response to subdermal implantation of textured microimplants in humans. Aesth Plast Surg. 1992; 16:227-230.
[57] Haneke E. Polymethyl methacrylate microspheres in collagen. Seminars in Cutaneous Medicine and Surgery. 2004; 23(4): 227-232.
[58] Lemperle G, Hazan-Gauthier N, Lemperle M. PMMA microspheres (Arte cool) for skin and soft tissue augmentation. II. Clinical investigations. Plast Reconstr Surg. 1995; 96(1):627-34.
[59] Munhoz O, Serra M, Trope B, Keiko L, Telline RMC. Tratamento da lipoatrofia facial em pacientes de HIV/AIDS com polimetilmetacrilato (PMMA). Ministério da Saúde. Secretaria de Vigilância em Saúde. Programa Nacional de DST/AIDS. 2006.
[60] Gelfer A, Carruthers A, Carruthers J, Jang F, Berstein S. The natural History of Polymethylmethacrylate Microspheres Granulomas. Dermatol Drug. 2007; 33(5): 614-20.

[61] Carruthers A, Carruthers J. Polymethylmethacrylate Microspheres / Collagen as an tissue augmentation agent: Personal experience over 5 years. Dermatol Surg. 2005; 31(11): 1561-65.

[62] Pinheiro AMC, Oliveira Filho J, Costa IMC. Preenchimentos Cutâneos: Principais Preenchedores Cutâneos: Indicações e Técnicas. In: GADELHA, A. R.; COSTA, I. M. C. Cirurgia Dermatológica em Consultório. São Paulo: Atheneu, 2009. p. 527-548.

[63] Orentreich D, Leone AS. A case of HIV-associated facial lipoatrophy treated with 1000-cs liquid injectable silicone. Dermatol Surg. 2004; 30(4):548-51.

[64] Loutfy MR, Raboud JM, Antoniou T, Kovacs C, Shen S, Halpenny R, et al. Immediate versus delayed polyalkylimide gel injections to correct facial lipoatrophy in HIV-positive patients. AIDS. 2007; 21(9): 1147-55.

[65] Jones DH, Carruthers A, Fitzgerald R et al. Late-Appearing Abscesses after Injections of Nonabsorbable Hidrogel for HIV-Associated Facial Lipoatrophy. Dermatol Surg. 2007;33(Supp2):S193-S198.

[66] Carruthers J, Carruthers A. Facial and Tissue Augmentation. Dermatol Surg. 2005; 31(1): 1604-1612.

[67] Carey DL, Baker D, Rogers GD et al. A randomized, open-label study of poly-L-lactic acid for HIV-1 facial lipoatrophy. J Acquir Immune Defic Syndr. 2007;46(5): 581-89.

[68] Denton AB, Tsaparas Y. Injectable hyaluronic acid for the correction of HIV-associated facial lipoatrophy. Otolaryngology-Head and Neck Surgery. 2007; 136(4): 563-67.

[69] Skeie L, Bugge H, Negaard A et al. Large particle hyaluronic acid for the treatment of facial lipoatrophy in HIV-positive patients: 3-year follow-up study. HIV Med. 2010;11(3):170-7.

[70] Hornberger J, Rajagopalan R, Shewade A et al. Cost consequences of HIV-associated lipoatrophy. AIDS Care. 2009;21(5):664-71.

[71] Soares, FMG. Polimetilmetacrilato no tratamento da lipoatrofia facial associada ao HIV/AIDS: impacto na contagem de CD4 e na qualidade de vida. [dissertação]. Brasília: Universidade de Brasília; 2011.

5

Update on the Royal Perth Hospital Anogenital Wart Database

McCloskey J.C.[1], Phillips M.[2], French M.A.H.[3], Flexman J.[4], McCallum D.[5] and Metcalf C.[5]

[1]*Sexual Health Service, Royal Perth Hospital, School of Biomolecular Sciences and Chemistry, and School of Pharmacology and Medicine, University of Western Australia*

[2]*Royal Perth Hospital, Western Australian Institute for Medical research, University of Western Australia*

[3]*School of Pathology and Laboratory Medicine, University of Western Australia and Department of Clinical Immunology, Royal Perth Hospital and PathWest Laboratory Medicine, Perth*

[4]*Department of Microbiology and Infectious Diseases, Royal Perth Hospital; PathWest Laboratory Medicine WA; Pathology and Laboratory Medicine and Microbiology & Immunology, University of Western Australia*

[5]*Department of Anatomical Pathology, Royal Perth Hospital, Australia*

1. Introduction

Genital warts are still thought to be a benign cosmetic problem despite increasing evidence that they may harbour high-grade intra-epithelial neoplasia (IN). We have previously published high rates of high-grade IN in surgically excised warts from December 1995 to December 2004 in a retrospective review of 115 men and 38 women, 29 of whom had HIV infection. The rates of IN were 78% (52% high-grade) in men with HIV, and 33% (20% high-grade) in men without HIV. In women the IN rate was 8.3% (2.8% high-grade).(McCloskey et al. 2007) Since reporting the data initially, the database has continued to accrue cases and we have analysed the data to see if the previous findings have held and to see if there has been a change in the frequency of reported IN over time.

2. Materials and methods

The patient population, surgical and specimen handling process has been previously reported.(McCloskey et al. 2007) The population consists of patients referred to the Sexual Health Clinic at Royal Perth Hospital from December 1995 to December 2010. Anal or perianal warts were treated by scissor excision by a single sexual health physician if they were large or multiple or located within the anal canal by scissor excision. Patients who were immunosuppressed or who had only mapping biopsies performed or whose HIV status was unknown were excluded from the main analysis.

3. Data analysis

Descriptive analysis used percentages for categorical and ordinal variables and means for continuous variables. Viral load and CD4 counts and percentages for HIV positive patients were found to follow a skewed log-normal distribution (Shapiro-Wilk's test, $p > 0.05$ for all variables) and the geometric mean was reported as an unbiased estimate of the mean. These variables were transformed using a natural logarithm for further analysis that was based upon an assumption of normality. For bivariable analysis of categorical and ordinal variables the likelihood ratio χ^2 test was used. For these analyses with continuous variables the Wilcoxon rank-sum test was used. Multivariable linear logistic regression analysis was used to examine associations with HIV status and other dichotomous variables and ordinal logistic regression was used to examine associations with the degree of IN. The validity of these latter statistical models depends upon an assumption of proportional odds across the outcome categories and this was assessed using the Brant test(Brant 1990). In every case the analysis was found to be valid. The assumption of linearity for continuous independent variables was assessed using restricted cubic splines and where non-linearity was found a spline regression was used to model the association.(Harrell 2001) Analysis of the degree of IN used operation as the unit of investigation and because operations are clustered within patients the assumption of independent sampling is violated. Estimates of standard error and p values were based upon a robust estimation of the clustered data. A p value less than 0.05 was regarded as statistically significant for all analysis. The analysis was conducted using the Stata statistical package (Version 11.1).(Corp 2009).

4. Results

4.1 Patient characteristics and operative procedures

Removal of anal and/or perianal warts was performed during 461 operations in 343 patients, 255 (74%) men and 88 (26%) women) of whom 278 (81%) of patients and 378 (82%) of operations were eligible to be included in the analysis. Reasons for exclusion included lack of histology results because of insufficient surgical material (total 44 patients, 30 men and 14 women), unknown HIV status (9 patients), operations performed for mapping biopsies (19 operations) and immunosuppression other than HIV (16 patients). In some instances there were multiple reasons for exclusion. Table 1.1 shows demographic data HIV antibody status for males, and Table 1.2 shows demographic data by HIV antibody status for females. Sixty-one eligible patients had HIV infection (59 men and two women). Men with HIV were significantly older than men without HIV (mean 8.7 years, 95% CI: 7.7-9.67, $p<0.00001$ rank sum test) (see Figure 1: Age distribution by HIV status).

A spline regression analysis showed that the likelihood of being HIV positive increased non-linearly with age in this population. The proportion positive increased at a significantly greater rate with each increasing year of age until about 30 years after which the proportion increases at a statistically significant but slower rate of increase (see Figure 2: HIV risk for men by age).

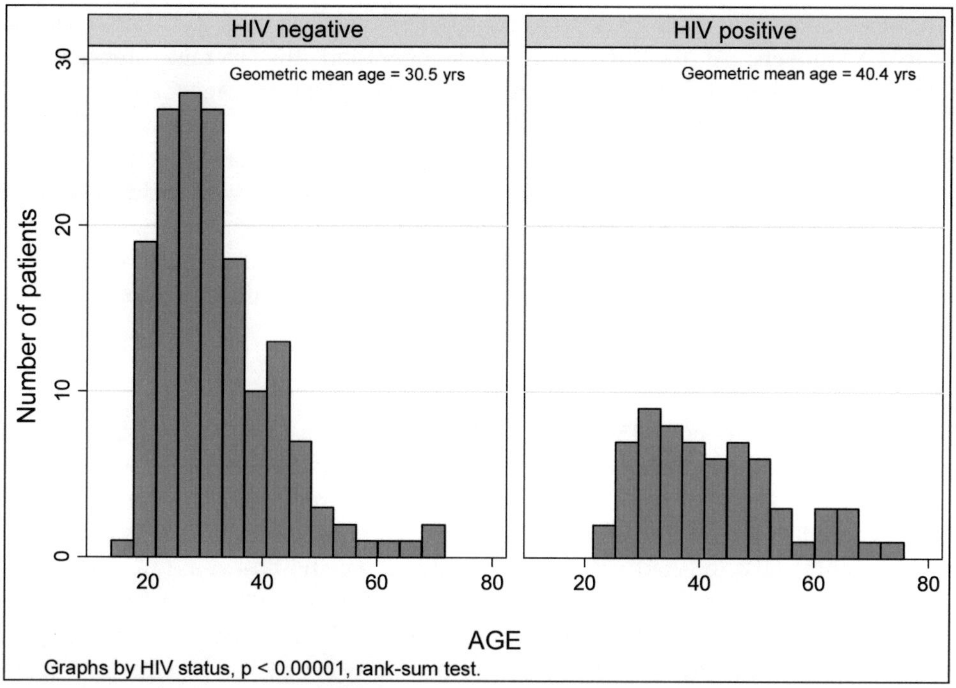

Fig. 1. Age distribution by HIV status.

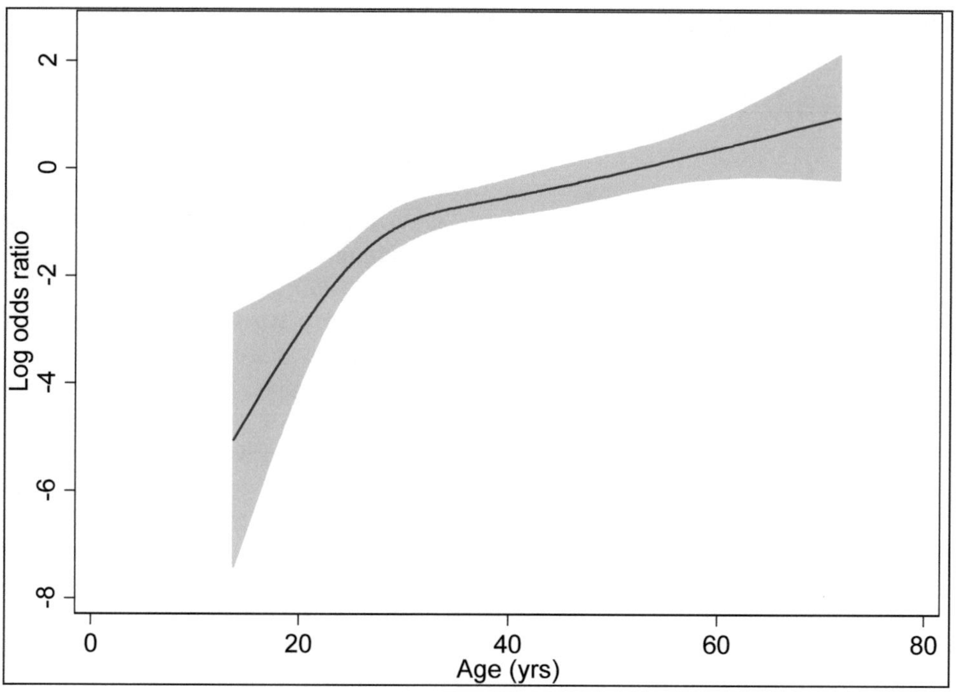

Note: Shaded area shows the 95% confidence interval.

Fig. 2. HIV risk for men by age, results of a non-linear spline regression

Seventy-three percent of male patients were homosexual/bisexual, 27% heterosexual and 47% current smokers. At the time of the first operation, the average duration of HIV infection was 3.4 years (95% CI: 2.4-5.0, geometric mean); the average CD4 T-cell count at first surgery was 329 $x10^6/L$ (95% CI: 258–420 $x10^6/L$, geometric mean) and the average nadir CD4 T-cell count prior to surgery was 96 $x10^6/L$ (95% CI: 66–139 $x10^6/L$, geometric mean). The HIV viral loads ranged from 40 to 135,000 viral copies/mL with 50% having a viral load less than 395, 25%, 395–20,400 and 15%, 20,400 –38,000). Sixty-four% of men without HIV were homosexual/bisexual, 36% heterosexual and 43.5% current smokers. The number of operations performed ranged from one to five for both HIV -positive men and HIV-negative men.

4.2 Change over time

Differences between the period December 1995-December 2004 and January 2005-December 2010 shows that there has been significant change in the patient population in the period December 2004 to Jan 2005 compared to the previously reported period of 1995 to 2004 (Table 2). Variables that show the change are age (3.0 years older, p=0.033), almost half as many (57% more) HIV infected patients (p =0.032), fewer homosexual (7% less) but more bisexual men (39% more), the number of lifetime partners is increased in males but not females, a greater proportion of patients have a history of chlamydia, there is less perianal disease and more anal disease. Importantly however between the two periods there has been no significant change in AIN or perianal intraepithelial neoplasia (PAIN).

4.3 Rates of IN were highest in patients with HIV infection

When all the operations are considered men with HIV infection and for whom histological data was available, 45 (44.1%) had AIN 2-3 (high-grade AIN) and 19 (58.1%) had PAIN 2-3 (Table 3). Overall, men with HIV had some form of high-grade IN in 68 (57.8%), with 85 (78%) having any grade of abnormality (AIN or PAIN 1-3). HIV negative men had high-grade IN in 49 (24.7%), 25 (5.7%) had high-grade PAIN, and 32 (21.4%) had high-grade AIN. The risk of IN was 2.9 times higher for HIV positive men than those without HIV for AIN ($p<0.0001$, ordinal logistic regression analysis) and 4.0 times higher than men without HIV for PAIN ($p<0.0001$, ordinal logistic regression analysis). The rate of AIN 2-3 was 10.7% for HIV-negative women and 1.8% for PAIN. Except for a few perianal lesions with classical features of Bowen's disease, none of the IN was evident at operation and was only discovered with histopathological examination.

The rate of PAIN or AIN 2–3 was significantly higher 64.7% (66/36) for homosexual/bisexual men with HIV and 33.3% (45/90) in those without HIV infection ($P<0.0001$). The rate of IN was consistently higher in the anal canal compared with the perianal area ($p < 0.00001$) (Table 3.1 and 3.2). Table 4 shows this difference for all operations, the samples would fall diagonally in the table if there were no difference between anal and perianal samples (see Table 4). Of the patients with PAIN or AIN, there is a statistically significant interaction between HIV status and current smoking, with those who are HIV positive and current smokers being 6.0 times more likely to have a higher grade of IN than those who are HIV negative and have never smoked ($P=0.010$, ordinal logistic regression).

Men	HIV positive n = 64 (%)	HIV negative n = 153 (%)	*P*
Mean age (years)	40.4	30.1	<0.0001
Range	22.9 - 71.8	13.7 - 71.7	
Sexual preference			
Heterosexual	3 (4.7)	55 (36.0)	<0.001
Homosexual	50 (78.1)	77 (50.3)	
Bisexual	11 (17.2)	21 (13.7)	
Lifetime Number of Sexual Partners			
1 - 10	4 (8.2)	32 (30.2)	0.002
11 - 50	17 (34.7)	39 (36.8)	
>50	28 (57.1)	35 (33.0)	
Smoking status			0.445
Current	34 (53.1)	67 (43.8)	
Ex-smoker	5 (7.8)	13 (8.5)	
Never smoked	25 (39.1)	73 (47.7)	
History of STDs			
Syphilis	8 (12.5)	4 (2.6)	0.006
Gonorrhoea	20 (31.3)	14 (9.2)	<0.001
Chlamydia	9 (14.1)	18 (11.8)	0.643
NSU	5 (7.8)	9 (5.9)	0.604
History of genital herpes	17 (26.6)	12 (8.0)	<0.001
HSV-2 seropositive	22 (42.3)	20 (18.2)	0.001
Hepatitis C antibody positive	5 (8.8)	4 (3.1)	0.107
Wart site first operation			
Perianal only	3 (4.7)	34 (22.2)	<0.001
Anal only	21 (32.8)	35 (22.98)	
Perianal & anal	38 (59.4)	74 (48.4)	
Perianal & penile	0	9 (5.9)	
Perianal, anal & penile	1 (0.7)	2 (3.1)	
Number of operations			
1	38 (59.4)	118 (77.1)	0.029
2	13 (20.3)	26 (17.0)	
3	8 (12.5)	6 (3.9)	
4	4 (6.3)	2 (1.3)	
5	1 (1.6)	1 (0.7)	

Table 1.1. Demographic data by HIV antibody status for males

Women	n = 2	n = 59	
Mean age (years)	22.2	27.4	0.352
Range	19.5-25.4	16.9 -65.0	
Sexual preference			0.723
Heterosexual	2 (100)	57 (96.6)	
Homosexual/bisexual	0	2 (3.4)	
Lifetime number of sexual partners			0.562
1 - 10	2 (100)	32 (74.4)	
11 - 50	0	6 (14.0)	
>50	0	5 (11.6)	
Smoking status			0.160
Current	0	31 (52.5)	
Ex-smoker	0	5 (8.5)	
Never smoked	2 (100)	23 (39.0)	
History of STDs			
Syphilis	0	0	
Gonorrhoea	1 (50.0)	3 (5.1)	0.081
Chlamydia	1 (50.0)	5 (8.5)	0.138
NSU	0	1 (1.7)	0.795
History of genital herpes	0	3 (5.4)	0.642
HSV-2 seropositive	0	4 (9.5)	
Hepatitis C Antibody positive	0	0	
Wart site first operation			0.732
Perianal only	0	11 (18.6)	
Anal only	0	4 (6.8)	
Perianal and anal	0	11 (18.6)	
Perianal, anal and vulval	1 (50.0)	13 (22.0)	
Perianal and vulval	1 (50.0)	16 (27.1)	
Number of operations			0.138
1	1 (50.0)	54 (91.5)	
2	1 (50.0)	5 (8.5)	

Table 1.2. Demographic data by sex and HIV antibody status for females

Variable	Coefficient	95% confidence interval		p
		LCL	UCL	
Age	3.04	0.25	5.84	0.033
HIV status	0.57	0.01	1.12	0.046
Sexual preference (male)				
Heterosexual	0 (reference)			
Homosexual	0.93	0.26	1.59	0.006
Bisexual	1.39	0.48	2.30	0.003
Sexual preference (female)				
Heterosexual	0 (reference)			
Lesbian	0.45	-2.37	3.27	0.756
Lifetime sexual partners				
Male	0.73	0.11	1.34	0.020
Female	-0.02	-1.37	1.33	0.976
Smoking status				
Never	0 (reference)			
Current	-0.41	-0.91	0.08	0.102
Ex-smoker	0.28	-0.62	1.18	0.543
History of:				
Syphilis	1.33	0.005	2.66	0.049
Gonorrhoea	0.34	-0.35	1.03	0.332
Chlamydia	1.00	0.23	1.76	0.011
HSV2	-0.12	-.086	0.63	0.756
NSU	0.06	-0.99	1.10	0.914
Warts	-1.90	-2.76	-1.04	<0.001
HAV	0.26	-0.29	0.82	0.349
HCV	-0.33	-1.67	1.02	0.634
HSV serology	-0.50	-1.16	0.16	0.140
Prior wart treatment	-0.93	-1.41	-0.44	<0.001
Number of operations	-0.20	-0.41	0.00	0.051
Site perianal	-0.86	-1.38	-0.35	0.001
Site anal	1.48	0.89	2.08	<0.001
PAIN	-0.23	-0.93	0.47	0.528
AIN	0.17	-0.31	0.65	0.488
IN	0.28	-0.19	0.74	0.246
CD4 count at surgery (ln)	-0.28	-0.76	0.21	0.262
Viral load at surgery (ln)	-1.63	-2.85	-0.41	0.010
CD4 count at nadir (ln)	-0.06	-0.35	0.23	0.681

Table 2. Differences between the period December 1995-December 2004 and January 2005-December 2010

5. Discussion

The data is consistent with our earlier observations of high rates of any IN men with HIV infection. Approximately 25% of HIV negative men had high-grade IN, indicating that anal/perianal warts in HIV negative men cannot be assumed to be benign lesions. Conversely anogenital warts in men with HIV have a high likelihood of containing some degree of IN with 62% having high-grade. The consistency of the data over the longer time period it highlights the importance of treating anal/perianal warts to remove IN that may eventually progress to invasive cancer as has previously been reported in the literature.(Scholefield, Castle and Watson 2005, Siegel 1962, Sturm et al. 1975) In particular the rates of anal cancer are rapidly rising in men with HIV(Crum-Cianflone et al. 2010) and it may be that men with warts represent a population of men at increased risk especially given the relatively common findings of anal cancer in men with warts (8.8%). Genital warts are recognised as a risk factor for the development of IN in renal transplant recipients.(Patel et al. 2010) AIN has been reported to progress to anal cancer with 10% progression at 5 years with higher rates in immunosuppressed individuals or those with multifocal disease.(Scholefield, Harris and Radcliffe 2011) Unlike other authors(Schlect et al. 2010) we did not detect anal cancer in any of the anal warts excised, but in our population, men with warts are referred early for surgery soon after the warts are diagnosed in the clinic. Schlect et al(Schlect et al. 2010) have similarly found high rates of IN in anal condylomata in 75/159 (47%) HIV positive men. In particular, given the increasing rates of anal cancer in men (Daling et al. 1982, Goedert et al. 1998)with HIV, further studies to explore the role of 'low-risk' HPV genotypes associated with warts and their possible role in anal cancer development should be undertaken. The fact that genotyping studies of anal cancer are

Men	**HIV positive**	**HIV negative**	*P*
Anal and/or perianal IN	n= 109	n= 199	
None	24 (22.0)	112 (56.3)	<0.001
IN 1	17 (15.6)	38 (19.1)	
IN 2	20 (18.4)	27 (13.6)	
IN 3	48 (44.0)	22 (11.1)	
Total IN	85 (78.0)	87 (43.7)	
Anal	n = 102	n = 150	
None	36 (35.3)	87 (58.0)	<0.001
IN 1	21 (20.6)	31 (20.7)	
IN 2	20 (19.6)	22 (14.7)	
IN 3	25 (24.5)	10 (6.7)	
Total AIN	66 (64.7)	63 (42.0)	
Perianal	n=67	n=140	<0.001
None	42 (61.2)	119 (85.0)	
IN 1	7 (10.5)	13 (9.3)	
IN 2	4 (6.0)	2 (1.4)	
IN 3	15 (22.4)	6 (4.3)	
Total IN	26 (38.8)	21 (15.0)	

Table 3.1 IN by HIV antibody status , and anatomical site- perianal/anal for all operations for males

sometimes finding only HPV 6 indicate this 'low –risk' HPV genotype may not in fact be 'low risk' in the anal canal in men.(Hillman et al. 2010, Abramowitz et al. 2010) Vaccination of boys to prevent infection of HPV with both low and high-risk HPV types should be promoted.

Anal and/or perianal IN			
n = 3	n = 62		
None	2 (66.7)	45 (72.6)	0.308
IN 1	0	12 (19.4)	
IN 2	0	1 (1.6)	
IN 3	1 (33.3)	4 (6.5)	
Total IN	1 (33.3)	17 (27.5)	
Anal	n = 1	n = 33	0.298
None	0	17 (60.7)	
IN 1	0	8 (28.6)	
IN 2	0	0	
IN 3	1 (100)	3 (10.7)	
Total IN	1 (100)	11 (33.3)	
Perianal	n = 3	n = 56	0.088
None	2 (66.7)	53 (94.6)	
IN 1	0	2 (3.6)	
IN 2	0	1 (1.8)	
IN 3	1 (50.0)	0	
Total IN	1 (50.0)	3 (5.4)	

Table 3.2 IN by HIV antibody status , and anatomical site- perianal/anal for all operations for females

PAIN	PAIN	PAIN	PAIN	PAIN	PAIN
AIN	Negative	IN 1	IN 2	IN 3	Total
Negative	86	3	1	1	91
%	49.7	1.7	0.6	0.6	52.6
IN 1	29	6	1	2	38
%	16.8	3.5	0.6	1.2	22.0
IN 2	17	6	3	0	26
%	9.8	3.5	1.7	0.0	15.0
IN 3	7	0	1	10	18
%	4.1	0.0	0.6	5.85	9.7
Total	139	15	6	13	173
%	80.4	8.7	3.5	7.5	100.0

Asymptotic symmetry test: $\chi 2 = 46.4$, d.f. = 6, $p < 0.00001$

Table 4. Contrast of AIN and PAIN

6. References

Abramowitz, L., A. Jacquard, J. Pretet, J. Haesebaert, L. Siproudhis, P. Pradat, O. Aynaud, Y. Leocmach, B. Soubeyrand, D. Riethmuller, C. Mougin & F. Denis. 2010. Human papillomavirus genotype distribution in anal cancer in France: The Edith V Study. In *Eurogin 2010 Congress*, 161. Monte Carlo.

Brant, R. (1990) Assessing proportionality in the proportional odds model for ordinal logistic regression. *Biometrics*, 46, 1171-1178.

Corp 2009. Stata Statistical Software: Release 11. College Station, TX :StataCoorp LP.

Crum-Cianflone, N., K. Hullsiek, V. Marconi, G. A, A. Weintrob, R. Barthel, B. Agan & The Infectious Disease Clinical Research Program HIV Working Group (2010) Anal cancers among HIV-infected persons: HAART is not slowing rising incidence. *AIDS*, 24, 535-543.

Daling, J. R., N. S. Weiss, L. L. Klopfenstein, L. E. Cochran, W. H. Chow & R. Daifuku (1982) Correlates of homosexual behaviour and the incidence of anal cancer. *JAMA*, 247, 1988-1990.

Goedert, J., T. Coté, P. Virgo, S. Scoppa, D. Kingma, M. Gail, E. Jaffe & R. Biggar (1998) Spectrum of AIDS-associated malignant disorders. *Lancet*, 351, 1833-39.

Harrell, F. J. 2001. *Regression Modelling Strategies*. New York: Springer.

Hillman, R., M. Steven, S. Tabrizi, N. Kumaradevan, S. Garland, C. Lemech, R. Ward, A. Meagher, L. McHugh, J. Jin, S. Carroll & D. Goldstein. 2010. The detection of human papillomavirus genotypes in anal cancer biopsy specimens from Sydney. In *Australasian Sexual Health Conference 2010*. Sydney.

McCloskey, J., C. Metcalf, M. French, J. Flexman, V. Burke & L. Beilin (2007) The frequency of high-grade intraepithelial neoplasia in anal/perianal warts is higher than previously recognised *Int J STD & AIDS*, 18, 538-542.

Patel, H., A. Silver, T. Levine, G. Williams & J. Northover (2010) Human papillomavirus infectin and anal dsplasia in renal transplant recipients. *Br J Surgery*, 97, 1716-1721.

Schlect, H., D. Fugelso, R. Murphy, K. Wagner, J. Doweiko, J. Proper, B. Dezube & L. Panther (2010) Frequency of occult high-grade squamous intraepithelial neoplasia and invasive cancer withing anal condylomata in men who have sex with men. *CID*, 51, 107-110.

Scholefield, J., M. Castle & N. Watson (2005) Malignant transformation of high-grade anal intraepithelial neoplasia. *British Journal of Surgery*, 92, 1133-1136.

Scholefield, J., D. Harris & A. Radcliffe (2011) Guidelines fo management of anal intraepithelial neoplasia. *Colorectal disease*, 13, 3-10.

Siegel, A. (1962) Malignant transformation of condyloma acuminatum. Review of the literature and report of a case. *Am J Surg*, 103, 613-17.

Sturm, J. T., C. E. Christenson, J. H. Uecker & D. J. Perry Jr (1975) Squamous-cell carcinoma of the anus arising in a giant condyloma acuminatum- report of a case. *Dis Colon Rectum*, 18, 147-51.

6

Kidney Involvement in HIV Infection

Naheed Ansari
Department of Medicine, Jacobi Medical Center, Division of Nephrology
Assistant Professor of Medicine, Albert Einstein College of Medicine
United States of America

1. Introduction

Human immunodeficiency virus (HIV) infection can involve various organs of the body. Kidney involvement is frequently seen during course of human immunodeficiency virus infection and it has become fourth leading condition contributing to death in acquired immunodeficiency virus (AIDS) patients after sepsis, pneumonia, and liver disease. Rao first described the presence of focal segmental glomerulosclerosis and renal failure with HIV infection in 1984. This entity is now known as HIV-associated nephropathy (HIVAN). Renal involvement in HIV infection can manifest in a variety of clinical presentations. Renal manifestations can range from acute kidney injury to chronic kidney disease to end stage kidney disease. Various fluid and electrolyte disorders and acid base disturbances can also occur. Immune complex mediated glomerular involvement is also seen in these patients (see Table). HIVAN remains the most common form of kidney disease among HIV infected individuals which is usually associated with nephrotic range proteinuria. Treatment for HIVAN includes use of highly active anti-retroviral therapy (HAART), Angiotensin converting enzyme inhibitors and systemic steroid administration. End stage renal disease (ESRD) is common in HIV infected individuals and accounts for 1% of patients receiving dialysis in USA. Survival of ESRD patients with HIV disease has improved dramatically over last one decade due to use of HAART. Both hemodialysis and peritoneal dialysis can be dialysis options for ESRD patients due to HIV disease. One year survival rate of HIV infected patients is equivalent to that of general population. Renal transplantation recently has become a viable option for renal replacement therapy in patients with well controlled HIV disease.

Renal involvement can occur at all stages of HIV infection and can be initial clue to the presence of HIV infection in an undiagnosed patient. Renal involvement in HIV disease can also occur due to other causes seen in non -HIV infected population like exposure to nephrotoxic medications, hemodynamic changes during an acute illness, and obstruction. Treatment of HIV infection with highly active anti-retroviral agents itself can induce various renal abnormalities. Therefore, evaluation of renal abnormalities should be part of the comprehensive work up of a patient with newly diagnosed HIV infection and it should be periodically ruled out on subsequent follow up. Usually urinalysis, random protein to creatinine ratio, and comprehensive metabolic panel should be obtained as part of the initial work up. Patients on HAART should be monitored for potential renal toxicity of these agents.

This chapter reviews details of various renal manifestations of HIV disease with special focus on presence of chronic kidney disease, pathogenesis and treatment of HIVAN, and renal toxicity associated with use of HAART. Various options of renal replacement therapy including renal transplantion will also be discussed.

Acute kidney injury	Pre-renal azotemia Renal due to Acute tubular toxicity Acute interstitial nephritis Glomerulonephritis Vasculitis HUS/TTP Obstruction due to crystalluria, stones, papillary necrosis, BPH, and urethral strictures
Chronic kidney disease	HIVAN Can present as proteinuria only with or without renal failure. Degree of kidney disease can vary from stage 1-5. MDRD equation can be used to estimate eGFR. CKD related to other co morbid conditions like Hypertension, Diabetes Mellitus, or due to use of recreational drug use like cocaine and heroin.
End Stage Kidney Disease	Options for renal replacement therapy
Disorders of Potassium	Hyperkalemia or Hypokalemia
Disorders of Sodium and Osmolality	Hyponatremia and Hypernatremia Syndrome of inappropriate ADH secretion
Disorders of Calcium	Hypocalcemia and Hypercalcemia
Disorders of Magnesium	Hypomagnesemia
Disorders of Phosphate	Hypophosphatemia or Hyperphosphatemia
Disorders of acid-base disturbances	High anion gap metabolic acidosis Non anion gap metabolic acidosis
Immune complex mediated Glomerulonephritis	Membranoproliferative GN Membranous Nephropathy Minimal Change Disease SLE like GN Post infectious GN
Renal toxicity of HAART	Fanconi's syndrome Renal failure Diabetes insipidus Lactic acidosis

Table 1. Renal Manifestations of HIV

2. Acute Kidney Injury

Acute kidney injury (AKI) is abrupt impairment of renal function and is commonly seen in patients infected with HIV both in inpatient and outpatient settings. In era prior to HAART,

AKI was commonly due to opportunistic infections and heralded a poor outcome in hospitalized patients. The incidence of AKI defined as peak serum creatinine level of ≥2mg/dl was reported to be 20%.

An increased risk of inpatient AKI among HIV infected individuals has been reported in the modern era of highly active antiretroviral therapy (HAART). One study reported incidence of AKI in hospitalized patients with HIV to be 6% as compared with 2.7% in HIV uninfected patients. In a large population of hospitalized HIV-infected patients, incidence of cardiovascular disease and heart failure increased linearly with severity of AKI. Among HIV patients requiring dialysis for AKI, the risk for cardiovascular disease and heart failure were 1.96 and 4.20 fold greater than individuals who did not develop AKI during their hospitalization. The development of AKI in these patients is associated with high mortality rate. AKI is also seen in ambulatory HIV infected patients and its incidence has been reported to be 5.9/100 person years.

2.1 Causes of AKI

No study has assessed etiology of AKI in hospitalized HIV infected patients. The usual causes of AKI are commonly encountered in HIV infected individuals as in other hospitalized non- HIV infected patients (Table 1).

The causes of AKI can be divided into prerenal, renal, and post renal causes. Pre-renal azotemia and acute tubular necrosis (ATN) remain most common cause of AKI in HIV infected individuals (38% and 35% respectively). Patients with AIDS are at high risk of prerenal azotemia which results from vomiting, fever, and poor po intake due to underlying illness. ATN results from sepsis causing ischemic ATN in up to 50% of cases. Use of nephrotoxic agents like aminoglycosides, amphotericin, pentamidine, and intravenous administration of contrast agent can cause ATN in 25% of cases.

Acute interstitial nephritis can result from hypersensitivity reaction to use of certain medications or can be caused by certain infections in AIDS patients. Infections associated with interstitial disease in immunocompromised patients include cytomegalovirus, candida, tuberculosis, and histoplasmosis. Common medications associated with acute interstitial nephritis are penicillins, cephalosporins, macrolides, ciprofloxacin, cotrimoxazole, rifampin, and nonsteroidal anti-inflammatory drugs. Acute interstitial nephritis secondary to use of HAART is very rare. One study found 2/60 biopsy specimens had drug related interstitial nephritis. Cessation of offending agent usually leads to renal recovery. Sometimes a short course of corticosteroids may need to be given in patients with severe acute interstitial nephritis where withdrawl of offending agent fails to improve kidney function.

Vacular causes of AKI include hemolytic uremic syndrome/thrombotic thrombocytopenic purpura can be encountered in HIV seropositive patients. The clinical manifestations are similar to that seen in HIV seronegative patients. Laboratory examination reveals microangiopathic hemolytic anemia, thrombocytopenia, and impaired kidney function. Kidney biopsy reveals platelet and fibrin thrombi in renal and glomerular capillaries. Treatment with plasmaphresis and fresh frozen plasma replacement may be effective.

Obstruction should be considered in differential diagnosis of AKI among HIV infected patients. Certain drugs are associated with obstructive nephropathy. These include sulfadiazine, acyclovir, atazanavir, and indinavir. Volume depletion with sluggish urine flow is the most important risk factor allowing crystallization. Reduced glomerular filtration rate is also a risk factor for crystallization. Normal dosing of drugs in patients with reduced

GFR is associated with high urinary concentration of insoluble drug and pH of urine. Sulfadiazine can cause intratubular obstruction by causing crystal formation. It can also cause stone formation which may give rise to ureteral obstruction. Acyclovir can cause crystalluria and AKI especially when given intravenously rapidly without concomitant hydration. Protease inhibitor indinavir has been reported to cause crystalluria in 20% of the patients receiving indinavir at normal dose. The use of this medication has declined significantly and has been replaced by less nephrotoxic protease inhibitors. Atazanavir can cause nephrolithiasis in up to 0.97% of the individuals taking the drug. Atazanavir stones appear to form in alkaline urine. No risk factors have been associated with stone formation from atazanavir use. One should keep in mind possibility of atazanavir stones in HIV patient who develops renal colic. Ciprofloxacin associated crystal formation commonly occurs in HIV infected patients and should be considered as cause of AKI in patients taking this antibiotic. Ciprofloxacin induced nephropathy occurs usually in patients with reduced renal function with hypovolemia and having urine pH above 6.0. One should adjust dose of ciprofloxacin in patients with reduced renal function and urine alkalinization should be avoided. Treatment of obstructive nephropathy secondary to crystalluria requires discontinuation of offending agent, intravenous hydration, and close monitoring of renal function.

Treatment of AKI in HIV positive individuals is similar to HIV seronegative individuals with renal failure. Indications of renal replacement therapy remain the same for both groups of patients.

3. Chronic Kidney Disease

Chronic kidney disease (CKD) is an important complication of HIV infection. The prevalence of impaired renal function defined as estimated glomerular filtration rate (eGFR) of <60ml/min/ 1.73m2 varies from 2.4 to 10% depending upon the social and demographic characteristics of the studied population. 10-30% of HIV- infected individuals have microalbuminuria or proteinuria. A variety of renal abnormalities on renal biopsy have been described in these patients. These abnormalities seen on renal biopsy can be HIV associated Nephropathy (HIVAN), HIV associated immune complex kidney disease (HIVICK), non collapsing focal and segmental glomerulosclerosis, thrombotic microangiopathy, nephropathy secondary to use of HAART, and diseases related to common comorbidities such as amyloidosis, diabetic nephropathy, hypertensive renal disease etc can be seen on renal biopsy.

HIV infected individuals with glomerular disease present clinically with significant proteinuria, hematuria, or reduced kidney function. Work up should focus on work up for possible secondary causes of glomerular diseases along with good history and physical examination. The work up should focus on evidence of hepatitis B or C infection, syphilis, evidence of malignancy or collagen vascular disease. A kidney biopsy is usually indicated in for tissue diagnosis and future management of the disease.

3.1 Epidemiology

HIVAN is a histopathological diagnosis based on kidney biopsy only. The true prevalence of HIVAN is unknown as many patients with HIV infection do not undergo renal biopsy routinely in clinical practice. In kidney biopsy series among HIV infected individuals;

HIVAN is seen in 40-60% of renal biopsy specimens. Autopsy studies on organs from HIV infected persons have reported prevalence of HIVAN to be 6.9%. HIVAN is the most important cause of milder forms of kidney disease in South Africa where it is commonly manifested clinically by microalbuminuria. Infectious Diseases Society of America (IDSA) guideline recommends urinalysis and estimation of kidney function for all HIV-infected persons at the time of HIV diagnosis.
HIVAN commonly occurs in African American individuals. With 90% of cases of HIVAN occuring in African Americans. The remaining 10% of cases are observed in mixed heritage or Hispanic patients. This entity is rarely seen in HIV seropositive white patients. HIVAN progresses very fast in African Americans and risk of End Stage Renal Disease (ESRD) is similar to diabetes in African American patients with HIVAN. In Caucasians, the risk of ESRD associated with HIV is not increased.

3.2 Pathogenesis

HIV is pathogenic through direct infection of epithelial cells of the nephron including the glomerulus, the tubules and the collecting duct. In situ hybridization studies have found the HIV genome in the tubular and glomerular epithelial cells in patients with HIVAN. The pattern of epithelial cell infection determines histological abnormalities seen with HIVAN. Transgenic mice expressing a replication-defective HIV-1 construct develop proteinuria, reduced renal function, and histologically characteristic HIVAN. Reciprocal transplantation studies using this mouse model demonstrate that HIVAN develops only in kidneys expressing the transgene. HIV RNA and DNA have been detected in podocytes and renal tubular epithelial cells of patients with HIVAN. The mechanism of entry of HIV into renal epithelial cells is unknown. Studies have shown that renal epithelial cell is able to support a productive viral life cycle, and renal epithelium is an important reservoir for HIV infection. Despite undetectable viral load in the serum, HIV can still be present in renal epithelial cells where it may undergo rapid replication. This may produce HIV stains in the kidney microenvironment that differ from HIV circulating in the blood.

3.3 Clinical features

Patients with HIVAN typically present with proteinuria. This proteinuria is variable in magnitude, usually is heavy in nephrotic range (>3gm/day), but can be mild and sometimes present only as microalbuminuria. HIVAN is associated with rapidly deteriorating renal function with high rate of progression to ESRD. These patients usually have poorly controlled HIV infection characterized by low CD4 count and high HIV RNA load. Besides heavy proteinuria, many patients with HIVAN do not exhibit significant edema or Hypertension. A recent study noted that 43% of patients with biopsy proven HIVAN did not have Hypertension. The serum albumin levels remain above 3 gm/dl besides heavy proteinuria. On the contrary, patients with early HIVAN lesions may have normal renal function, microalbuminuria or mild proteinuria. Renal function may remain stable for many years in these patients. Urinalysis usually shows bland sediment with varying number of proteinaceous casts, oval fat bodies, and renal tubular epithelial cells. Abdominal ultrasound reveals relatively large, echogenic kidneys. Ultrasound findings are limited predictive value. Serologic markers are usually negative in these patients on work up. A diagnostic renal biopsy is usually indicated for diagnosis.

3.4 Histopathology

HIVAN is associated with characteristic glomerular, tubulointerstitial, and electron micrographic lesions. The characteristic findings on histopathology include presence of focal segmental glomerulosclerosis, cystic tubular dilatation, interstitial edema, cellular infiltrates, and dilated tubules filled with pale staining amorphous casts. Collapsing glomerulosclerosis is a common variant in patients with HIVAN due to hypercellularity of the cells lining the Bowman's capsule. Proliferation of tubular epithelial cells contributes to micro cyst formation and may account for the bigger size of the kidneys. Increased proliferation of podocytes is also present and plays an important role in lesions of collapsing FSGS found in HIVAN. Immunoflorescence staining is non specific. Electron microscopy reveals tubuloreticular inclusions in the endothelial cells of glomerular capillaries. Collapsing FSGS is not pathognomonic of HIVAN and can be seen in non- HIV related collapsing focal segmental glomerulosclerosis, heroin nephropathy, and as complication of bisphosphonate therapy.

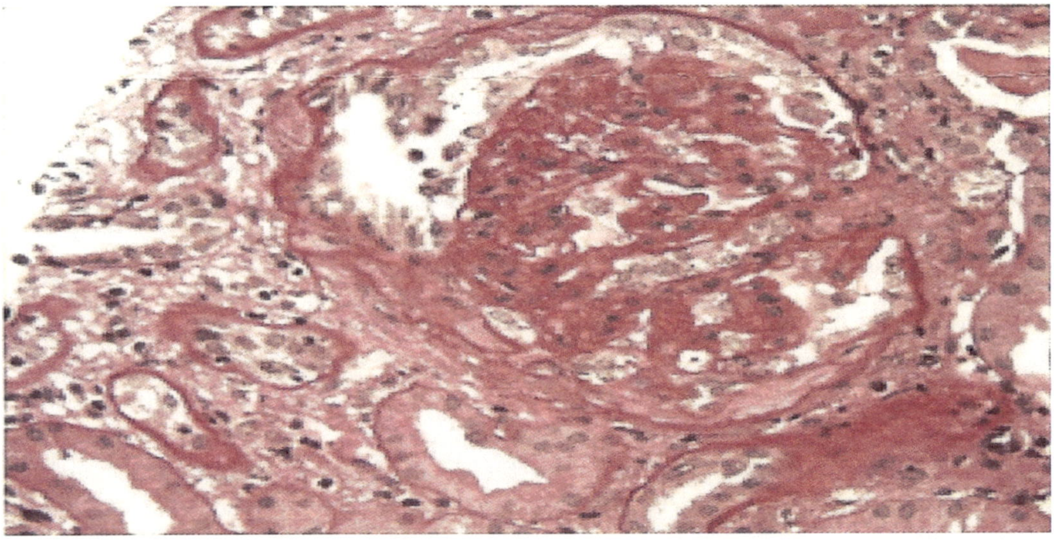

Fig. 1. Collapsing FSGS

It shows collapsing focal segmental glomerulosclerosis in a patient with HIV showing global collapse of the glomerular capillary loops and proliferation of visceral epithelial cells.

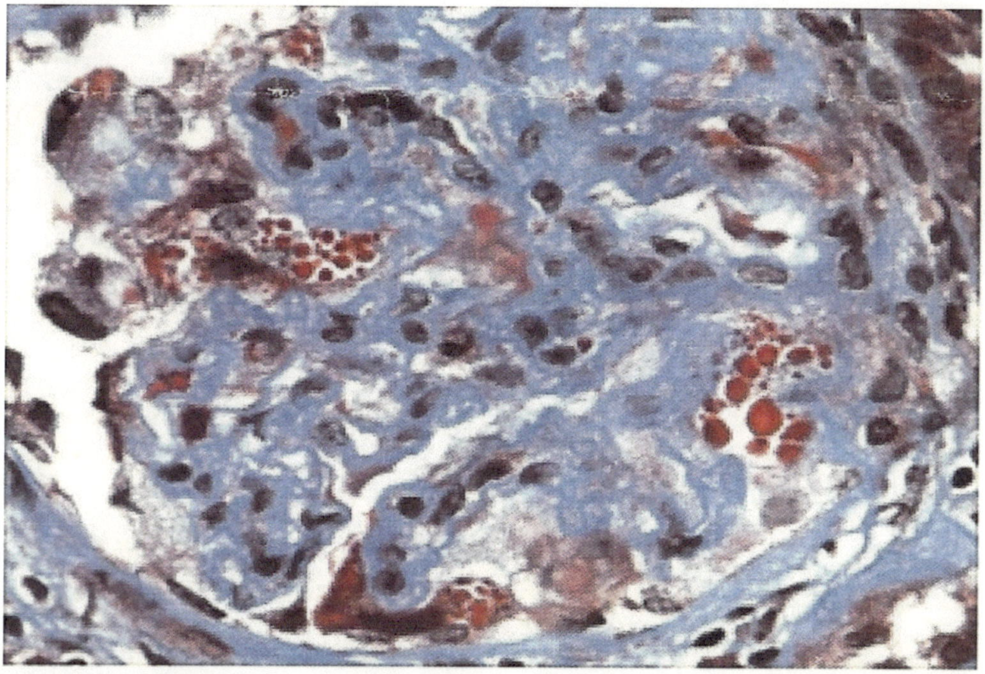

Fig. 2. Collapsing FSGS

It shows podocyte hypertrophy.

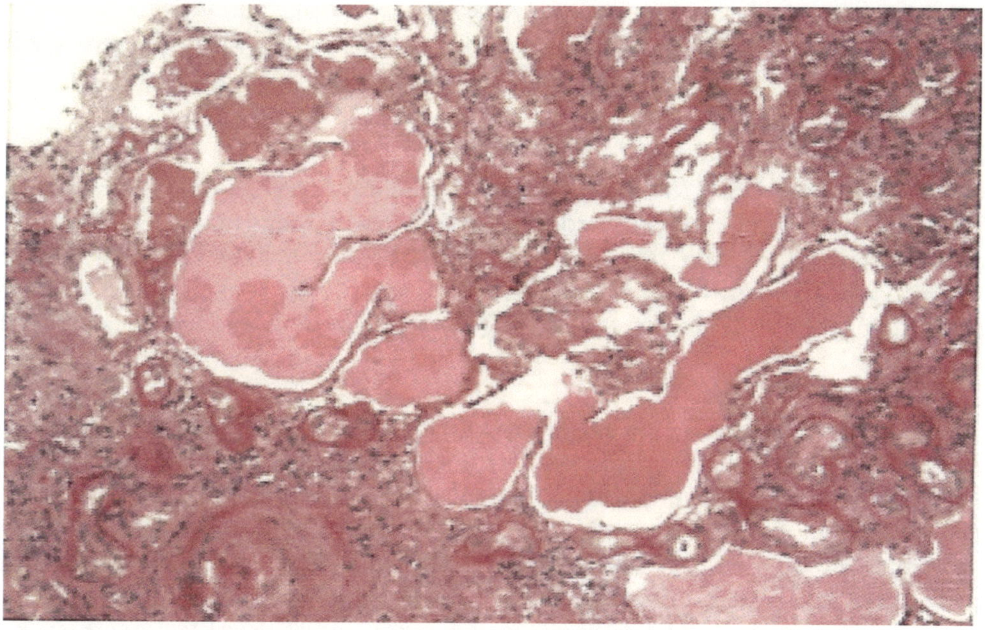

Fig. 3. Tubulointerstitial involvement in HIV associated Nephropathy

It shows microcystic dilatation of tubules, proteinaceous material casts within tubular lumina, and interstitial inflammation.

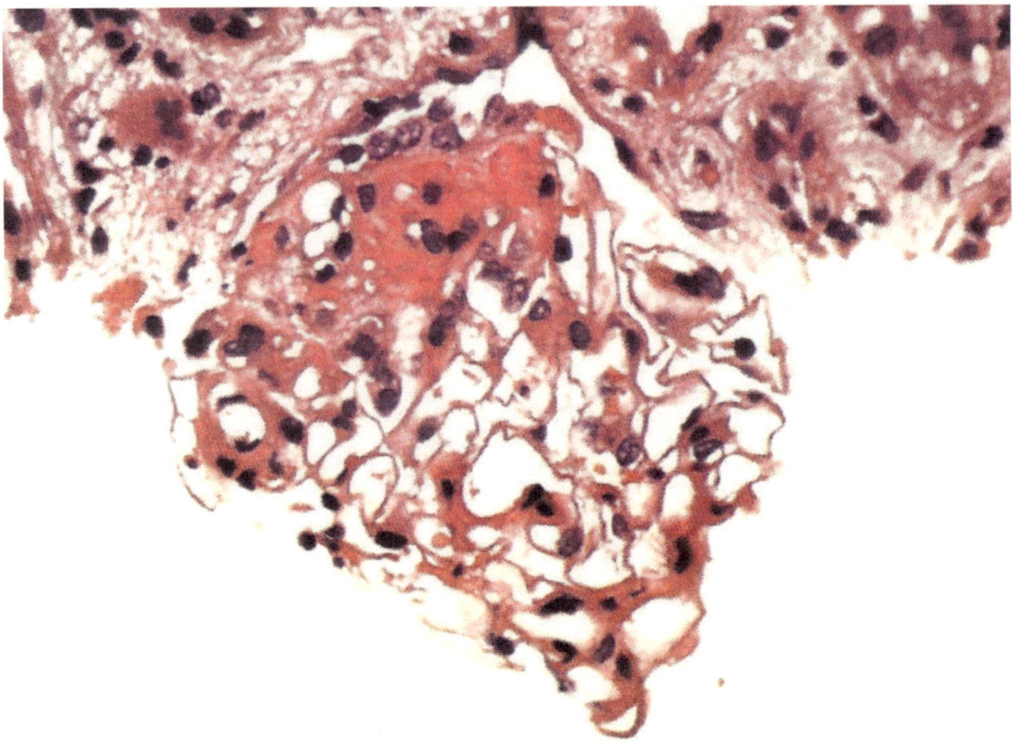

Fig. 4. Non-Collapsing FSGS

It shows focal segmental glomerulosclerosis at 12 o'clock position in an HIV infected patient.

3.5 Treatment

There have been no randomized controlled trials with any type of therapy in treatment of HIVAN. US department of Health and Human Services recommends use of HAART for diagnosis of HIVAN regardless of CD4 count. Other medications used in the treatment of HIVAN in patients with suboptimal response to HAART include angiotensin converting enzyme inhibitors and corticosteroids. A summary of the trials conducted in HIVAN is given in Table 2.

3.5.1 Highly Active Antiretroviral Agents (HAART)

The use of antiretroviral agents has slowed down progression of HIVAN to ESRD and reports of patients dependent on dialysis becoming dialysis free have been published after use of HAART. In one study, a patient with HIVAN and dialysis dependent renal failure became dialysis free after 15 weeks of HAART. Repeat renal biopsy revealed significant histologic recovery from fibrosis and infrequent collapsing glomerulosclerosis.

The rationale for using HAART is based on the direct role of the HIV virus itself in the pathogenesis of HIVAN. The effect of HAART on kidney disease progression has been characterized by observational studies. The evidence for effectiveness of HAART is from the retrospective cohort of biopsy proven HIVAN. In this study, renal survival benefit was noted in 26 patients treated with antiretroviral agents compared with ten patients who did not receive anti-retroviral therapy. Median renal survival was significantly improved for the treated group compared with the untreated group (18.4 months vs. 3.9 months respectively). Complete viral suppression was associated with better renal outcome than partial viral suppression. Continuous therapy with HAART is recommended in preventing and slowing the progression of kidney disease due to HIVAN as evidenced by Strategies for Management of Antiretroviral Therapy (SMART) study.

3.5.2 Corticosteroids

The rationale for using corticosteroids is based on presence of significant tubulointerstitial inflammation seen in histology of renal biopsy of patients with HIVAN. In vitro studies have shown up regulation of proinflammatory genes in renal tubular cells of individuals with HIVAN as a possible explanation for development of tubulointerstitial disease. The use of corticosteroids decreases this inflammation markedly in these patients. There is improvement in kidney function and reduction in mean urinary protein excretion in patients with HIVAN with use of corticosteroids. There are no long term studies supporting efficiency and safety of corticosteroid use in patients with HIVAN. Most of the studies supporting use of corticosteroids in patients with HIVAN have been short term, non randomized and retrospective in design. In a single center cohort study, 20 patients with HIVAN were prospectively enrolled to receive treatment with corticosteroids. 17 out of 20 patients manifested improvement in kidney function and had significant reduction in proteinuria. Another study of steroid therapy employed control group and found similar results with no increased risk of infection in the steroid group. Based on this evidence, steroids are considered as second line of therapy for patients with HIVAN especially in patients with a rapidly deteriorating renal function despite use of HAART. Usually a dose of 1mg/kg (up to maximum dose of 60mg/day) with a taper over 2 months is recommended. Simultaneous use of HAART is essential to suppress viral replication.

3.5.3 Inhibition of the renin-Angiotensin – Aldosterone system

Angiotensin- Aldosterone system activation has been shown to play a role in development and progression of HIVAN in animal models. The rationale for the use of ACE-inhibitors in HIVAN is based on their favorable efficacy in most other renal glomerular diseases, resulting from their renal hemodynamic effect and their modulation of profibrotic cytokines such as transforming growth factor-beta. Two prospective studies support use of ACEI for the treatment of HIVAN. In a case control study of 18 patients with HIVAN prior to discovery of HAART, 9 were treated with captopril , and matched with 9 controls. The captopril treated group had improved renal survival compared with controls. Another prospective single center study of 34 patients with HIVAN was treated with fosinopril 10mg/day and was compared with group of patients who refused treatment over a period of 5 years. The patients treated with fosinopril had better median renal survival as compared to untreated patients. All untreated patients progressed to ESRD over a median period of 5 months. This is limited data showing efficacy of ACEI in these non randomized trials. There are no trials on use of angiotensin receptor blockers. Usually ACEI may be used in halting the progression of HIVAN especially as first choice therapy in a patient with coexisting hypertension.

Medication used	Study Name	Number of patients	Study Design	Diagnosis of HIVAN (Biopsy proven or clinical diagnosis)	Outcome (change in renal function, effect on proteinuria)
HAART	Cosgrove	23 13 patients received HAART and remaining 10 patients received nothing	retrospective	Clinical and biopsy proven HIVAN	S/Cr stabilized in treated group as compared to untreated group
HAART	Szczech	42 patients with HIVAN. 27 patients with HIVAN took HAART	retrospective	Biopsy proven HIVAN.	Slower progression to ESRD in HAART treated group
Corticosteroids	Eustace	21 patients of which 13 patients received steroids	Retrospective Systemic steroids in dose of 60mg for one month followed by several month taper	Biopsy proven HIVAN	Reduction in proteinuria and stabilization of renal function at 3, 6, and 12 months
	Smith 1994	4 patients	Case series of Systemic corticosteroids given at dose of 60mg/day for 2-6 weeks	Biopsy proven HIVAN	Improvement of renal function but no effect on proteinuria
	Smith 1996	20 patients Given systemic steroids at 60mg/day for 2-11 weeks followed by taper over 2-26 weeks	Prospective, no control group	Clinical and biopsy diagnosis of HIVAN	Improvement in serum creatinine and improvement in proteinuria. Serum albumin increased. 25% rate of relapse seen on withdrawl of steroids
Angiotensin converting enzyme inhibitors	Wei	44 patients Fosinopril 10mg/day was given for HIVAN	Single center prospective with control group which received nothing	Clinical and biopsy proven HIVAN	Improvement of renal function with reduction in risk of kidney failure
	Kimmel	18 9 patients treated with captopril three times daily and 9 patients were untreated	Single center prospective	Biopsy proven HIVAN	Stabilization of renal function

Table 2. Trials of Various Agents Used in Treatment of HIVAN

3.6 Other glomerular diseases in HIV infection

HIV-related immune complex mediated kidney disease (HIVICK) can occur in HIV infected individuals of non-African descent due to deposition of or in situ development of HIV antigen specific immune complexes. HIV infected individuals are likely to develop non-HIV related kidney diseases related to various comorbidities as their age matched counterparts in the general population. Due to use of HAART, the aging HIV infected individuals with Diabetes Mellitus (DM) and Hypertension (HTN) can develop renal disease due to Diabetic Nephropathy or Hypertensive Nephrosclerosis. The incidence of diabetes mellitus, hypertension, and dyslipidemia is increased fourfold in HIV infected individuals on HAART as compared with HIV uninfected persons. The treatment of CKD due to either DM or HTN is similar to treatment of CKD due to these co morbid conditions in non- HIV infected individuals.

Hepatitis C related kidney disease can also occur in patients with HIV who are co infected with Hepatitis C virus. This is commonly seen in intravenous drug users. Approximately a third of HIV infected individuals are co infected with Hepatitis C. Membranoproliferative glomerulonephritis(usually with cryoglobulins) is seen on histopathology of kidney biopsy of the coinfected patients. These patients have circulating immune complexes of antigen-antibody with low complement levels and circulating cryoglobulins. They present clinically with proteinuria, hematuria, renal insufficiency, and maculopapular non blanching rash usually over the lower extremities. The treatment includes treatment of underlying Hepatitis C infection with interferon and Ribavarin.

Other glomerular diseases can be seen in HIV infected individuals which includes classic FSGS, IgA Nephropathy, Lupus like glomerulopathy, AA amyloidosis, Membranous Nephropathy, and immune complex mediated Glomerulonephritis.

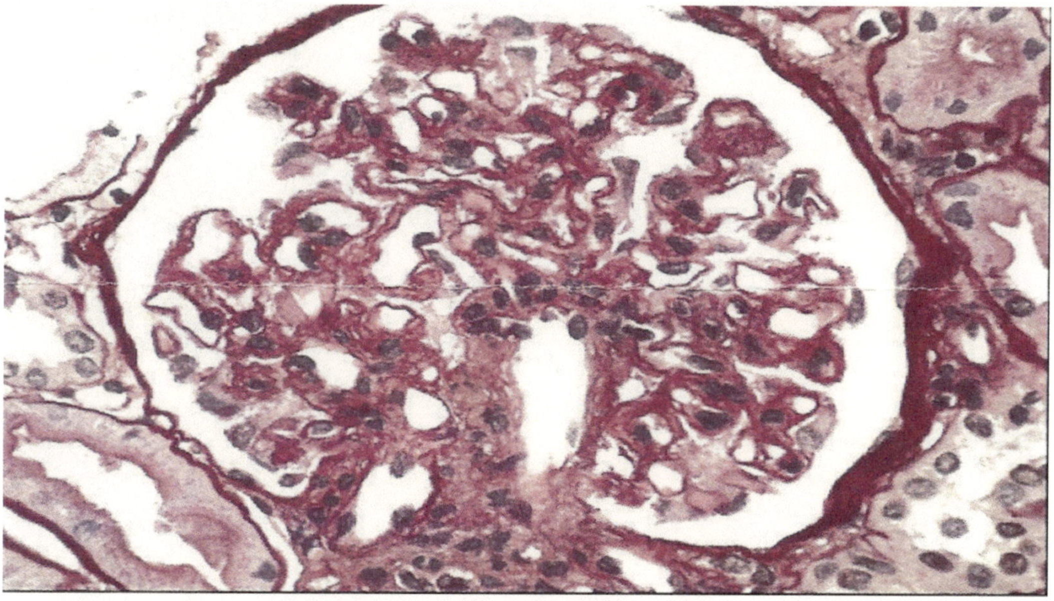

Fig. 5. Membranoproliferative Glomerulonephritis in HIV patient

It shows segmental glomerular basement duplication of Membranoproliferative glomerulonephritis seen in a patient coinfected with HIV and Hepatitis C.

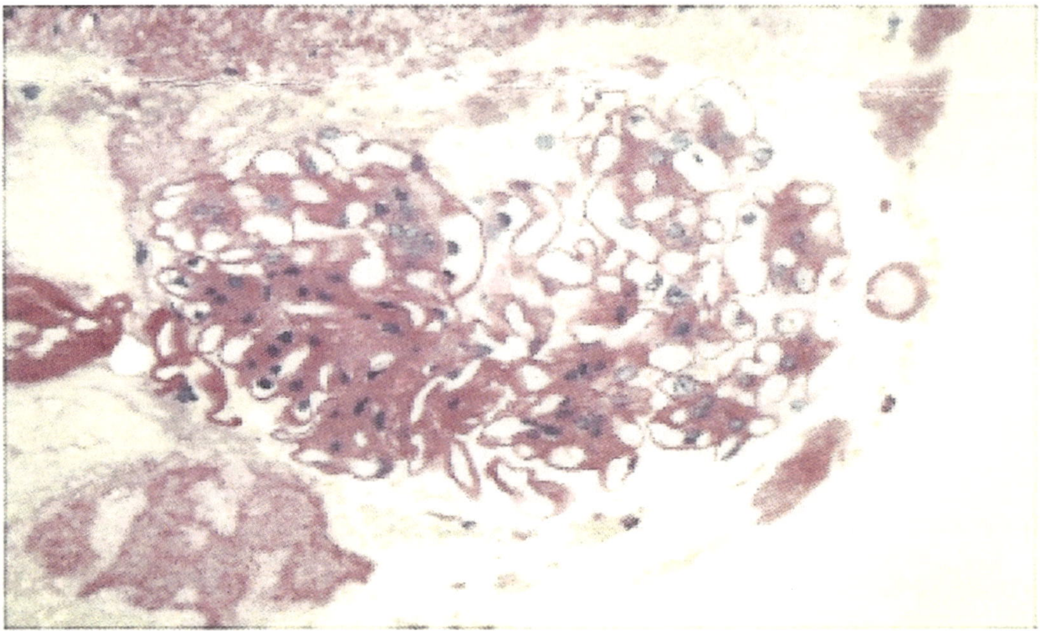

Fig. 6. Nodular Diabetic Nephropathy

It shows mesangial sclerosis consistent with Diabetic Nephropathy in an HIV infected patient with Diabetes Mellitus.

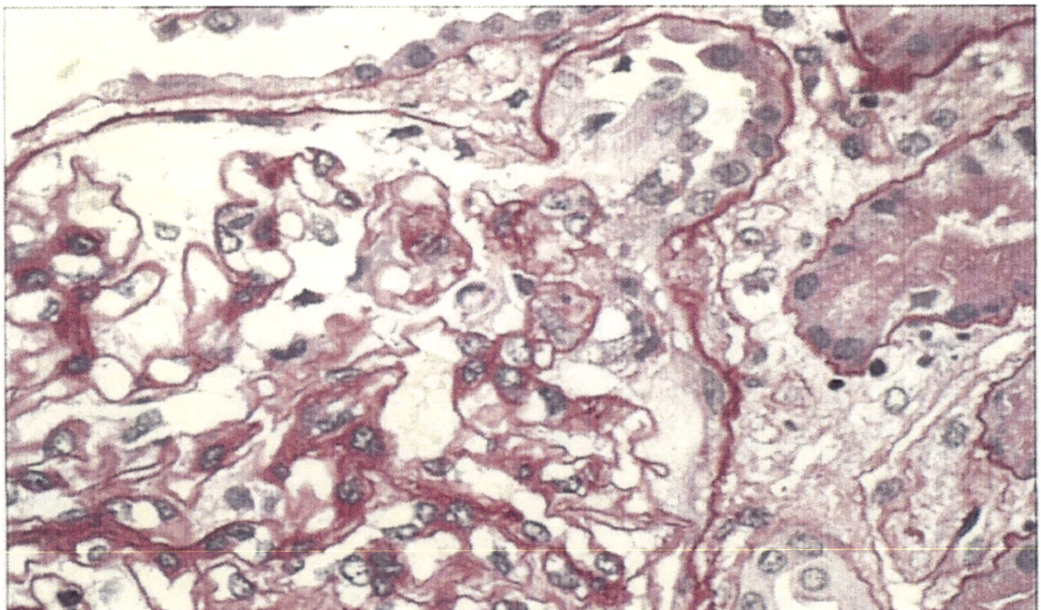

Fig. 7. FSGS with Tip lesion

It shows glomerular tip lesion of FSGS in a patient with HIV.

3.7 Supportive measures in chronic kidney disease

All supportive measures need to be employed to halt the progression of renal disease in patients with chronic kidney disease due to HIVAN. These measures include strict blood pressure control especially with blockade of renin angiotensin system in proteinuric patients. Use of nephrotoxic agents like aminoglycosides, non-steroidal anti-inflammatory drugs (NSAIDs), and radiocontrast agent for computerized tomography should be minimized. Hyperlipidemia should be treated with lipid lowering drugs with target goal of low density lipoprotein level to <100mg/dl. Cessation of smoking should be emphasized. Complications of CKD like anemia, hyperparathyroidism should be treated accordingly to Dialysis Outcome Quality Initiative (DOQI) guidelines. Options for renal replacement therapy should be discussed with the patients and appropriate referrals made during chronic kidney disease stage 4. Option for renal transplantation should be discussed with HIV infected patients with CKD.

4. End Stage Renal Disease (ESRD)

End Stage Renal Disease is common in HIV infected African Americans. According to Unites States Renal Data System (USRDS) more than 4000 incident cases of ESRD secondary to AIDS Nephropathy were reported to initiate dialysis from 2000-2004. Epidemiological studies have characterized the marked racial differences in the ESRD incidence among HIV-infected individuals. Blacks are the largest and fastest growing racial group with HIV in the United States. African Americans account for 63% of all persons with HIV infection in Africa. Prevalence of ESRD may rise very high in future.

4.1 Survival of HIV infected ESRD patient

Patients with HIV and ESRD had very high mortality rate in early 1980s before era of highly reactive anti-retroviral agents (HAART). These patients had advanced HIV disease with multiple opportunistic infections. Currently, with use of HAART, survival of HIV patients with ESRD has improved drastically over past decade. One year survival rate of HIV-infected patients was equivalent to that of general population in both US and French database.

All options of renal replacement therapy (RRT) should be offered to a patient who develops ESRD with HIV infection due to any etiology. This includes hemodialysis, peritoneal dialysis, and renal transplantation. Each modality of RRT has its own advantages and disadvantages.

4.2 Hemodialysis

It is the most commonly utilized modality of renal replacement therapy in HIV infected patients. Indications of initiation of hemodialysis are the same as in non-HIV infected individuals with kidney disease. Early surgical referral for placement of an arteriovenous fistula should be made so that a working access is available for use at time of initiation of chronic hemodialysis. Arteriovenous grafts (AVG) and permanent catheters are less favorable accesses in HIV infected individuals. AVG infection rate is high in patients with AIDS, asymptomatic HIV infection as compared to HIV negative patients. AVF survival rates are similar between HIV seropositive and HIV negative individuals with ESRD. Usually isolation of HIV infected patient with ESRD is not needed in dialysis unit. Reuse of properly sanitized dialyzer is permissible in HIV infected ESRD individuals. There is risk of transmission of HIV to dialysis staff through blood and needle stick exposure. Universal precautions of infection control need to be observed by the dialysis staff taking care of HIV ESRD patients. Routine cleaning with sodium hypochlorite solution of dialysis equipment and commonly touched surfaces are sufficient measures with regard to treating HIV infected individuals on hemodialysis. There is very small removal of HIV particle during hemodialysis to dialysate and hence dialysate should be handled as a potentially contaminated body fluid.

4.3 Peritoneal dialysis

This modality is preferred mode of dialytic therapy due to greater independence of life style and preservation of residual renal function as compared to patients on hemodialysis. Outcome of patients between hemodialysis and peritoneal dialysis is similar and therefore should be offered to HIV patients with ESRD. This modality minimizes exposure of healthcare workers to contaminated blood and needles. Peritoneal dialysis is associated with increased losses of protein in the dialysate and can cause protein malnutrition. Peritonitis is seen in patients on peritoneal dialysis. The risk of peritonitis in HIV infected with ESRD is higher than the HIV negative individuals on peritoneal dialysis particularly peritonitis caused by pseudomonas species and fungi. HIV is eliminated in the peritoneal dialysate is handled as a contaminated body fluid product. Peritoneal dialysis patients are instructed to pour dialysate into the home toilet. They should dispose off dialysate bags and lines by tying them in plastic bags and disposing these bags with conventional home garbage.

4.4 Kidney transplantation

It is an available modality for RRT in HIV infected individuals with well controlled HIV infection. HIV RNA must be undetectable using an ultra-sensitive assay. Individual and graft kidney survival rates are comparable with those of other population groups. Usually HIV infected individuals have high incidence of acute rejection after kidney transplantation. Studies have shown a 94% 3-year kidney transplant recipient survival but 67% of the patients in the study experienced acute rejection. The high incidence of acute rejection has not affected the graft survival rate due to use of immunosuppressive therapy. HIV disease does not progress in patients with kidney transplantation due to use of immunosuppressive therapy. HIV RNA levels and CD4 counts remain stable with use of immunosuppressive drugs. There is drug interaction of HAART with immunosuppressive drugs like Cyclosporin, Tacrolimus, and Sirolimus. These drugs are metabolized by cytochrome P450 system in the liver and hence raise level of immunosuppressive drugs. Usually doses of immunosuppressive agents used are usually 20% of the immunosuppressive dose administered to renal transplant recipients without HIV because concomitant HAART tends to raise serum levels of Cyclosporin and Tacrolimus.

5. Disorders of potassium

Both hyperkalemia and hypokalemia can be seen in HIV infected individuals. Hyperkalemia is very common in HIV infected patients and can be due to multiple

causes. It can be medication induced (see Table 3) due to use of Trimethoprim/ Sulphamethoxazole or Pentamidine use for Pneumocytis Carinii pneumonia prophylaxis or treatment respectively.
Hyperkalemia can also occur due to mineralocorticoid deficiency resulting from adrenal insufficiency or the syndrome of hyporenin hypoaldosteronism. Hyperkalemia can also occur with acute or chronic kidney disease. Usually treatment of Hyperkalemia includes discontinuation of any offending drug if possible, dietary potassium restriction especially in advanced kidney disease, and treatment of underlying cause of Hyperkalemia. Administration of certain medications like loop diuretics, fludrocortisones, and administration of corticosteroids in patients with adrenal insufficiency can be considered.
Hypokalemia is usually seen in conditions of gastrointestinal secretory losses like vomiting, diarrhea or nasogastric tube drainage. It is also seen in patients with severe wasting syndrome in advanced HIV disease. Certain medications also can cause hypokalemia like diuretics, amphotericin, foscarnet, and use of anti-retroviral agents like tenofovir and cidofovir. Some HIV infected patients have distal tubular renal tubular acidosis and can present with severe hypokalemia with metabolic acidosis.

PCP prophylaxis or treatment	Trimethoprim/ Sulphamethoxazole Pentamidine
Potassium sparing diuretics	Amiloride or Triamterene
Mineralocorticoid antagonists	Spironolactone and Epleronone
Renin angiotensin blockade with angiotensin converting enzyme inhibitors or angiotensin receptor blockers	Captopril, Fosinopril, Lisinopril, Losartan, Telmisartan
Non steroidal anti-inflammatory medications	Ibuprofen, Naproxen, Indomethacin
Immunosuppressive drugs especially in patients who undergo renal transplantation	Cyclosporin, Tacrolimus
DVT prophylaxis or treatment	Heparin(both unfractionated and low molecular weight heparin)
Congestive Heart failure	Digoxin

Table 3. Drugs Causing Hyperkalemia in HIV Infected Patients

6. Disorders of osmolality

Hyponatremia is very common in HIV infected patients and can be seen in 30-60% of hospitalized patients. It is a marker of severe illness which is associated with increased mortality in HIV- infected patients. In one study of 212 HIV infected patients hospitalized patients, the mortality rate was higher in hyponatemic group as compared to patients with normal serum sodium (36% vs. 19%).
Hyponatremia is usually due to multiple reasons in HIV infected patients. The commonest causes are volume depletion, syndrome of inappropriate antidiuretc hormone secretion (SIADH), and adrenal insufficiency. Volume depletion causing hyponatremia is usually due to gastrointestinal losses in HIV infected patients like vomiting or severe diarrhea. Volume

depletion is associated with low urinary sodium, high urine osmolality, increased BUN/Cr ratio. Hypovolemia usually responds well to intravenous hydration, along with measures to treat the underlying cause of volume losses. Syndrome of inappropriate antidiuretic hormone secretion can occur due to variety of intrapulmonary or intracranial causes like pneumocystis carini pneumonia, pulmonary tuberculosis, cerebral toxoplasmosis, and histoplasmosis etc. SIADH is treated with free water restriction and treatment of underlying infection or malignancy. In some cases, one may have to use specific medications to treat SIADH like demeclocycine or ADH receptor antagonists like conivaptan.

Adrenal insufficiency is an uncommon cause of hyponatremia as compared to hypovolemia and SIADH. Hyponatremia results from cortisol deficiency leading to urinary salt wasting. The adrenal insufficiency can result from adrenalitis, an abnormality that may be infectious in etiology caused by cytomegalovirus, mycobacterium avium intracellulare, or HIV itself. Adrenal hemorrhage and infiltration with Kaposi's sarcoma may also be seen.

Hypernatremia is seen uncommonly and results from loss of water from the body in excess of salt. This is seen usually in HIV infected patients admitted to the hospital due to opportunistic infections accompanied by high fevers. It occasionally can occur as consequence of loss of massive amounts of water in the urine due to development of Diabetes Insipidus or adipsia.

7. Disorders of acid-base disturbances

Acid base disturbances in HIV infected patients are commonly caused by infections or drugs. Both metabolic and respiratory acid base disorders are encountered in HIV infected patients. Respiratory alkalosis and respiratory acidosis may occur in opportunistic infections of the lungs or central nervous system. Metabolic acidosis can be of both anion and nonanion type. Nonanion gap metabolic acidosis can occur as a result of several different processes taking place in the body. These include gastrointestinal losses due to diarrhea, renal acid loss due to adrenal insufficiency or syndrome of hyporeninemic hypoaldosteronism, or nephrotoxicity of the drugs used to treat HIV infected patients.

High anion gap metabolic acidosis in HIV infected patients occur due to multiple causes. These patients are prone to multiple opportunistic infections especially in untreated HIV individuals which can be serious and can result in sepsis induced lactic acidosis (type A lactic acidosis). Type B lactic acidosis can result from mitochondrial dysfunction in the absence of sepsis, hypoperfusion or hypoxia. Type B Lactic Acidosis has been reported with use of nucleoside reverse transcriptase inhibitors like zidovudine, didanosine, zalcitabine, and stavudine. Life threatening lactic acidosis is rare; 5-25% of HAART treated patients may develop mildly elevated lactate levels without acidosis. It is not recommended to screen HIV positive patients for presence of lactic acidosis, but lactic acid level should be measured in patients who present with low bicarbonate level, an elevated anion gap, or abnormal liver enzymes.

8. Disorders of calcium

Both hypercalcemia and hypocalcemia can be seen in patients infected with HIV. It is present in 6.5% of HIV infected patients. Hypocalcemia is usually due to presence of vitamin D deficiency, pancreatitis, hypoparathyroidism, use of certain drugs like foscarnet,

tenofovir, pentamidine for treatment of pneumocystis carinii pneumonia. Hypomagnesemia can accompany hypocalcemia in these patients.
Hypercalcemia can occur due to use of certain drugs like high doses of vitamin D and calcium supplements. Certain diseases like pulmonary tuberculosis, sarcoidosis, Mycobactrium avium intracellulare infection, Hyperparathyroidism, monoclonal gammopathy, human T lymphotropic virus (HTLV-1) associated Lymphoma, and other malignancies have been associated with hypercalcemia in HIV infected individuals. Hypercalcemia can be severe in HTLV -1 associated lymphoma which needs urgent treatment. Hypercalcemia may be associated with kidney failure due to its vasoconstrictive effects which is often reversible. Hypercalcemia is managed usually with IV hydration followed by forced diuresis, calcitonin, and bisphosphonates. Hemodialysis against low calcium bath may be needed in patients presenting with severe hypercalcemia with CNS manifestations.

9. Disorders of magnesium

Hypomagnesemia is encountered frequently in HIV infected individuals. It usually results from the use of certain medications like foscarnet or pentamidine especially if both are used together. Hypomagnesemia has been associated with nonrecovery of renal function and high inpatient mortality in AIDS patients with acute kidney injury.

10. Disorders of phosphate

Hypophosphatemia is seen usually as a result of drug therapy in HIV infected patients. The drugs usually involved with hypophosphatemia are tenofovir, foscarnet and other antiretroviral agents. Hypophosphatemia results from fanconi's syndrome in these patients which cause phosphaturia and hence hypophosphatemia.
Hyperphosphatemia is seen usually in patients who develop chronic kidney disease due to HIV related or non-HIV related causes. It is usually seen in advanced stages of chronic kidney disease usually stage 4 &5. The management of hyperphosphatemia includes dietary phosphate restriction, use of non calcium based phosphate binders etc. Hyperparathryroidism resulting from chronic kidney disease is managed on the same principles as in non-HIVrelated CKD.

11. Nephrotoxicity of anti-retroviral agents

Nephrotoxicity is commonly encountered with use of anti-retroviral medications used for treatment of HIV infected individuals. Kidneys are involved in the excretion of these drugs and hence are exposed to high concentrations of these drugs, their metabolites or both. These medications require dose adjustment in patients with reduced GFR. Drug induced nephrotoxicity is seen in clinical practice and accounts for 2-15% cases of acute kidney injury (AKI). The exact frequency of nephrotoxicity induced by anti-retroviral agents in HIV infected patients is unknown. The dose recommendations by the pharmaceutical manufacturers are based on creatinine clearance and clinical validity of Modification of Diet in Renal Disease (MDRD) and Cockroft-Gault equations in HIV patients is not available. A brief overview of commonly used groups of drugs is given below.

11.1 PI (Protease Inhibitors)

Protease inhibitors are metabolized primarily in the liver. Urinary excretion accounts for approximately 10% of parent drug clearance for indinavir and 5% or less for other drugs in this class. PI's are highly protein bound (60-90%) and have large volume of distribution. None of the currently available PI requires dose adjustment for patients with reduced GFR. These medications are not cleared significantly by dialysis (both hemodialysis and peritoneal dialysis) although studies supporting this evidence recruited small number of patients. Some of the commonly used protease inhibitors are given in Table 4.
No adjustment of dose is needed in patients with reduced GFR or on dialysis.

Brand Name	Generic Name	Normal Dose
crixivan	Indinavir	800mg q8hour
Invirase	Saquinavir	1000mg bid with ritonavir 100mg bid
Norvir	Ritonavir	600mg bid
Viracept	Nelfinavir	750mg tid
Kaletra	Lopinavir/Ritonavir	Lopinavir 400mg/ritonavir 100mg bid
Reyatas	Atazanavir	1400mg bid
Lexiva	Fos-amprenavir	1400mg bid
Fortovase	Saquinavir(soft gel)	1200mg tid

Table 4. Commonly Used Protease Inhibitors with Doses in HIV

11.2 NRTI (Nucleoside /Nucleotide Reverse Transcriptase Inhibitors)

These drugs are eliminated by the kidney except abacavir which is mostly metabolized by the liver (Table 5 & 6). Urinary excretion ranges from 20-70% for various formulations except abacavir which is eliminated by 1% through the kidney. All the agents need dose

Brand Name	Generic Name	Normal Dose	Dose Adjustment Needed for Reduced GFR
Emtriva	Emtricitabine	200mg qd	Dose interval needs to be increased depending on GFR
Epivir	Lamivudine	150mg bid or 300mg /day	Dose needs to be decreased based on level of GFR
Hivid	Zalcitabine	0.75mg tid	Dose interval needs to be increased based on GFR
Retrovir	Zidovudine	300mg bid or 200mg tid	Dose needs to be decreased in dialysis patients
Videx	Didanosine	≥60kg: 200mg bid ≤ 60kg:125mg bid	Dose needs to be reduced in patients with compromised GFR
Viread	Tenofovir	300mg /day	Dose interval needs to be increased in patients with reduced GFR
Ziagen	abacavir	300mg bid	No dosage adjustment needed
Zerit	Stavudine	≥60kg:40mg q12h ≤60kg:30mg q12h	Dose needs to be reduced in patients with reduced GFR

Table 5. Nucleoside/Nucleotide Reverse Transcriptase Inhibitors Dosing in Patients with Normal and Impaired Renal Function

adjustment except abacavir in patients with reduced GFR. In dialysis patients, these drugs should be given after dialysis session. Unlike PI, these drugs have low protein binding and small volume of distribution. These drugs are eliminated by both glomerular filtration and tubular secretion. Nucleoside RTIs are less nephrotoxic than Nucleotide RTIs.

Other drugs such as Cimetidine and Trimethoprim can reduce their elimination by competing for tubular secretion by organic cation pathway.

Fixed drug combination should be avoided in patients with GFR <50ml/min. The reader should refer to individual package inserts for guidance with dosing of antiretroviral combinations.

Brand Name	Generic Name	Usual Dose
Combivir	Lamivudine/ Zidovudine	One tablet bid
Trizivir	Abacavir, Lamivudine, Zidovudine	One tablet bid
Truvada	Emtricitabine, Tenofovir	One tablet daily
Epzicom	Abacavir, Lamivudine	One tablet daily

Table 6. Nucleoside Reverse Transcriptase Inhibitors Fixed Dose Combinations

11.3 NNRTI (Non-Nucleoside Reverse Transcriptase Inhibitors)

These drugs are eliminated primarily by the liver. These drugs are protein bound and they do not require drug adjustment in patients with reduced GFR. These drugs are removed to some extent by dialysis and should be dosed after hemodialysis. Nevirapine is removed significantly by peritoneal dialysis but it remains unclear if a dosage adjustment is needed for patients on peritoneal dialysis as its trough plasma level remains unaffected.

Efavorenz and Delavirdine have not been studied in patients with reduced GFR or on dialysis.

11.4 Pathogenesis of nephrotoxicity

Nephrotoxicity results from mitochondrial dysfunction induced by NRTIs since they inhibit nuclear or mitochondrial DNA polymerase from host cell along with inhibition of reverse transcriptase of HIV. NRTIs affects DNA polymerase of mitochondria with subsequent deficits in mitochondrial DNA encoded enzymes of the mitochondrial respiratory chain. Oxidative phosphorylation is disrupted with deficits in energy production. This leads to production of lactate from anaerobic respiration which results in clinical effects like lactic acidosis, cardiomyopathy, peripheral neuropathy, fatty liver, and pancreatitis. Clinically it manifests as tubular injury to proximal tubular cells. Histologically is characterized by tubulointerstitial nephropathy with mitochondrial cytopathy. Protease inhibitors induce kidney injury by causing crystalluria, renal stones, and tubulointerstitial disease.

11.5 Renal manifestations of toxicity of antiretroviral agents

Various lesions caused by anti-retroviral agents as cause of AKI are acute tubular necrosis (ATN), crystalluria, Fanconi's syndrome, distal tubular acidosis (RTA), nephrogenic diabetes insipidus (NDI), and lactic acidosis. Chronic kidney disease can also result from long term HAART use.

AKI secondary to acute tubular necrosis (ATN) is commonly seen in patients with HIVinfection(up to 10%) and regarding HAART, tenofovir and indinavir are most commonly associated with nephrotoxicity.

Tenofovir is taken up into renal epithelial cells by basolateral membrane human organic anion transporters, then secreted into the urine across the apical membrane by transporters called multidrug resistance associated protein. Tenofovir toxicity was first reported by Verhelst et al in 2002. Tenofovir is associated with reversible Fanconi's syndrome, nephrogenic diabetes insipidus and they occur within 5-12 months after starting therapy with tenofovir. These abnormalities resolve within few months of discontinuation of tenofovir. Renal biopsy reveals cytoplasmic vacuolization, apical localization of nuclei, and reduction of brush border on proximal tubular cells. Clinically, it is manifested by glucosuria, aminoaciduria, hyperuricosuria, hypouricemia and hypophosphatemia due to phosphaturia. Most patients who develop tenofovir related renal dysfunction also have concomitant use of ritonavir. Patients taking tenofovir should have close monitoring of renal function especially if ritonavir is used concomitantly. Glucosuria and hypophosphatemia are early manifestations of tenofovir induced injury and tenofovir should be discontinued promptly. Nephrotoxicity improves upon discontinuation of tenofovir in most cases although in some patients serum creatinine levels remain above baseline levels.

Indinavir has been associated with crystalluria, nephrolithiasis, and obstructive nephropathy which can occur anytime after initiation of drug and has been reported in as many as 33% of patients on chronic therapy. Obstructive nephropathy may be mild to severe and may need urologic intervention. It is recommended to monitor patients on indinavir periodically during the first 6 months of therapy and then biannually. The use of indinavir has declined recently in patients with HIV.

Renal calculi have been reported with use of nelfinavir and saquinavir. Ritonavir has been associated with AKI in few reports. Atazanavir can induce AKI secondary to interstitial nephritis.

Some NRTI can induce interstitial nephritis and proximal tubular dysfunction like abacavir. Fanconi's syndrome has also been reported in patients using DDI and stavudine/lamivudine.

Lactic Acidosis has been described with use of NRTI. The development of lactic acidosis can range from asymptomatic chronic hyperlactemia to acute life threatening lactic acidosis. Lactic acidosis was first described with didanosine and zidovudine. It is believed to be caused by inhibition of mitochondrial DNA polymerase by intracellularly generated triphosphate metabolites of these drugs. Approximately 20-30% of patients who are treated with these drugs can be found to have asymptomatic hyperlactemia that develops several months after institution of therapy. Severe lactic acidosis (lactate acid level >5mmol/L) is clinically characterized by fatigue, nausea, vomiting, anorexia, and abdominal pain is rare and is associated with 80% mortality rate. Risk factors associated with lactic acidosis include longer duration of treatment with HAART, older age, female, pregnancy, hypertriglyceridemia, impaired renal function, and use of alcohol. Most patients with asymptomatic hyperlactemia remain stable. Stavudine and didanosine (alone or in combination) have been associated with hyperlactinemia and lactic acidosis, although all of NRTI have been implicated. Routine monitoring of lactic acid is not recommended except in patients with symptoms of lactic acidosis.

NNRTI can rarely be associated with AKI in association with rash and eosinophilia. HAART treated patients may develop chronic kidney disease especially in patients with partial recovery of renal function after an episode of AKI. These medications are excreted through kidneys and may be involved in causation of chronic kidney disease in HIV patients.

12. References

Abbott et al: Human immunodeficiency virus infection and kidney transplantation in the era of highly active antiretroviral therapy and modern immunosuppression. J Am Soc Nephrol 2004; 15:1633-9

Ahuja et al: Changing trends in the survival of dialysis patients with human immunodeficiency virus in the United States. J Am Soc Nephrol 2002; 13:1889-93.

Ahuja et al: Effect of hemodialysis and antiretroviral therapy on plasma viral load in HIV-1 infected hemodialysis patients. Clin Nephrol 1999:51: 40-4.

AIDS Surveillance--General Epidemiology: Estimated Number of Persons Living with AIDS by Race/Ethnicity, 1993-2003--United States. In: Centers for Disease Control and Prevention 2005.

Aly et al: Hypercalcaemia: a clue to Mycobacterium avium intracellulare infection in a patient with AIDS. Int J Clin Pract. 1999 Apr-May; 53(3):227-8.

Am J Kidney Dis. 1996; 28(2):202.

Andrieu et al: Effects of cyclosporin on T-cell subsets in human immunodeficiency virus disease. Clin Immunol Immunopathol 1988:47:181-98.

Berns et al: Renal aspects of therapy for human immunodeficiency virus and associated opportunistic infections. J Am Soc Nephrol 1991; 1:1061-80.

Bonnet et al: Risk factors for hyperlactataemia in HIV-infected patients, Aquitaine Cohort, 1999–2003. Antivir Chem Chemother 16: 63–67, 2005.

Boubaker et al: Hyperlactatemia and antiretroviral therapy: The Swiss HIV Cohort Study. Clin Infect Dis 33: 1931–1937, 2001.

Brock et al: The influence of human immunodeficiency virus infection and intravenous drug abuse on complications of hemodialysis access surgery. J Vasc Surg 1992; 16:904-10; discussion 911-2

Brodie et al: Variation in incidence of indinavir-associated nephrolithiasis among HIV-positive patients. AIDS 12 (18):2433–2437 (1998).

Brown et al.: Antiretroviral therapy and the prevalence and incidence of diabetes mellitus in the multicenter AIDS cohort study. Arch Intern Med; 165(10), 1179–1184 (2005).

Brown et al.: Antiretroviral therapy and the prevalence and incidence of diabetes mellitus in the multicenter AIDS cohort study. Arch. Intern. Med. 165(10):1179–1184(2005).

Burns et al: Effect of angiotensin-converting enzyme inhibition in HIV-associated nephropathy.

Calza et al: Tenofovir-induced renal toxicity in 324 HIV-infected, antiretroviral-naïve patients. Scand J Infect Dis. 2011 Apr 1.

Caramelo et al: Hyperkalemia in patients infected with the human immunodeficiency virus: involvement of a systemic mechanism. Kidney Int 1999; 56:198-205.

Chao et al: Two cases of hypocalcemia secondary to vitamin D deficiency in an urban HIV-positive pediatric population AIDS. 2003 Nov 7; 17(16):2401-3.

Chattha et al: Lactic acidosis complicating the acquired immunodeficiency syndrome. Ann Intern Med 1993; 118:37-9.

Choi et al. Long-term clinical consequences of acute kidney injury in the HIV-infected. Kidney Int. 2010 Sep; 78 (5):478-85.

Choi et al: HIV-infected persons continue to lose kidney function despite successful antiretroviral therapy. AIDS 23(16):2143–2149(2009).

Choi et al: HIV-infected persons continue to lose kidney function despite successful antiretroviral therapy. AIDS 23(16): 2143–2149(2009).

Cortés et al: Hypocalcemia and hypomagnesemia associated with the treatment with pentamidine in 2 patients with HIV infection.Med Clin (Barc). 1996 May 11; 106(18):717.

Curi et al: 2nd. Hemodialysis access: influence of the human immunodeficiency virus on patency and infection rates. J Vasc Surg 1999; 29: 608-16.

Dial Transplant 16: 643, 2001.

Dieleman et al: Persistent leukocyturia and loss of renal function in a prospectively monitored cohort of HIV-infected patients treated with indinavir. J Acquir Immune Defic Syndr 2003; 32:135-42.

Dinleyici et al: Adrenal insufficiency associated with cytomegalovirus infection in two infants. Int J Infect Dis. 2009 Jul; 13(4):e181-4.

Dong et al: Sulfadiazine-induced crystalluria and renal failure in a patient with AIDS. J Am Board Fam Pract 1999; 12:243-8.

Earle et al: Fanconi's syndrome in HIV+ adults: report of three cases and literature review. J. Bone Miner. Res. 19(5):714–721 (2004).

Earle et al: Fanconi's syndrome in HIV+ adults: report of three cases and literature review. J Bone Miner Res. 2004 May; 19(5):714-21.

Eggers et al: Is there an epidemic of HIV Infection in the US ESRD program? J Am Soc Nephrol 2004; 15:2477-85.

Estrella et al.: HIV type 1 RNA level as a clinical indicator of renal pathology in HIV-infected patients. Clin. Infect.Dis. 43(3):377–380(2006).

Estrella et al.: HIV type 1 RNA level as a clinical indicator of renal pathology in HIV-infected patients. Clin. Infect.Dis: 43(3), 377–380 (2006).

Eustace et al: Cohort study of the treatment of severe HIV-associated nephropathy with corticosteroids. Kidney Int. 58(3):1253–1260 (2000).

Eustace et al: Cohort study of the treatment of severe HIV-associated nephropathy with corticosteroids. Kidney Int. 2000; 58 (3):1253.

Fernando et al: Prevalence of chronic kidney disease in an urban HIV infected population. Am. J.Med.Sci. 335(2):89–94(2008).

Franceschini et al: Incidence and etiology of acute renal failure among ambulatory HIV-infected patients. Kidney Int. 67(4):1526–1531(2005).

Garg et al Incidence and Predictors of Acute Kidney Injury in an Urban Cohort of Subjects with HIV and Hepatitis C Virus Coinfection AIDS Patient Care STDS. 2011 Mar; 25(3):135-41.

Gearhart MO, Sorg TB. Foscarnet-induced severe hypomagnesemia and other electrolyte disorders Ann Pharmacother. 1993 Mar; 27(3):285-9.

Geusau et al: Primary adrenal insufficiency in two patients with the acquired immunodeficiency syndrome associated with disseminated cytomegaloviral infection Wien Klin Wochenschr. 1997 Nov 14; 109 (21):845-9.

Gorski et al: Complications of hemodialysis access in HIV-positive patients. Am Surg 2002; 68:1104-6.

Hammer et al.: Antiretroviral treatment of adult HIV infection: 2008 recommendations of the International AIDS Society-USA panel.JAMA 300(5), 555–570(2008).

Isnard Bagnis C et al: Changing electrolyte and acid-basic profile in HIV-infected patients in the HAART era Nephron Physiol. 2006; 103(3):p131-8. Epub 2006 Mar 23.

Izzedine et al: Atazanavir: A novel inhibitor of HIV-protease in haemodialysis. Nephrol Dial Transplant 20: 852–853, 2005.

Izzedine et al: Indinavir pharmacokinetics in haemodialysis. Nephrol Dial Transplant 15: 1102–1103, 2000.

Izzedine et al: Pharmacokinetic of nevirapine in haemodialysis. Nephrol Dial Transplant 16: 192–193, 2001.

Izzedine et al: Pharmacokinetics of ritonavir and nevirapine in peritoneal dialysis. Nephrol Izzedine et al: Pharmacokinetics of ritonavir and saquinavir in a haemodialysis patient. Nephron 87: 186– 187, 2001.

Izzedine et al: Renal tubular transporters and antiviral drugs: An update. AIDS 19: 455–462, 2005.

J Am Soc Nephrol. 1997; 8(7):1140.

Jones et al.: Cystatin C and creatinine in an HIV cohort: the Nutrition for Healthy Living Study. Am.J. Kidney Dis. 51(6):914–924 (2008).

Kalin et al: Hyporeninemic hypoaldosteronism associated with acquired immune deficiency syndrome. Am J Med 1987; 82:1035-8.

Kalin et al: Hyporeninemic hypoaldosteronism associated with acquired immune deficiency syndrome.Am J Med 1987; 82:1035-8.

Karras et al: Tenofovir-related nephrotoxicity in human immunodeficiency virus-infected patients: three cases of renal failure, Fanconi syndrome, and nephrogenic diabetes insipidus. Clin Infect Dis 2003; 36:1070-3.

Keuneke et al: Adipsic hypernatremia in two patients with AIDS and cytomegalovirus encephalitis Am J Kidney Dis. 1999 Feb; 33(2):379-82.

Kimmel et al: Captopril and renal survival in patients with human immunodeficiency virus nephropathy.

Kimmel et al: Continuous ambulatory peritoneal dialysis and survival of HIV infected patients with end-stage renal disease. Kidney Int .1993; 44:373-8.

Kimmel et al: HIV-associated immune-mediated renal disease. Kidney Int. 44(6): 1327–1340(1993).

Kimmel et al: HIV-associated immune-mediated renal disease. Kidney Int. 44(6), 1327–1340 (1993).

Kleyman et al: A mechanism for pentamidine-induced hyperkalemia: inhibition of distal nephron sodium transport. Ann Intern Med 1995; 122:103-6.

Kopp et al: Crystalluria and urinary tract abnormalities associated with indinavir. Ann Intern Med 1997; 127:119-25.

Kumar et al: Safety and success of kidney transplantation and concomitant immunosuppression in HIV-positive patients. Kidney Int 2005; 67:1622-9.

Lavae-Mokhtari et al: Acute renal failure and hypercalcemia in an AIDS patient on tenofovir and low-dose vitamin D therapy with immune reconstitution inflammatory syndrome. Med Klin (Munich). 2009 Oct 15; 104(10):810-3.

Lucas et al: Highly active antiretroviral therapy and the incidence of HIV-1-associated nephropathy: a 12-year cohort study.AIDS 18(3), 541–546 (2004).

Marks et al: Endocrine manifestations of human immunodeficiency virus (HIV) infection. Am J Med Sci 1991; 302:110-7.

Marks et al: Endocrine manifestations of human immunodeficiency virus (HIV) infection. Am J Med Sci 1991; 302:110-7.

Marroni et al: Acute interstitial nephritis secondary to the administration of indinavir. Ann. Pharmacother. 32 (7–8):843–844 (1998).

Mathew G, Knaus SJ: Acquired Fanconi's syndrome associated with tenofovir therapy. J. Gen. Intern. Med. 21(11):C3–C5 (2006).

Mitchell et al: Arteriovenous access outcomes in haemodialysis patients with HIV infection. Nephrol Dial Transplant 2007; 22:465-70.

Moreno et al: Magnesium deficiency in patients with HIV-AIDS. Nutr Hosp. 1997 Nov-Dec; 12(6):304-8.

Moyle et al: Hyperlactataemia and lactic acidosis during antiretroviral therapy: relevance, reproducibility and possible risk factors. Aids 2002; 16:1341-9.

Navarro et al: Nephrogenic diabetes insipidus and renal tubular acidosis secondary to foscarnet therapy. Am J Kidney Dis. 1996 Mar; 27(3):431-4.

Obialo et al: Hem dialysis vascular access: variable thrombus-free survival in three subpopulations of black patients. Am J Kidney Dis 1998; 31:250-6.

Osler et al: Risk factors for and clinical characteristics of severe hyperlactataemia in patients receiving antiretroviral therapy: a case-control study. HIV Med. 2010 Feb; 11(2):121-9. Epub 2009 Aug 20.

Parkhie et al: Characteristics of patients with HIV and biopsy-proven acute interstitial nephritis. Clin. J.Am. Soc. Nephrol. 5(5):798–804 (2010).

Peyriere et al: Renal tubular dysfunction associated with tenofovir therapy: report of 7 cases. J. Acquir. Immune Defic. Syndr. 35(3):269–273(2004).

Prasanthai et al: Prevalence of adrenal insufficiency in critically ill patients with AIDS.Med.Assoc Thai. 2007 Sep; 90 (9):1768-74.

Rao et al. Associated focal and segmental glomerulosclerosis in the acquired immunodeficiency syndrome. N Engl J Med 1984; 310:669-73.

Roubaud-Baudron et al: Hyperpnoea and ketonuria in an HIV-infected patient Nephrol Dial Transplant. 2007 Feb; 22(2):649-51.

Santos et al: Hypomagnesemia is a risk factor for nonrecovery of renal function and mortality in AIDS patients with acute kidney injury.. Braz J Med Biol Res. 2010 Mar; 43(3):316-23.

Schambelan et al: Management of metabolic complications associated with antiretroviral therapy for HIV-1 infection: Recommendations of an International AIDS Society – USA panel. J Acquir Immune Defic Syndr 31: 257–275, 2002.

Smith Effect of corticosteroid therapy on human immunodeficiency virus-associated nephropathy. Am J Med.1994; 97(2):145.

Smith et al: Clinical pharmacokinetics of non-nucleoside reverse transcriptase inhibitors. Clin Pharmacokinet 40: 893–905, 2001.

Smith et al: Prednisone improves renal function and proteinuria in human immunodeficiency virus-associated nephropathy.Am J Med. 1996:101(1):41.

Stengel B, Couchoud C: Chronic kidney disease prevalence and treated end-stage renal disease incidence: a complex relationship.J.Am.Soc.Nephrol.17 (8), 2094–2096(2006).

Stengel B, Couchoud C: Chronic kidney disease prevalence and treated end-stage renal disease incidence: a complex relationship. J. Am. Soc. Nephrol. 17(8):2094–2096(2006).

Stock et al: Evolving clinical strategies for transplantation in the HIV-positive recipient. Transplantation 2007; 84:563-71.

Szczech et al.: Microalbuminuria in HIV infection.AIDS 21(8), 1003–1009 (2007).

Szczech et al.: The clinical epidemiology and course of the spectrum of renal diseases associated with HIV infection. Kidney Int. 66(3):1145–1152(2004).

Szczech et al: Protease inhibitors are associated with a slowed progression of HIV-related renal diseases. Clin Nephrol. 2002; 57(5):336.

Tabure et al: Antiretroviral drug removal by haemodialysis. AIDS 14: 902–903, 2000

Taylor et al: Pharmacokinetics of nelfinavir and nevirapine in a patient with end stage renal failure on continuous ambulatory peritoneal dialysis. J Antimicrob Chemother 45: 716–717, 2000.

Thoden et al: Highly active antiretroviral HIV therapy-associated fatal lactic acidosis: quantitative and qualitative mitochondrial DNA lesions with mitochondrial dysfunction in multiple organs. AIDS 2008 May 31; 22 (9):1093-4.

Tuon et al: Vitamin D intoxication: a cause of hypocalcaemia and acute renal failure in a HIV patient. Int J STD AIDS. 2008 Feb; 19(2):137-8.

UNAIDS.AIDS Epidemic Update: December 2006. Geneva: Joint United Nations Programme on HIV/AIDS (UNAIDS) and World Health Organization (WHO); 2006. Report No.: UNAIDS/06.29E.

United States Renal Data System 2006 Annual Data Report. Bethesda, MD: National Institutes of Health, National Institute of Diabetes and Digestive and Kidney Diseases; 2006

Uno K et al: Fatal cytomegalovirus-associated adrenal insufficiency in an AIDS patient receiving corticosteroid therapy Intern Med. 2007; 46 (9):617-20.

Velazquez et al: Renal mechanism of trimethoprim-induced hyperkalemia. Ann Intern Med 1993; 119:296-301.

Velazquez et al: Renal mechanism of trimethoprim-induced hyperkalemia. Ann Intern Med 1993; 119:296-301.

Wali et al: HIV-1-associated nephropathy and response to highly-active antiretroviral therapy. Lancet.1998; 352(9130):783.

Williams J, Chadwick DR: Tenofovir-induced renal tubular dysfunction presenting with hypocalcaemia. Jnfect. 2006 Apr; 52 (4):107-8.

Winston et al: HIV-associated nephropathy is a late, not early, manifestation of HIV infection.Kidney Int: 55(3), 1036–1040 (1999).

Yahaya et al: Interventions for HIV-associated nephropathy.Cochrane Database Syst. Rev. 4, CD007183 (2009).

7

Oral Health-Related Quality of Life Among People Living with HIV/AIDS

Norkhafizah Saddki and Wan Majdiah Wan Mohamad
School of Dental Sciences, Universiti Sains Malaysia, Health Campus, Kubang Kerian, Kelantan, Malaysia

1. Introduction

Since it was first recognized in early 1980s, the Acquired Immunodeficiency Syndrome (AIDS) has been one of the most destructive diseases recorded in the world history. The devastating impact of HIV/AIDS on individual patient, family, community and the nation is vast. The disease not only robs a country of its monetary resources in covering for the costs of HIV prevention and treatment, but also of the nation's human resources when young productive lives are affected. The latest statistics suggested that the overall growth of the disease has stabilised with declining number of new HIV cases since the last decade. However, the number of people living with HIV/AIDS (PLWHA) remained high and appeared to be still on the rise (UNAIDS, 2010).

With increasing availability and use of highly active antiretroviral therapy (HAART) in 1996, fewer deaths due to AIDS-related diseases have been observed. Worldwide, about 1.8 million HIV-related deaths were reported in 2009 as compared to the peak 2.1 million in 2004. In Southern Alberta, Canada, analysis of AIDS death records between pre-HAART (1984-1996) and HAART (1997-2003) periods revealed reduction in crude mortality rate from 117 deaths per 1000 patient-years pre-HAART to 24 in the HAART period (Krentz et al., 2005). Across Europe, the HIV-related death rates reduced substantially between September, 1995, and March, 1998, in a large cohort of 4270 HIV-infected patients to less than a fifth of their previous level (Mocroft et al., 1998). A study in Taiwan compared the mortality rate of 10,162 HIV-infected patients whose diagnosis was made in three different periods: the pre-HAART period, from 1 January 1984 to 31 March 1997; the early HAART period, from 1 April 1997 to 31 December 2001; and the late HAART period, from 1 January 2002 to 31 December 2005 (Yang et al., 2008). Results showed that the mortality rate of HIV-infected patients declined significantly from 10.2 deaths per 100 person-years in the pre-HAART period to 6.5 deaths and 3.7 deaths per 100 person-years in the early and late HAART periods, respectively. This increase in survival rates contributes to the increasing number of PLWHA as AIDS is no longer a lethal disease but has been transformed into a chronic condition.

Oral lesions are common in PLWHA. Some oral manifestations have been documented as early markers of HIV infection and as predictors of disease progression. Among the most common oral manifestations of HIV include oral candidiasis, oral hairy leukoplakia and necrotizing ulcerative periodontitis (Coogan et al., 2005; Ranganathan & Hemalatha, 2006).

Oral problems may give rise to physical, functional and emotional discomfort, dysfunction, or disability which in turn has been shown to affect the overall quality of life (QOL) of PLWHA (Coulter et al., 2002; Yengopal & Naidoo, 2008). As people are living longer with HIV, the study on QOL has emerged as an important factor in management of HIV infection (Grossman et al., 2003). This chapter aims to describe the epidemiology and manifestations of oral lesions commonly associated with HIV/AIDS and the impact of oral health problems on the QOL of PLWHA.

2. Epidemiology of HIV-associated oral manifestations

Oral lesions are common in individuals with HIV infection. Many epidemiologic studies have been conducted around the world to study the prevalence of oral lesions among PLWHA not long after the virus was first discovered and reported in the United States in 1981. Bhayat et al. (2010) reported that oral manifestations of HIV/AIDS occurred in more than 60% of HIV-positive patients and were often the first sign of underlying immunosuppression. Another study by Nittayananta et al. (2002) found that more than 90% of HIV-infected individuals will have at least one oral manifestation during the illness. Not only HIV-related oral lesions are among the early clinical features of the infection, but can also indicate the stage and progress of the disease. Prevalence of oral lesions has been shown to be significantly higher in individuals with a CD4+ count less than 200 cells/mm^3 and a viral load greater than 3000 copies/mL (Bravo et al., 2006; Greenspan et al., 2000; Tappuni & Fleming, 2001). The importance of oral lesions as clinical indicators of HIV infections and markers of clinical progression to AIDS has been demonstrated in many studies that reported their association with CD4+ depletion and high viral load (Bravo et al., 2006; Campo et al., 2002; Chattopadhyay et al., 2005; Glick et al., 1994; Greenspan et al., 2000; Patton, 2000; Ramírez-Amador et al., 2003; Shiboski et al., 2001).

A comprehensive review of epidemiologic studies on HIV-related oral lesions reported from developed and developing countries over more than a decade, encompassing the pre-HAART and early-HAART period from 1986 to 2000, revealed oral candidiasis as the most common lesion found in all ages across the world (Patton et al., 2002). Prevalence of the lesion, however, ranged considerably from as low as 5% found in two separate studies in Minnesota (Little et al., 1994; Melnick et al., 1991) to as high as 94% among those with AIDS-defining illnesses in Zaire (Tukutuku et al., 1990). This review paper by Patton et al. (2002), which was the outcome of an International Workshop that addressed the prevalence and classification of HIV/AIDS associated oral lesions, identified hairy leukoplakia as the second most reported oral lesion with prevalence that ranged from 2% in Nairobi, Kenya (Wanzala et al., 1989) to 43% in Mexico (Gillespie & Mariño, 1993). This wide-ranged prevalence was due to variations in the populations studied, including differences in the prevalence of AIDS diagnoses, CD4+ count, or diagnostic techniques used.

Prevalence of other oral lesions commonly associated with HIV also varies according to region of the world and the population examined (Patton et al., 2002). According to the review by Patton et al. (2002), Kaposi's sarcoma was reported to be present in 12% of 83 heterosexual AIDS patients in Kinshasa, Zaire (Tukutuku et al., 1990), while higher frequency of 38% was found among 84 AIDS patients in the United States (Roberts et al., 1988). HIV-related periodontal lesions, namely linear gingival erythema, necrotizing ulcerative gingivitis and necrotizing ulcerative periodontitis were found in up to 22% of patients in New York (Lamster et al., 1994), 24% in Argentina (Gillespie & Mariño, 1993), and 23% in India (Anil & Challacombe, 1997), respectively. Of these periodontal lesions, necrotizing ulcerative periodontitis is the most severe form. Lower prevalence was reported for non-Hodgkin's lymphoma which was detected in 5% of 124 AIDS patients in Thailand (Nittayananta & Chungpanich, 1997) and 2% in San Francisco (Silverman Jr et al., 1986).

The introduction of HAART has not only resulted in significant decline in mortality associated with HIV across the world, significant reduction was also seen in the prevalence of most AIDS-defining illnesses and opportunistic infections (Buchacz et al., 2010; Kaplan et al., 2000; Mocroft et al., 2004). Similarly, there has been a downward trend in the prevalence of oral opportunistic lesions in response to the use of HAART (Franceschi et al., 2008; Patton et al., 2000; Ramírez-Amador et al., 2003; Shiboski, 2002; Yang et al., 2010). Notable reduction was reported in the prevalence of two most common HIV-associated lesions, oral candidiasis and hairy leukoplakia (Eyeson et al., 2002; Nicolatou-Galitis et al., 2004; Patton et al., 2000; Ramírez-Amador et al., 2003). Despite the great success of HAART, the therapy remains an expensive option that may be unaffordable to many, especially those living in low-income countries (WHO et al., 2009). It was reported that at least 5 million PLWHA in need of treatment are not able to have access to the life-prolonging therapy although the availability of HAART has increased rapidly from 7% in 2003 to 42% in 2008 to reach over four million people in low- and middle-income countries.

Nevertheless, even when HAART is available to reduce the viral load, many other factors have been suggested to predispose to oral lesions in HIV-infected individuals such as cigarette smoking, heroin/methadone use, poor oral hygiene, and socio-demographic factors such as older age, lower education level and lower household income (Chattopadhyay et al., 2005; Ferreira et al., 2007; Greenspan et al., 2000; Nittayananta et al., 2001; Noce et al., 2009; Shiboski et al., 1999a). In addition, studies have suggested that HIV disease progression can be influenced by psychological factors (Leserman, 2003; Leserman, 2008). Specifically, feelings of hopelessness, depressed mood, and avoidant coping have been shown to be associated with reduced CD4+ cell count and increased viral load in a study among 177 HIV-positive patients (Ironson et al., 2005). Owing to the established association of CD4+ count and viral load with prevalence of oral lesions, it is possible that psychosocial factors may also have an effect on the incidence of oral lesions in HIV patients.

Besides, related psychological and social impact including stigma of HIV infection should also be considered in general management of PLWHA as these may further influence health-seeking behaviour, diagnosis, quality of care provided, treatment and its outcomes, and adherence to therapy (Carr & Gramling, 2004; WHO, 2008). There have been several reports that suggested while the oral health needs among HIV-infected patients are high, utilization of care unfortunately has been poor (Dobalian et al., 2003; Mascarenhas & Smith, 1999; Patton et al., 2003; Shiboski et al., 1999b). These circumstances can develop a vicious cycle as poor use of services will undoubtedly create greater unmet needs which in turn further deteriorate oral conditions and increase the oral health impact among PLWHA. On the whole, although the prevalence of oral health conditions among PLWHA has mainly reduced, the problem remains as a fundamental component of disease progression. It is important that clinicians are able to diagnose oral lesions related to the infection, recognise the predisposing and risk factors, and initiate appropriate therapy.

3. Oral manifestations strongly associated with HIV

In 1993, the EC-Clearinghouse on Oral Problems Related to HIV Infection and the World Health Organization (WHO) Collaborating Centre on Oral Manifestations of the

Immunodeficiency Virus (EC-Clearinghouse & WHO, 1993) published a consensus on the classification of oral manifestations related with HIV infection and their diagnostic criteria. The lesions were grouped into three categories depending on their strength of association with the infection. Oral candidiasis, hairy leukoplakia, specific forms of periodontal disease (linear gingival erythema, necrotizing ulcerative gingivitis and necrotizing ulcerative periodontitis), Kaposi's sarcoma and non-Hodgkin's lymphoma have been classified as oral lesions strongly associated with HIV infection.

3.1 Oral candidiasis

Oral candidiasis is predominantly caused by *Candida albicans* (Laskaris, 2000). It is an early manifestation of HIV that can occur in patients who appear otherwise healthy. In HIV-infected patients, candidal infection can occur in two major forms, pseudomembranous and erythematous. The pseudomembranous type presents as white or yellowish spots or plaque that can be wiped off, revealing an erythematous surface. The soft palate, buccal mucosa, lateral borders of the tongue, commisures, lips and gingival are more frequently affected (Laskaris, 2000). On the other hand, the erythematous form presents as red area usually on the palate and the dorsum of the tongue although occasionally it can be located on the buccal mucosa (EC-Clearinghouse & WHO, 1993; Laskaris, 2000). White spots and plaque may be seen, but these are not usually conspicuous (Laskaris, 2000).

Clinical diagnosis of oral candidiasis is confirmed with the presence of candidal hypae in oral smears of the affected oral mucosa (Ramírez-Amador et al., 2006). The treatment of oral candidiasis includes azole (ketoconazole, fluconazole, itraconazole) and polyene drugs (nystatin and amphotericine B). However, resistance to these drugs and recurrences are frequent (Laskaris, 2000).

3.2 Oral hairy leukoplakia

Oral hairy leukoplakia is commonly found in patients at the late stage of HIV infection (Greenspan & Greenspan, 1992). It usually appears when CD4+ T cell count drops below 150 cells/mm3 (Glick et al., 1994). Although the actual cause and pathogenesis of the lesion is unclear, Epstein-Barr virus seems to play an important role (Cruchley et al., 1997; Tüzün et al., 2005). It is usually diagnosed clinically as asymptomatic, non-removable, flat or vertically correlated bilateral whitish or gray lesions on the lateral margins of the tongue (EC-Clearinghouse & WHO, 1993; Laskaris, 2000). Sometimes it occurs on the dorsum of the tongue and occasionally on the buccal mucosa. Appearance of the lesion may vary from subtle translucent white to dense white plaque, and Epstein-Barr virus has been detected by *in situ* hybridization of the lesion (Webster-Cyriaque et al., 1997). Oral hairy leukoplakia is almost always asymptomatic, self-limiting and often requires no treatment. Antifungal therapy may resolve the symptoms of superimposed candidosis but the lesion will not resolve completely. High dose acyclovir, zidovudine and podophyllin are the drugs of choice while surgical excision can be offered to patients who request for removal of the lesion (Scully & McCarthy, 1992). Oral hairy leukoplakia tends to recur when treatment is discontinued (Laskaris, 2000).

3.3 Linear gingival eythema

Linear gingival erythema appears as distinct fiery red band about 2-3 mm width along the free gingival margin (EC-Clearinghouse & WHO, 1993). Initially, the lesion was thought to be directly associated with HIV, and was thus previously called HIV-associated gingivitis.

However, subsequent evidence showed that the lesion is not specific to HIV infection. It also occurs in HIV negative immunocompromised patients and was renamed as linear gingival erythema. Clinical oral examination will reveal inflamed gingival tissues which bleed easily upon manipulation. There is absence of ulceration, periodontal pocket, or attachment loss. Unlike conventional periodontal disease, linear gingival erythema is not associated with the amount of plaque. It does not respond well to oral hygiene measures, removal of dental plaque and calculus. However, plaque and calculus should be removed in these patients to help reduce the erythema and possibly accelerate the healing. This procedure should be done very carefully to avoid excessive bleeding. Therapeutic protocol for linear gingival erythema includes 0.12% chlorexidine gluconate mouth rinse twice daily and systemic antibiotics such as metronidazole (Flagyl) if the lesion persists despite the preceding therapy.

3.4 Necrotizing ulcerative gingivitis

Clinically, necrotizing ulcerative gingivitis may present with fiery red and swollen gingiva as well as destruction of one or more interdental papillae. The onset of the disease is either acute or subacute. In acute stage, ulceration, necrosis and sloughing of both gingival margin and the top of interdental papillae are common findings. The anterior gingiva is most frequently affected. Pain, bleeding and halitosis are the common symptoms. Subacute stage is characterized by localized or generalized acute, painful ulceronecrotic lesions of the oral mucosa beyond the gingiva. In acute phase, treatment includes metronidazole, 500mg three times daily for 6 to 8 days and topical mouthwashes. Conventional periodontal treatment (plaque control measures, root planing, scaling) should follow (Laskaris, 2000).

3.5 Necrotizing ulcerative periodontitis

HIV-associated periodontitis is a serious and rapidly progressive condition, usually occur in severe immunosuppression when CD4+ T cell count is less than 100 cells/mm^3 (Glick et al., 1994). Clinically, necrotizing ulcerative periodontitis is characterized by gingival ulceration and necrosis as well as rapid and progressive destruction of the periodontal attachment and loosening of teeth (EC-Clearinghouse & WHO, 1993; Patton, 2003). Spontaneous bleeding, deep-seated pain, halitosis, erythema and edema are the prominent features (Laskaris, 2000). This condition can be treated with systemic administration of metronidazole or tetracycline for 8 to 12 days in conjunction with topical antibacterial mouthwashes. Conventional periodontal treatment maintenance and prevention should follow (Robinson, 1997). However, relapses are common.

3.6 Kaposi's sarcoma

Kaposi's sarcoma is the most common malignancies in HIV-infected patients (Wood & Harrington Jr, 2005). Human Herpes Virus-8 has been found to be necessary but not sufficient for its development because other factors such as immunosuppression are also required (Boshoff et al., 1995; Laskaris, 2000; Whitby et al., 1995; Wood & Harrington Jr, 2005). Clinically, in the early phase, patients with oral Kaposi's sarcoma may present with a blue, red or purple macules on the palate, gingival and/or tongue (Casiglia & Woo, 2000; Glick et al., 1994). The lesion may progress to become raised and nodular, and subsequently may result in ulceration, bleeding and pain (Casiglia & Woo, 2000; Laskaris, 1996). Biopsy of the lesion is required to confirm the diagnosis (Laskaris, 2000). Histopathologically, it is characterized by proliferation of spindle-shaped cells that form the vascular channels (Casiglia & Woo, 2000; Wang et al., 2007). The differential diagnoses of oral Kaposi's sarcoma include bacillary angiomatosis, pyogenic granuloma, peripheral giant cell granuloma, leiomyoma, angiosarcoma, nevi, malignant melanoma and oral lesions of amyloidosis (Laskaris, 2000).

Treatment for Kaposi's sarcoma mainly focus on palliation and local control since chemotherapy may further suppress the immune system and favor the proliferation of the lesion (Gascón & Schwartz, 2000). Local measures include excision, laser ablation, radiation or intralesional injection. A small lesion may be completely excised or ablated. Radiotherapy reduces the pain and results in regression of the lesion. However, it may give rise to potential side effects such as taste loss, mucositis as well as superimposed candidal infection. Prophylactic antifungal therapy with amphotericin B rinses and ketoconazole is beneficial to minimize this complication (Piedbois et al., 1994). Systemic involvement of Kaposi's sarcoma is usually treated with chemotherapy. Regimens include the use of vinblastine as a single agent or combination of adriamycin, bleomycin and vincristine (Casiglia & Woo, 2000).

3.7 Non-Hodgkin's lymphoma

Non-Hodgkin's lymphoma is the second most common intraoral neoplasm in patients with HIV infection, particularly those with CD4+ count less than 100 cells/mm^3 (Laskaris, 2000). As compared with healthy individuals, HIV patients have 60 to 70 times greater risk of developing the malignancy (Reynolds et al., 1993). Epstein Barr virus is a known risk factor for HIV-related non-Hodgkin's lymphoma (Wood & Harrington Jr, 2005). Factors such as viral infection can precipitate either chronic antigenic stimulation or immunosuppression which may provide a preferential environment for the development of non-Hodgkin's lymphoma (Fisher & Fisher, 2004).

Clinically, patients may present with intraoral ulcerations or soft tissue masses which are painful and rapidly enlarged. The most common sites include palate, retromolar pad, tonsillar pillars and tongue (Green & Eversole, 1989). However, most HIV patients presented with oral non-Hodgkin's lymphoma may already have nodal and extranodal involvement at the time of diagnosis (Carbone et al., 1995). Patients with localized disease are treated with radiotherapy. Chemotherapy is another treatment option. However, chemotherapy can induce profound neutropenia which can be treated effectively with concomitant administration of granulocyte-macrophage colony-stimulating factor (Kaplan et al., 1991). Complete remission occurs in approximately 65% of patients with the median survival time between 4 and 11 months (Carbone et al., 1995). Low CD4+ count and involvement of bone and extranodal site indicate poor prognosis (Levine et al., 1991).

4. Oral health-related quality of life among PLWHA

The effects of HIV infection on the QOL of those who live with it are substantial and have been well documented. While the symptoms of HIV vary according to the stage of infection, studies have shown that health-related QOL (HRQOL) of PLWHA declines as the disease progresses and as the number of symptoms increase (Hays et al., 2000; Lorenz et al., 2006; Lorenz et al., 2001). In view of the fact that oral manifestations are among the most common symptoms of HIV which may provide strong indication of the disease progress (Bravo et al., 2006; Greenspan et al., 2000; Lewis et al., 2003 ; Patton, 2000; Pedreira et al., 2008), the presence of oral lesions can therefore have significant impact on the general well-being of individuals affected (Lorenz et al., 2001).

Coulter et al. (2002) conducted a longitudinal study to determine the association between self-perceived oral health and general health in a sample of adults receiving medical care for HIV in the United States. Data was obtained via personal interviews that were conducted in three phases on a cohort that initially consisted of 2,864 patients. Oral health was assessed using seven items with a five-point scale on oral-related pain and discomfort, worry, appearance, and function, which were adapted from the General Oral Health Assessment Index (GOHAI) developed originally to measure oral health problems of older adults (Atchison & Dolan, 1990), while the general health was assessed using 28 items on a 0 to 100 scale that measure physical functioning and emotional well-being of the patients. In both measures, higher score indicated better health. Results of the study suggested that oral health was strongly associated with physical and mental health of individuals with HIV. The authors concluded that oral health is indeed an essential component of general health and thus should be included in the assessment of HRQOL among PLWHA.

To date, available evidence on the association between oral symptoms and HRQOL among PLWHA is scarce. The impact of oral conditions in PLWHA was first reported by Coates et al. (1996) in a study among 54 HIV positive dental patients. The oral health status of patients with HIV, as measured by the Decayed, Missing, and Filled Teeth (DMFT) Index for measuring dental caries and the Community Periodontal Index of Treatment Needs (CPITN) for measuring periodontal disease, was compared with general dental patients receiving public-funded care in Adelaide, South Australia, while the impact on HRQOL was evaluated against another sample of Adelaide residents. The results showed that the CPITN scores were higher among the HIV group compared with the control group although dental caries experience did not differ significantly. More importantly, HIV patients have reported greater impact on HRQOL aspects due to disabling oral conditions than the comparison group. The impact of oral conditions was measured using the Oral Health Impact Profile (OHIP) questionnaire (Slade & Spencer, 1994).

The OHIP questionnaire has been used to measure the impact of oral diseases on life experiences in various groups of patients and individuals. Originally developed in English, the OHIP questionnaire has been translated into other languages including Japanese, Korean, Malay, and Chinese (Bae et al., 2007; Ide et al., 2006; Saub et al., 2007; Wong et al., 2002). The questionnaire measures individual perceptions of impact, with questions divided into seven domains, namely functional limitation, physical pain, psychological discomfort, physical disability, psychological disability, social disability, and handicap. The original version contains 49 items (OHIP-49) as shown in Table 1.

The OHIP questionnaire has been the most commonly used instrument for assessing the oral health-related QOL (OHRQOL) among PLWHA. A five-point Likert scale response format is used to assess the frequency of impact caused by oral conditions during the previous 12 months, ranging from 'never' to 'very often'. From the results, the prevalence of impact can be determined which is the percentage of respondents reporting 1 or more impacts 'fairly often' or 'very often' (Slade et al., 2005). This information enables identification of those whose oral health impacts are chronic rather than transitory. A shorter version of the OHIP questionnaire with 14 items (OHIP-14) is also available to be used in settings where the use of 49 items is not suitable (Slade, 1997).

Yengopal & Naidoo (2008) used the OHIP questionnaire to assess the impact of oral lesions in a convenient sample of 150 HIV infected adults seen at HIV clinics in Cape Town, South Africa. Two groups of HIV-positive patients were compared, a case group of 71 patients with HIV-associated oral manifestations, and a control group of 79 patients who had no

Functional Limitation	Physical Disability
• Had difficulty chewing any foods • Trouble pronouncing words • Noticed a tooth which doesn't look right • Felt that appearance has been affected • Felt that breath has been stale • Felt that sense of taste has worsened • Had food catching in teeth or dentures • Felt that digestion has worsened • Felt that dentures have not been fitting properly **Physical Pain** • Had painful aching in mouth • Had a sore jaw • Had headaches • Had sensitive teeth with hot or cold food or drinks • Had toothache • Had painful gums • Found it uncomfortable to eat any foods • Had sore spots in mouth • Had uncomfortable dentures **Psychological discomfort** • Been worried by dental problems • Been self-conscious • Been miserable • Felt uncomfortable about appearance • Felt tense	• Speech has been unclear • People misunderstood some words • Felt there has been less flavour in food • Been unable to brush teeth properly • Had to avoid eating some foods • Had an unsatisfactory diet • Been unable to eat with dentures • Avoided smiling • Had to interrupt meals **Psychological Disability** • Sleep has been interrupted • Been upset • Found it difficult to relax • Felt depressed • Concentration has been affected • Been embarrassed **Social Disability** • Avoided going out • Been less tolerant of spouse or partner • Had trouble getting on with other people • Been a bit irritable with other people • Had difficulty doing usual job **Handicap** • Felt that general health has worsened • Suffered any financial loss • Been unable to enjoy other people's company • Felt that life in general was less satisfying • Been totally unable to function • Been unable to work to full capacity

Table 1. Dimensions and items of the full version of the OHIP questionnaire (OHIP-49).

associated oral lesions. Results of the study revealed that oral candidiasis, angular cheilitis, and hairy leukoplakia were the most common oral lesions found among the cases, who also had significantly higher prevalence of other oral problems such as dental caries, periodontitis, dry mouth, and taste problems compared with patients in the control group. Data for assessment of impact obtained using the full version of the OHIP questionnaire was analysed by simple frequency count and by the use of item weights for each question. In general, the frequency count analysis showed that patients with HIV-associated oral lesions had higher impact scores in all oral health domains measured than those in the group without associated lesion. Further investigations using item weights showed that patients with associated oral lesions appeared to be more affected in terms of their functional limitation, physical pain, psychological discomfort, physical disability, and psychological disability compared with the other two dimensions, social disability and handicap. In total, the impact scores remain significantly different between the two groups with the case group reporting higher impact than the control group.

Similar results were found in a study by Mulligan et al. (2008) that compared a group of HIV-infected women (n = 597) with another group of at-risk HIV-negative women (n = 92). All the participants were part of the Women's Interagency HIV Study (WIHS) cohort that investigated manifestations of HIV in women at six sites throughout the United States (Chicago, Los Angeles, Bronx, Brooklyn, San Francisco and Washington). However, for the OHRQOL study, the participants were selected among women from only four WIHS sites (excluding Brooklyn and Washington). The shorter version of OHIP questionnaire was used in this study. The OHRQOL were determined at the beginning, during, and end of the study. Results showed that HIV-infected women had higher OHIP-14 scores, both at the baseline and during the study, than women at-risk. The difference between the two groups however was not significant at the last measurement. All things considered, the WIHS oral cohort study concluded that HIV-positive women had significantly poorer OHRQOL than HIV-negative women with an average of 10% difference in impact scores measured repeatedly over 5.5 years between the two groups. In addition, the HIV-positive group showed poorer oral health status than the control group as indicated by some dental caries and periodontal parameters measured clinically at the baseline.

Oral health status of HIV-infected patients was also found to be poor in a study among a sample of 101 HIV-positive adult patients, 32 women and 69 men, seen at the Immunodeficiency Unit of the Cascais Hospital Center, Portugal (Santo et al., 2010). Clinical examinations of dental caries status, periodontal health, oral hygiene, and dental prosthesis status were done. The mean DMFT for the whole sample was 16.4 (SD 8.42), which was higher than that found among general adult populations reported in other studies. The mean DMFT of general adults was 11.4 (SD 7.87) in Istanbul, Turkey (Namal et al., 2008), 12.5 (SD 7.1) in Oviedo, Spain (Alvarez-Arenal et al., 1996), and 12.8 in Australia (Do & Roberts-Thomson, 2007). For the age group of 35-44 years old, the mean DMFT was higher in the HIV infected Portuguese patients which was 15.8 (SD 8.32) compared with that found in general population of similar age group. In Athens, Greece, the mean DMFT was 14.6 (SD 6.30) (Athanassouli et al., 1990), while in Pomerania, Germany, the mean DMFT was notably lower at 9.5 (SD 2.6) and 8.2 (SD 2.9) for female and male patients, respectively (Splieth et al., 2003). Further, examination of the periodontium showed that only 6.9% of the HIV-positive patients presented with healthy periodontium, while the majority of them (77.2%) had periodontal pockets of at least 4-5mm depth. Oral hygiene was also poor among the majority of patients (63.4%) as determined by the Oral Hygiene Index that assessed the amount of plaque on six index teeth (Greene & Vermillion, 1960). With regard to dental prosthesis status and perceived needs, while 28.8% of the patients were wearing dental prosthesis, 51.4% claimed that they needed dentures in the maxilla and 49.5% in the mandible. The OHRQOL among the HIV-positive Portuguese patients was assessed using the OHIP-14 questionnaire. Common oral health impact reported by the patients include discomfort when eating any foods (58.4%), self-conscious because of teeth, mouth or dentures (45.5%), painful aching in mouth (38.6%), embarrassed because of oral problems (38.6%), and felt tense because of problems with teeth, mouth or dentures (34.7%).

Of 33.3 million PLWHA around the world in year 2009, 2.5 million were children under 15 years (UNAIDS, 2010), the prevalence and percentage of which has increased from 2.3 million of 40.3 million PLWHA in year 2005 (UNAIDS, 2005). Similar to adults, oral manifestations are common in children infected with HIV and have been found to be directly associated with the degree of immunosuppression and disease progression (Fonseca et al., 2000; Santos et al., 2001). In addition, oral candidiasis has also been the most commonly reported lesion in children, although the distributions of other oral lesions are somewhat different between children adults (Greenspan & Greenspan, 2002; Patton et al., 2002; Ranganathan & Hemalatha, 2006). While there is a need to update and revise the classification of HIV-associated oral lesions in the paediatric population (Coogan et al., 2005), the relevant documents seem to be inadequate. Studies on the oral health impact of children with HIV are also lacking although they suffer a higher prevalence of oral health problems like untreated dental caries than their peers (Flaitz et al., 2001; Massarente et al., 2009; Pongsiriwet et al., 2003).

A recent study on OHRQOL of 88 HIV-positive children in Brazil who had developed AIDS symptoms further highlighted the dismal picture (Massarente et al., 2011). Measurement of OHRQOL was done using the Brazilian Portuguese version of the Child Perceptions Questionnaire for children aged 11 to 14 years (CPQ 11-14) (Goursand et al., 2008). The CPQ11-14 is a 37-item measure of OHRQOL encompassing four domains: oral symptoms, functional limitations, emotional and social well-being (Jokovic et al., 2006). It is designed specifically for children in the particular age group, taking into account their cognitive abilities and lifestyles. Besides, there is another version of the questionnaire, CPQ 8-10, developed for an age range from 8 to 10 years (Jokovic et al., 2004). Results showed that higher viral load was associated with poorer OHRQOL where children with more severe AIDS manifestations ranked lower in all domains of OHRQOL measured.

5. Summary

Oral manifestations are common in PLWHA. Oral lesions, that may be seen as early clinical features of HIV infection, has been used to evaluate the immunological status of HIV-infected patients as measured by reduced CD4+ T cell count and increased HIV RNA quantity in plasma. Besides being important indicators of HIV infection, oral lesions may predict progression of the disease to AIDS. Therefore it is imperative that health care providers, particularly oral health professionals, are able to identify the signs and symptoms of HIV-related oral lesions and recognize the significant role of these lesions in diagnosis and management of HIV infection.

Introduction of HAART has resulted in considerable reduction in prevalence of oral lesions in HIV-infected individuals. However, as the HAART regimens may not be available or accessible to those in need, oral lesions thus remain as indispensable component of HIV infection. While there is continuing interest to investigate oral manifestations and immunologic responses among PLWHA, the study on OHRQOL has emerged as an important focus in HIV research. The social impact of HIV-related oral lesions and other oral health problems is recognised as an important attribute used to assess the outcomes of oral health services, to assist in cost-benefit analysis, and to monitor individual patient care. Although to date, studies on the OHRQOL among HIV-infected individuals are not many, the current available evidence suggested that the impact is substantial. Collectively, this chapter highlights the important role of dentists in the interdisciplinary management of PLWHA.

6. References

Alvarez-Arenal A., Alvarez-Riesgo J., Pena Lopez J., Fernandez Vazquez J. & Villa Vigil M. (1996). DMFT and treatment needs in adult population of Oviedo, Spain. *Community Dent Oral Epidemiol* 24: 17-20

Anil S. & Challacombe S. (1997). Oral lesions of HIV and AIDS in Asia: an overview. *Oral Dis* 3 Suppl 1: S36-40

Atchison K. & Dolan T. (1990). Development of the Geriatric Oral Health Assessment Index. *J Dent Educ* 54: 680-7

Athanassouli T., Koletsi-Kounari H., Mamai-Homata H. & Panagopoulos H. (1990). Oral health status of adult population in Athens, Greece. *Community Dent Oral Epidemiol* 18: 82-4

Bae K., Kim H., Jung S., Park D., Kim J., Paik D. & Chung S. (2007). Validation of the Korean version of the oral health impact profile among the Korean elderly. *Community Dent Oral Epidemiol* 35: 73-9

Bhayat A., Yengopal V. & Rudolph M. (2010). Predictive value of group I oral lesions for HIV infection. *Oral Surg Oral Med Oral Pathol Oral Radiol Endod* 109: 720-3

Boshoff C., Schulz T., Kennedy M., Graham A., Fisher C., Thomas A., McGee J., Weiss R. & O'Leary J. (1995). Kaposi's sarcoma-associated herpesvirus infects endothelial and spindle cells. *Nat Med* 1: 1274-8

Bravo I., Correnti M., Escalona L., Perrone M., Brito A., Tovar V. & Rivera H. (2006). Prevalence of oral lesions in HIV patients related to CD4 cell count and viral load in a Venezuelan population. *Med Oral Patol Oral Cir Bucal* 11: E33-9

Buchacz K., Baker R., Palella Jr F., Chmiel J., Lichtenstein K., Novak R., Wood K., Brooks J. & HOPS Investigators (2010). AIDS-defining opportunistic illnesses in US patients, 1994-2007: a cohort study. *AIDS Care* 24: 1549-59

Campo J., Del Romero J., Castilla J., García S., Rodríguez C. & Bascones A. (2002). Oral candidiasis as a clinical marker related to viral load, CD4 lymphocyte count and CD4 lymphocyte percentage in HIV-infected patients. *J Oral Pathol Med* 31: 5-10

Carbone A., Vaccher E., Barzan L., Gloghini A., Volpe R., De Re V., Boiocchi M., Monfardini S. & Tirelli U. (1995). Head and neck lymphomas associated with human immunodeficiency virus infection. *Arch Otolaryngol Head Neck Surg* 121: 210-8

Carr R. & Gramling L. (2004). Stigma: a health barrier for women with HIV/AIDS. *J Assoc Nurses AIDS Care* 15: 30-9

Casiglia J. & Woo S. (2000). Oral manifestations of HIV infection. *Clin Dermatol* 18: 541-51

Chattopadhyay A., Caplan D., Slade G., Shugars D., Tien H. & Patton L. (2005). Risk indicators for oral candidiasis and oral hairy leukoplakia in HIV-infected adults. *Community Dent Oral Epidemiol* 33: 35-44

Coates E., Slade G., Goss A. & Gorkic E. (1996). Oral conditions and their social impact among HIV dental patients. *Aust Dent J* 41: 33-6

Coogan M., Greenspan J. & Challacombe S. (2005). Oral lesions in infection with human immunodeficiency virus. *Bull World Health Organ* 83: 700-6

Coulter I., Heslin K., Marcus M., Hays R., Freed J., Der-Martirosia C., Guzmán-Becerra N., Cunningham W., Andersen R. & Shapiro M. (2002). Associations of self-reported oral health with physical and mental health in a nationally representative sample of HIV persons receiving medical care. *Qual Life Res* 11: 57-70

Cruchley A., Williams D., Niedobitek G. & Young L. (1997). Epstein-Barr virus: biology and disease. *Oral Dis* 3 Suppl 1: S156-63

Do L. & Roberts-Thomson K. (2007). Dental caries experience in the Australian adult population. *Aust Dent J* 52: 249-51

Dobalian A., Andersen R., Stein J., Hays R., Cunningham W. & Marcus M. (2003). The impact of HIV on oral health and subsequent use of dental services. *J Public Health Dent* 63: 78-85

EC-Clearinghouse & WHO (1993). EC-Clearinghouse on Oral Problems Related to HIV Infection and WHO Collaborating Centre on Oral Manifestations of the Immunodeficiency Virus. Classification and diagnostic criteria for oral lesions in HIV infection. *J Oral Pathol Med* 22: 289-91

Eyeson J., Tenant-Flowers M., Cooper D., Johnson N. & Warnakulasuriya K. (2002). Oral manifestations of an HIV positive cohort in the era of highly active anti-retroviral therapy (HAART) in South London. *J Oral Pathol Med* 31: 169-74

Ferreira S., Noce C., Júnior A., Gonçalves L., Torres S., Meeks V., Luiz R. & Dias E. (2007). Prevalence of oral manifestations of HIV infection in Rio De Janeiro, Brazil from 1988 to 2004. *AIDS Patient Care STDS* 21: 724-31

Fisher S. & Fisher R. (2004). The epidemiology of non-Hodgkin's lymphoma. *Oncogene* 23: 6524-34

Flaitz C., Wullbrandt B., Sexton J., Bourdon T. & Hicks J. (2001). Prevalence of orodental findings in HIV-infected Romanian children. *Pediatr Dent* 23: 44-50

Fonseca R., Cardoso A. & Pomarico I. (2000). Frequency of oral manifestations in children infected with human immunodeficiency virus. *Quintessence Int* 31: 419-22

Franceschi S., Maso L., Rickenbach M., Polesel J., Hirschel B., Cavassini M., Bordoni A., Elzi L., Ess S., Jundt G., Mueller N. & Clifford G. (2008). Kaposi sarcoma incidence in the Swiss HIV Cohort Study before and after highly active antiretroviral therapy. *Br J Cancer* 99: 800-4

Gascón P. & Schwartz R. (2000). Kaposi's sarcoma. New treatment modalities. *Dermatol Clin* 18: 169-75

Gillespie G. & Mariño R. (1993). Oral manifestations of HIV infection: a Panamerican perspective. *J Oral Pathol Med* 22: 2-7

Glick M., Muzyka B., Lurie D. & Salkin L. (1994). Oral manifestations associated with HIV-related disease as markers for immune suppression and AIDS. *Oral Surg Oral Med Oral Pathol Oral Radiol Endod* 77: 344-9

Goursand D., Paiva S., Zarzar P., Ramos-Jorge M., Cornacchia G., Pordeus I. & Allison P. (2008). Cross-cultural adaptation of the Child Perceptions Questionnaire 11-14 (CPQ11-14) for the Brazilian Portuguese language. *Health Qual Life Outcomes* 6

Green T. & Eversole L. (1989). Oral lymphomas in HIV-infected patients: association with Epstein-Barr virus DNA. *Oral Surg Oral Med Oral Pathol* 67: 437-42

Greene J. & Vermillion J. (1960). The oral hygiene index: a method for classifying oral hygiene status. *JADA* 61: 29-35

Greenspan D. & Greenspan J. (1992). Significance of oral hairy leukoplakia. *Oral Surg Oral Med Oral Pathol Oral Radiol Endod* 73: 151-4

Greenspan D., Komaroff E., Redford M., Phelan J., Navazesh M., Alves M., Kamrath H., Mulligan R., Barr C. & Greenspan J. (2000). Oral mucosal lesions and HIV viral load in the Women's Interagency HIV Study (WIHS). *J Acquir Immune Defic Syndr* 25: 44-50

Greenspan J. & Greenspan D. (2002). The epidemiology of the oral lesions of HIV infection in the developed world. *Oral Dis* 8 Suppl 2: 34-9

Grossman H.A., Sullivan P.S. & Wu A.W. (2003). Quality of life and HIV: Current assessment tools and future directions for clinical practice. *The AIDS Reader* 12: 583-97

Hays R., Cunningham W., Sherbourne C., Wilson I., Wu A., Cleary P., McCaffrey D., Fleishman J., Crystal S., Collins R., Eggan F., Shapiro M. & Bozzette S. (2000). Health-related quality of life in patients with human immunodeficiency virus infection in the United States: results from the HIV Cost and Services Utilization Study. *Am J Med* 108: 714-22

Ide R., Yamamoto R. & Mizoue T. (2006). The Japanese version of the Oral Health Impact Profile (OHIP)--validation among young and middle-aged adults. *Community Dent Health* 23: 158-63

Ironson G., O'Cleirigh C., Fletcher M., Laurenceau J., Balbin E., Klimas N., Schneiderman N. & Solomon G. (2005). Psychosocial factors predict CD4 and viral load change in men and women with human immunodeficiency virus in the era of highly active antiretroviral treatment. *Psychosom Med* 67: 1013-21

Jokovic A., Locker D. & Guyatt G. (2006). Short forms of the Child Perceptions Questionnaire for 11-14-year-old children (CPQ11-14): development and initial evaluation. *Health Qual Life Outcomes* 4

Jokovic A., Locker D., Tompson B. & Guyatt G. (2004). Questionnaire for measuring oral health-related quality of life in eight- to ten-year-old children. *Pediatr Dent* 26: 512-8

Kaplan J., Hanson D., Dworkin M., Frederick T., Bertolli J., Lindegren M., Holmberg S. & Jones J. (2000). Epidemiology of human immunodeficiency virus-associated opportunistic infections in the United States in the era of highly active antiretroviral therapy. *Clin Infect Dis* 30 Suppl 1: S5-14

Kaplan L., Kahn J., Crowe S., Northfelt D., Neville P., Grossberg H., Abrams D., Tracey J., Mills J. & Volberding P. (1991). Clinical and virologic effects of recombinant human granulocyte-macrophage colony-stimulating factor in patients receiving chemotherapy for human immunodeficiency virus-associated non-Hodgkin's lymphoma: results of a randomized trial. *J Clin Oncol* 9: 929-40

Krentz H., Kliewer G. & Gill M. (2005). Changing mortality rates and causes of death for HIV-infected individuals living in Southern Alberta, Canada from 1984 to 2003. *HIV Med* 6: 99-106

Lamster I., Begg M., Mitchell-Lewis D., Fine J., Grbic J., Todak G., el-Sadr W., Gorman J., Zambon J. & Phelan J. (1994). Oral manifestations of HIV infection in homosexual men and intravenous drug users. Study design and relationship of epidemiologic, clinical, and immunologic parameters to oral lesions. *Oral Surg Oral Med Oral Pathol* 78: 163-74

Laskaris G. (1996). Oral manifestations of infectious diseases. *Dent Clin North Am* 40: 395-423

Laskaris G. (2000). Oral manifestations of HIV disease. *Clin Dermatol* 18: 447-55

Leserman J. (2003). HIV disease progression: depression, stress, and possible mechanisms. *Biol Psychiatry* 54: 295-306

Leserman J. (2008). Role of depression, stress, and trauma in HIV disease progression. *Psychosom Med* 70: 539-45

Levine A., Sullivan-Halley J., Pike M., Rarick M., Loureiro C., Bernstein-Singer M., Willson E., Brynes R., Parker J. & Rasheed S. (1991). Human immunodeficiency virus-related lymphoma. Prognostic factors predictive of survival. *Cancer* 68: 2466-72

Lewis D., Callaghan M., Phiri K., Chipwete J., Kublin J., Borgstein E. & Zijlstra E. (2003). Prevalence and indicators of HIV and AIDS among adults admitted to medical and surgical wards in Blantyre, Malawi. *Trans R Soc Trop Med Hyg* 97: 91-6

Little J., Melnick S., Rhame F., Balfour Jr H., Decher L., Rhodus N., Merry J., Walker P., Miller C. & Volberding P. (1994). Prevalence of oral lesions in symptomatic and asymptomatic HIV patients. *Gen Dent* 42: 446-50

Lorenz K., Cunningham W., Spritzer K. & Hays R. (2006). Changes in symptoms and health-related quality of life in a nationally representative sample of adults in treatment for HIV. *Qual Life Res* 15: 951-8

Lorenz K., Shapiro M., Asch S., Bozzette S. & Hays R. (2001). Associations of symptoms and health-related quality of life: findings from a national study of persons with HIV infection. *Ann Intern Med* 134: 854-60

Mascarenhas A.K. & Smith S.R. (1999). Factors associated with utilization of care for oral lesions in HIV disease. *Oral Surg Oral Med Oral Pathol Oral Radiol Endod* 87: 708-13

Massarente D., Domaneschi C. & Antunes J. (2009). Untreated dental caries in a Brazilian paediatric AIDS patient population. *Oral Health Prev Dent* 7: 403-10

Massarente D., Domaneschi C., Marques H., Andrade S., Goursand D. & Antunes J. (2011). Oral health-related quality of life of paediatric patients with AIDS. *BMC Oral Health* 11: 2

Melnick S., Hannan P., Decher L., Little J., Rhame F., Balfour Jr H. & Volberding P. (1991). Increasing CD8+ T lymphocytes predict subsequent development of intraoral lesions among individuals in the early stages of infection by the human immunodeficiency virus. *J Acquir Immune Defic Syndr* 4: 1199-207

Mocroft A., Kirk O., Clumeck N., Gargalianos-Kakolyris P., Trocha H., Chentsova N., Antunes F., Stellbrink H., Phillips A. & Lundgren J. (2004). The changing pattern of Kaposi sarcoma in patients with HIV, 1994-2003: the EuroSIDA Study. *Cancer* 100: 2644-54

Mocroft A., Vella S., Benfield T., Chiesi A., Miller V., Gargalianos P., d'Arminio Monforte A., Yust I., Bruun J., Phillips A. & Lundgren J. (1998). Changing patterns of mortality across Europe in patients infected with HIV-1. EuroSIDA Study Group. *Lancet* 352: 1725-30

Mulligan R., Seirawan H., Alves M., Navazesh M., Phelan J., Greenspan D., Greenspan J. & Mack W. (2008). Oral health-related quality of life among HIV-infected and at-risk women. *Community Dent Oral Epidemiol* 36: 549-57

Namal N., Can G., Vehid S., Koksal S. & Kaypmaz A. (2008). Dental health status and risk factors for dental caries in adults in Istanbul, Turkey. *East Mediterr Health J* 14: 110-8

Nicolatou-Galitis O., Velegraki A., Paikos S., Economopoulou P., Stefaniotis T., Papanikolaou I. & Kordossis T. (2004). Effect of PI-HAART on the prevalence of oral lesions in HIV-1 infected patients. A Greek study. *Oral Dis* 10: 145-50

Nittayananta W., Chanowanna N., Sripatanakul S. & Winn T. (2001). Risk factors associated with oral lesions in HIV-infected heterosexual people and intravenous drug users in Thailand. *J Oral Pathol Med* 30: 224-30

Nittayananta W., Chanowanna N., Winn T., Silpapojakul K., Rodklai A., Jaruratanasirikul S. & Liewchanpatana K. (2002). Co-existence between oral lesions and opportunistic systemic diseases among HIV-infected subjects in Thailand. *J Oral Pathol Med* 31: 163-8

Nittayananta W. & Chungpanich S. (1997). Oral lesions in a group of Thai people with AIDS. *Oral Dis* 3 Suppl 1

Noce C., Ferreira S., Silva Júnior A. & Dias E. (2009). Association between socioeconomic status and HIV-associated oral lesions in Rio de Janeiro from 1997 to 2004. *Braz Oral Res* 23: 149-54

Patton L. (2000). Sensitivity, specificity, and positive predictive value of oral opportunistic infections in adults with HIV/AIDS as markers of immune suppression and viral burden. *Oral Surg Oral Med Oral Pathol Oral Radiol Endod* 90: 182-8

Patton L. (2003). HIV disease. *Dent Clin North Am* 47: 467-92

Patton L., McKaig R., Strauss R., Rogers D. & Eron J.J. (2000). Changing prevalence of oral manifestations of human immuno-deficiency virus in the era of protease inhibitor therapy. *Oral Surg Oral Med Oral Pathol Oral Radiol Endod* 89: 299-304

Patton L., Phelan J., Ramos-Gomez F., Nittayananta W., Shiboski C. & Mbuguye T. (2002). Prevalence and classification of HIV-associated oral lesions. *Oral Dis* 8 Suppl 2: 98-109

Patton L., Strauss R., McKaig R., Porter D. & Eron J.J. (2003). Perceived oral health status, unmet needs, and barriers to dental care among HIV/AIDS patients in a North Carolina cohort: impacts of race. *J Public Health Dent* 63: 86-91

Pedreira E., Cardoso C., Barroso Edo C., Santos J., Fonseca F. & Taveira L. (2008). Epidemiological and oral manifestations of HIV-positive patients in a specialized service in Brazil. *J Appl Oral Sci* 16: 369-75

Piedbois P., Frikha H., Martin L., Levy E., Haddad E. & Le Bourgeois J. (1994). Radiotherapy in the management of epidemic Kaposi's sarcoma. *Int J Radiat Oncol Biol Phys* 30: 1207-11

Pongsiriwet S., Iamaroon A., Kanjanavanit S., Pattanaporn K. & Krisanaprakornkit S. (2003). Oral lesions and dental caries status in perinatally HIV-infected children in Northern Thailand. *Int J Paediatr Dent* 13: 180-5

Ramírez-Amador V., Anaya-Saavedra G., Calva J., Clemades-Pérez-de-Corcho T., López-Martínez C., González-Ramírez I. & Sierra-Madero J. (2006). HIV-related oral lesions, demographic factors, clinical staging and anti-retroviral use. *Arch Med Res* 37: 646-54

Ramírez-Amador V., Esquivel-Pedraza L., Sierra-Madero J., Anaya-Saavedra G., González-Ramírez I. & Ponce-de-León S. (2003). The Changing Clinical Spectrum of Human Immunodeficiency Virus (HIV)-Related Oral Lesions in 1,000 Consecutive Patients: A 12-Year Study in a Referral Center in Mexico. *Medicine (Baltimore)* 82: 39-50

Ranganathan K. & Hemalatha R. (2006). Oral lesions in HIV infection in developing countries: an overview. *Adv Dent Res* 19: 63-8

Roberts M., Brahim J. & Rinne N. (1988). Oral manifestations of AIDS: a study of 84 patients. *J Am Dent Assoc* 116: 863-6

Robinson P. (1997). Treatment of HIV-associated periodontal diseases. *Oral Dis* 3 Suppl 1: S238-40

Santo A., Tagliaferro E., Ambrosano G., Meneghim M. & Pereira A. (2010). Dental status of Portuguese HIV+ patients and related variables: a multivariate analysis. *Oral Dis* 16: 176-84

Santos L., Castro G., de Souza I. & Oliveira R. (2001). Oral manifestations related to immunosuppression degree in HIV-positive children. *Braz Dent J* 12: 135-8

Saub R., Locker D., Allison P. & Disman M. (2007). Cross-cultural adaptation of the Oral Health Impact Profile (OHIP) for the Malaysian adult population. *Community Dent Health* 24: 166-75

Scully C. & McCarthy G. (1992). Management of oral health in persons with HIV infection. *Oral Surg Oral Med Oral Pathol Oral Radiol Endod* 73: 215-25

Shiboski C. (2002). HIV-related oral disease epidemiology among women: year 2000 update. *Oral Dis* 8 Suppl 2: 44-8 ISSN 1354-523X

Shiboski C., Neuhaus J., Greenspan D. & Greenspan J. (1999a). Effect of receptive oral sex and smoking on the incidence of hairy leukoplakia in HIV-positive gay men. *J Acquir Immune Defic Syndr* 21: 236-42

Shiboski C., Wilson C., Greenspan D., Hilton J., Greenspan J., Moscicki A. & Adolescent Medicine HIV/AIDS Research Network (2001). HIV-related oral manifestations among adolescents in a multicenter cohort study. *J Adolesc Health* 29: 109-14

Shiboski C.H., Palacio H., Neuhaus J.M. & Greenblatt R.M. (1999b). Dental care access and use among HIV-infected women. *Am J Public Health* 89: 834-9

Silverman Jr S., Migliorati C., Lozada-Nur F., Greenspan D. & Conant M. (1986). Oral findings in people with or at high risk for AIDS: a study of 375 homosexual males. *J Am Dent Assoc* 112: 187-92

Slade G. (1997). Derivation and validation of a short-form oral health impact profile. *Community Dent Oral Epidemiol* 25: 284-90

Slade G., Nuttall N., Sanders A., Steele J., Allen P. & Lahti S. (2005). Impacts of oral disorders in the United Kingdom and Australia. *Br Dent J* 198: 489-93

Slade G. & Spencer A. (1994). Development and evaluation of the Oral Health Impact Profile. *Community Dent Health* 11: 3-11

Splieth C., Schwahn C., Bernhardt O., Kocher T., Born G., John U. & Hensel E. (2003). Caries prevalence in an adult population: results of the Study of Health in Pomerania, Germany (SHIP). *Oral Health Prev Dent* 1: 149-55

Tappuni A. & Fleming G. (2001). The effect of antiretroviral therapy on the prevalence of oral manifestations in HIV-infected patients: a UK study. *Oral Surg Oral Med Oral Pathol Oral Radiol Endod* 92: 623-8

Tüzün Y., Kalayciyan A., Engin B. & Tüzün B. (2005). Life-threatening disorders of mucous membranes. *Clin Dermatol* 23: 267-75

Tukutuku K., Muyembe-Tamfum L., Kayembe K., Odio W., Kandi K. & Ntumba M. (1990). Oral manifestations of AIDS in a heterosexual population in a Zaire hospital. *J Oral Pathol Med* 19: 232-4

UNAIDS (2005). AIDS epidemic update UNAIDS/WHO: Geneva.

UNAIDS (2010). Global Report: UNAIDS Report on the Global AIDS Epidemic. UNAIDS: Geneva.

Wang J., Stebbing J. & Bower M. (2007). HIV-associated Kaposi sarcoma and gender. *Gend Med* 4: 266-73

Wanzala P., Manji F., Pindborg J. & Plummer F. (1989). Low prevalence of oral mucosal lesions in HIV-1 seropositive African women. *J Oral Pathol Med* 18: 416-8

Webster-Cyriaque J., Edwards R., Quinlivan E., Patton L., Wohl D. & Raab-Traub N. (1997). Epstein-Barr virus and human herpesvirus 8 prevalence in human immunodeficiency virus-associated oral mucosal lesions. *J Infect Dis* 175: 1324-32

Whitby D., Howard M., Tenant-Flowers M., Brink N., Copas A., Boshoff C., Hatzioannou T., Suggett F., Aldam D. & Denton A. (1995). Detection of Kaposi sarcoma associated herpesvirus in peripheral blood of HIV-infected individuals and progression to Kaposi's sarcoma. *Lancet* 346: 799-802

WHO (2008). HIV/AIDS and mental health. Report by the Secretariat. World Health Organization: Geneva.

WHO, UNICEF & UNAIDS (2009). Towards universal access: scaling up priority HIV/AIDS interventions in the health sector. Progress report 2009. World Health Organization: Geneva.

Wong M., Lo E. & McMillan A. (2002). Validation of a Chinese version of the Oral Health Impact Profile (OHIP). *Community Dent Oral Epidemiol* 30: 423-30

Wood C. & Harrington Jr W. (2005). AIDS and associated malignancies. *Cell Res* 15: 947-52

Yang C., Chen M., Hsieh S., Sheng W., Sun H., Hung C. & Chang S. (2010). Non-Hodgkin's lymphoma in patients with human immunodeficiency virus infection in Taiwan. *J Microbiol Immunol Infect* 43: 278-84

Yang C., Huang Y., Hsiao C., Yeh Y., Liou H., Hung C. & Yang S. (2008). Trends of mortality and causes of death among HIV-infected patients in Taiwan, 1984-2005. *HIV Med* 9: 535-43

Yengopal V. & Naidoo S. (2008). Do oral lesions associated with HIV affect quality of life? *Oral Surg Oral Med Oral Pathol Oral Radiol Endod* 106: 66-73

8

HIV-Co Opportunistic Infections - A Current Picture in Tropical Climatic Eastern Indian Seropositive Population

Nilanjan Chakraborty
ICMR Virus Unit, Kolkata
India

1. Introduction

HIV or Human Immunodeficiency Virus, a RNA virus. On exposure to this virus, it directly attacks certain human organs, such as the heart, brain and kidneys. It plays a very significant role in weakening the immune system of its host. The immune system forms the framework in protecting the body from attack by any foreign agent like the bacteria, fungus, virus or any type of infection and even from some cancers by reacting accordingly. The primary cells attacked by HIV are the CD4+ lymphocytes, which are glycoprotein expressed on the surface of T_h cells, macrophages, monocytes, regulatory T cells and dendritic cells and plays a vital role in performing important immune responses in the body. It helps in direct immune function in the body. It is via this CD4 that HIV-1 enters into the host T-cells. A progressive reduction in the number of T cells expressing CD4 occurs on HIV infection. Since CD4+ plays a very important role in maintaining a proper immune system function, progressive loss of CD4+ lymphocytes as destroyed by HIV, the immune system barely works. With more active HIV infection or on prolonged exposure to HIV would deprive the host of its CD4 containing cells and this reduced CD4 count leading to reduced host immunity. Opportunistic infections take advantage of this weak host immune system and manifest their adverse effects. Many people especially during the advanced stage of HIV infection face problems resulting from opportunistic infections (OIs) and cancers.

The HIV/AIDS is a global epidemic and approximately 40 million people are living with HIV/AIDS worldwide (Quinn, 1996). Of all HIV/AIDS infected people, 95% are living in developing countries. Africa is the worst affected of all the continents. It consists of 19 countries worldwide with the highest prevalence of reported infections with more than 24.5 million, and more than 60% of the HIV-infected population. South Africa holds the record of being the country with the largest population living with the disease, at well over 5 million people infected. South Africa is followed by followed by Nigeria in 2nd place and India being the 3rd largest population of HIV infected people. Currently India about 5.134 million HIV infected cases are present in India which comprises of 65% cases of Southeast Asia. In India, HIV/ AIDS pandemic no longer belongs to the high-risk groups but now it is common among the general population (Ran & Hemalatha, 2006; Solomon *et al.*2006). Exponential growth of this epidemic is now at the threshold for India.

2. OIs associated with HIV

As mentioned earlier, taking advantage of this weakened immune system of its host with advanced HIV infection several infections and malignancies called 'opportunistic infections' appear.Opportunistic Infections (OIs) have been recognized as common complications of HIV infection due to immune deficiency which detoriates both the standard of life and life expectancy of the these HIV infected people. One of the main reasons behind hospitalization and substantial morbidity in HIV infected patients due to these OIs. OIs have been recognized as common complications of HIV infection since the beginning of the HIV epidemic (Kanabus *et al.* 2006; CDC, 1982; Selik *et al.*1984). These OIs develop several complicacies which lead to substantial morbidity and hospitalization. Several toxic and expensive therapies are required as a part of the treatment procedure. These ultimately lead to shorten the survival of people with HIV infection OI (Moore & Chassion, 1996; Finkelstein *et al.*1996). The decrease in the CD4 count in these HIV infected people is not doubt partially responsible for these various OIs (Talib *et al.*1993). A dramatic reduction in the incidence of OI among HIV-positive people who have received ART has been observed on introduction of antiretroviral therapy (ART); however, HIV/AIDS patients all around the world cannot afford or are not exposed to ART. Millions of people living with HIV in resource-poor communities/ countries donot get access to ART and in these cases especially the occurrence of OIs is very common (Kanabus *et al.* 2006). Even where ART drugs are available, they do not entirely remove the need for preventing and treating OI. Because of poor adherence, drug resistance or other factors measures to prevent and treat OIs become essential if ART stops working. However, providing prevention and treatment of OIs is of utmost importance to these people as it not only helps HIV-positive persons to live longer, healthier lives, but it can also help to prevent tuberculosis (TB) and other transmissible OIs from spreading to others. At present, the absolute CD4+ count determines the initiation of primary prophylactic therapies for OIs, which is an excellent predictor of the short-term overall risk of developing AIDS among HIV-infected patients (Stein *et al.*1992).

The spectrum and frequency of certain OIs highlight the urgency of studying HIV/AIDS in resource-limited countries like India where locally specific disease patterns may be observed. With the identification of such opportunistic pathogens in these HIV/AIDS patients, the HIV epidemic can be more effectively managed if physicians and health planners are aware of this information. The data may thus serve as a baseline, which can be implemented to the remote district level study as well and may further give an insight into the HIV related opportunistic infections would render help for subsequent HIV/AIDS care and management in a developing country like India.

2.1 Study carried out by our research group

In our study (published as *Current Trends of Opportunistic Infections among HIV- Seropositive patients from Eastern India* published in Jpn.J.Infect.Dis. 61, 49-53, 2008) the HIV-Co Opportunsitic infections from the cases reported from the various HIV-infected patients admitted Calcutta Medical College Hospital, Kolkata West Bengal, and of referred patients from Apex Clinic, Calcutta Medical College Hospital, a referral center for patients of HIV infection or AIDS were included. The patients admitted in the hospital were from different states of eastern India such as Bihar, Orissa, Jharkhand and from West Bengal. Their HIV status was confirmed by three ERS (Enzyme-linked immunosorbent assay [ELISA], Rapid, Simple), an ELISA (viz., HIV ELISA, Rapid test) and Western blot as recommended by the National AIDS Control Organization (NACO), Ministry of Health and Family Welfare, Government of India (NACO,2000).

For the diagnosis of OIs, routine microbiology smears, cultures and serology should be performed with utmost precaution. Different samples as directed by clinicians were collected depending on patient symptoms and clinical presentation under universal aseptic precautions in suitable sterile containers for the routine diagnosis. For the isolation, culture and identification of species of the pathogen in order to detect the OIs from blood samples, sputum and stool. OIs were diagnosed according to the criteria suggested by the Centers for Disease Control and Prevention (CDC) (CDC,1992). For isolation of *Candida* causing oral candidiasis to the HIV patients, Sabourand's dextrose agar (SDA) was used as transporting media. Pseudohyphae and budding yeast were characteristic findings. The appearance of the lesion and presence of yeast forms on microscopic examination of the oropharynix were sufficient evidence to confirm the diagnosis (Kolmer *et al.*1969). The most prevalent and obtained pure culture of yeast was compared with referral strain *Saccharomyces cerevisiae* ATCC 2601 and that of *Candida albicans* spp. was compared with referral strain *C. albicans* ATCC 10231. Cases of TB were classified as definite if the culture for *Mycobacterium tuberculosis* was positive for acid-fast bacilli. The decontaminated sputum sample from the diagnosed TB patients was further studied for obtaining a pure culture of *M. tuberculosis* growing on prepared LJ slants.The positive pure cultures grew yellow colonies on the slants. The isolated pure culture of *M. tuberculosis* spp. was compared with referral strain *M. tuberculosis* ATCC 25177. Stool specimens from all diarrhea patients (following WHO criteria of watery stool for at last 48 h prior to investigation) were processed (da Silva, & Pieniazek, 2003) and examined microscopically for the presence of *Cryptosporidium parvum*, a zoonotic pathogen that causes chronic watery diarrhea. The staining technique used for staining of *Cryptosporidium* was modified Ziehl-Neelsen (AFB staining). Cryptosporidia and other coccidia stained pink-red. The isolated pure culture of *Cryptosporidium* spp. was compared with a referral strain *Cryptosporidium* (Microbiology QC slides, Himedia SL45-10; Himedia).Enteric bacterial flora from the stool samples of diarrhea patients were isolated using differential selective screening media such as UTI agar (urinary tract infection agar; Himedia) after documenting their clinical manifestations, including intestinal flu, inflammation-associated cramping, abdominal pain, nausea and vomiting. Different enteric pathogens that exhibit a particular colony color facilitate the identity of particular microorganisms such as *Escherichia coli* (pink-magenta), *Proteus mirabilis* (light green), *Enterococcus fecalis* (bluish green), *Staphylococcus aureus* (cream), *Pseudomonas aureginosa* (colorless) and *C. albicans* (pin point white). For isolation of *Vibrio cholerae* and other enteropathogenic *Vibrio*, TCBS agar (thiosulfate citrate bile salt sucrose; SRL, Mumbai, India) was used. Cryptococcal meningitis was confirmed by clinical symptoms and signs as well as the detection of cryptococcal capsular antigen (*Cryptococcus* antigen latex agglutination Test; Remel, Lenexa, Kans., USA). Toxoplasmic encephalitis was diagnosed in the presence of at least two of the following findings: a history of neurological symptoms, neurological signs at admission or suggestive computed tomography scan or magnetic resonance imaging of the brain (Luft, & Remington,1988, 1992). A response to anti-*Toxoplasma* (IgM) antibodies, which was detected by a serological ELISA commercial kit gives a satisfactory result.

Characteristic	No. of Patients: (n=125) Male (%)	Female (%)
No. of HIV-seropositive patients	105 (84)	20 (16)
Age in years (mean ± standard deviation)	(35.6 ± 6.77)	(33.15 ± 6.68)
≤20	1 (0.8)	1 (0.8)
21 - 30	27 (21.6)	7 (5.6)
31 - 40	55 (44)	10(8)
≥41	22 (17.6)	2(1.6)
Mode of transmission of HIV		
Heterosexual transmission	80 (64)	-
Homosexual transmission	6 (4.8)	_
Blood transfusion	3 (2.4)	1 (0.8)
Intravenous drug abuse	20(16)	5(4)
Frequent needle prick	_	_
Vertical transmission	_	_
Unsterilized injection equipments	6 (4.8)	4 (3.2)
CD4+ lymphocyte count/µl (mean ± standard deviation)	(439.45 ± 222.11)	(12 ± 93.82)
≤50	18 (14.4)	4 (3.2)
51 - 100	25 (20)	3 (2.4)
101 - 200	38 (30.4)	8 (6.4)
≥201	24 (19.2)	5 (4)

Table 1. Patient Characteristic

In our study, 125 HIV (HIV-1 subtype) patients with OI were studied, of whom, 105 (84%) were male and 20 (16%) were female. The majority of patients (52%) were 31 - 40 years old followed by 27, 19 and 1% for the age groups 21 - 30, ≥41 and ≤20 years old, respectively. Heterosexual mode of transmission was obtained to be the predominant mode of transmission of HIV accounting for 64% of cases, followed by other routes (Table 1).

According to CD4 cell count/cu mm of blood ,the distribution of the study population was a maximum 36% of the population with 101-200 CD4+ cell count, followed by 23, 22 and 17% of patients with ≥201, 51 - 100 and ≤50 CD4 cell count, respectively. A significant finding from an epidemiological point of view was the complete absence of Yeast, HBV and venereal disease in female subjects. The follow-up of the case studies revealed that 7 cases (5.6%) out of 125 HIV-infected patients expired during the later period of their treatment. Ten (8%) of the study patients were receiving ART. Dermatological reactions were found as drug-related complications in patients with HIV infection. The most serious disorder, Steven-Johnson syndrome (SJS), was found to occur in 5 (4%) HIV-infected patients after intake of a combination of rifampicin-isoniazid after beginning treatment for recurrent Pulmonary TB occurring as an OI (Pitche *et al.* 2005).

2.1.1 Prevalence of different OIs

Oral candidiasis (OC) emerged as the most frequent infection to be associated with HIV infection in patients across the total range of CD4+ as studied by us among the spectrum of OIs observed. OC infection was found to be prevalent among 88% of these patients. Oral yeast (*Saccharomyces*)-infection was found in 5.6% of patients. TB emerged as the second most prevalent infection amongst the population as studied by us, developing in 57% of subjects. The diagnosis of TB was definite for all the suspected patients. Both pulmonary (69.4%) and extra pulmonary (16.6%) types were found to be prevalent. Amongst the HIV positive patients extra pulmonary TB was found to be prevalent amongst patients with lower median CD4+ counts (46/µl blood). But amongst the HIV/AIDS patients pulmonary TB was found amongst the patients having median CD4+ of 105/µl blood -which are the most common location of the disease.

HIV is driving the tuberculosis (TB) epidemic in many developing countries including India. During our study to determine the drug resistance pattern of pulmonary TB among HIV seropositive and HIV negative hospitalized patients from different states of Eastern India, (published as *Drug susceptibility profile of Mycobacterium tuberculosis isolated from HIV infected and uninfected pulmonary tuberculosis patients in Eastern India* in Transactions of the Royal Society of Tropical Medicine and Hygiene 104 (2010) 195–201) the TB positive isolates were screened and characterized by conventional laboratory methods followed by first- and second-line drug susceptibility testing on Lowenstein-Jensen medium by the proportion method. The drug susceptibility testing showed 17.7% and 6.6% multidrug-resistant (MDR) TB for the HIV positive and HIV negative patients, respectively. 22.2% of the isolated MDR-TB cases could be classified as extensively drug-resistant (XDR) TB isolates. 88.8% of all the MDR-TB isolates and all XDR-TB isolates were screened from HIV patients. 27.7% of the MDR-TB isolates showed resistance to all the first-line drugs. Mortality rate among the XDR-TB isolates was as high as 75%. Patients with interrupted anti-TB drug treatment were the ones most affected. These findings are critical and the risk to public health is high, particularly with HIV infected patients.

The pathogen most frequently isolated from the diarrheic patients was *C. parvum* (43.1%). In about 47% of the immunocompromised patients, various enteropathogenic species of *Vibrio* were found, while simultaneously the presence of bacterial pathogens from *Enterobacteriacae* was 40% and *E. coli* was found in 42% of cases.

Among the viral OIs, CMV infection was the most predominant; 45% of subjects were positive for CMV infection among 125 HIV-seropositive study subjects. The other viral infections found in the study population were HSV (7.2%) and HBV (5.6%) which were much less in comparison to the prevalence of CMV infection. The absence of any specific clinical symptoms of CMV amongst the patients was an important characteristic of CMV infection and was often indistinguishable from other types of infection. The common unifying feature of CMV disease in the immunocompromised patient was the presence of fever, and approximately 65% of cases developed hearing defects and perceptual organ damage such as optic atrophy and blindness.

The most common form of disseminated cryptococcosis was Meningitis, and it developed in 4% of the study patients. All cases were diagnosed by clinical and neurological symptoms with confirmation by laboratory investigations.

Very few other OIs were found, viz., herpes zoster virus (HZV) infection, syphilis from *T.pallidum*, etc., among the patients investigated. Interestingly, not even a single case of malignancy was found to occur among the investigated patients.

2.1.2 Highlights of our study

Our study highlights that candidial infection is the most common OI, followed by TB and diarrhea, all of which are presumed to result from our geographic, climatic and socio-economic conditions. Early diagnosis of OIs and prompt treatment definitely contributes to increased life expectancy among infected patients, delaying the progression to AIDS. Despite the moderate (n = 125) number of patients included in our study, we believe the data obtained here provide some important background information that can form the basis of future, more elaborative and systematic studies. Furthermore, the data shown can be a valuable means of determining the range and relative frequency of infectious diseases, and this can potentially have an immediate impact on patient care by suggesting appropriate interventions based on the results.

The following table (2) represents the cases of dual infection in these HIV infected patients:

Co-infection with Oral Candiditis	Number of cases	Percentage of Cases
Enteropathogenic *Vibrio*	47	37.6
Tuberculosis	50	40.0
Escherichia coli infection	42	33.6
Cryptosporidial diarrhea	40	32.0

Table 2. Represents the cases of dual infection in these HIV infected patients

As a part of our investigation, we also studied co-infection of Oral Candidiasis with other OIs among the different HIV/AIDS population:

The figures below demonstrate:

The Venn Diagrams below demonstrate the co-infections:

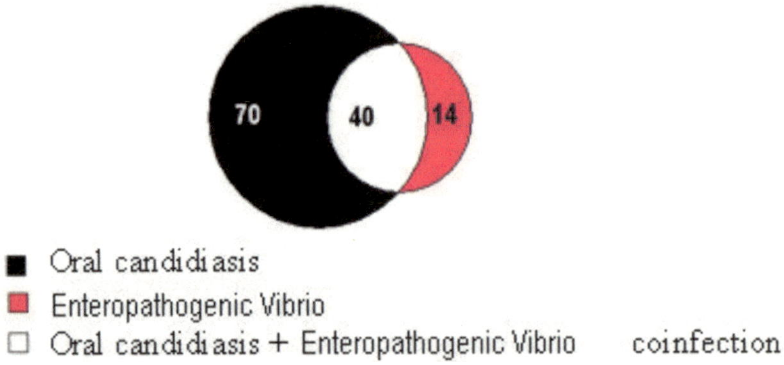

Fig. 1. Co-infection of Oral candidiasis with Enteropathogenic Vibrio

Oral candidiasis was found to be prevalent amongst 110 of the 125 HIV/AIDS infected patients. Enteropathogenic *Vibrio* was found to be prevalent amongst 54 of the AIDS/HIV infected patients. Amongst them, 40 developed co-infection of these two OIs. Thus, only 14 of the 54 patients infected with Enteropathogenic *Vibrio* did not develop any infection from Oral candidiasis.

From our study, it again becomes very prominent that HIV/AIDS patients suffering from Enteropathogenic *Vibrio* have high possibility of developing infection from Oral candidiasis.

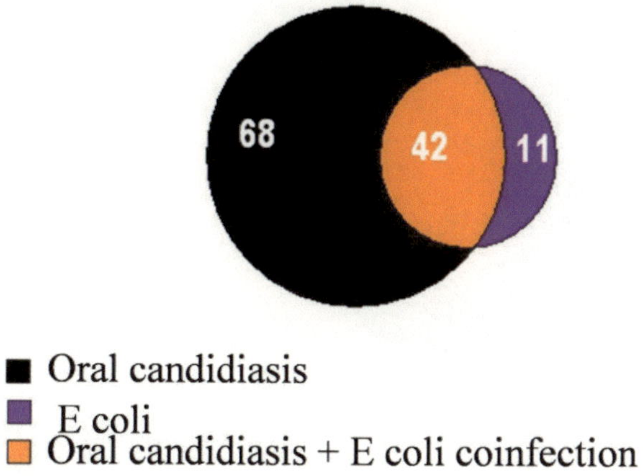

Fig. 2. Co-infection of Oral candidiasis with E coli

Oral candidiasis was found to be prevalent amongst 110 of the 125 HIV/AIDS infected patients as mentioned previously. E coli infection was found to be prevalent amongst 53 of the AIDS/HIV infected patients. Amongst them, 42 developed co-infection of these two OIs. Thus, only 11of the 53 patients infected with E coli did not develop any infection from Oral candidiasis.

From our study, it again becomes very prominent that HIV/AIDS patients suffering from E Coli develop high possibility of developing infection from Oral candidiasis.

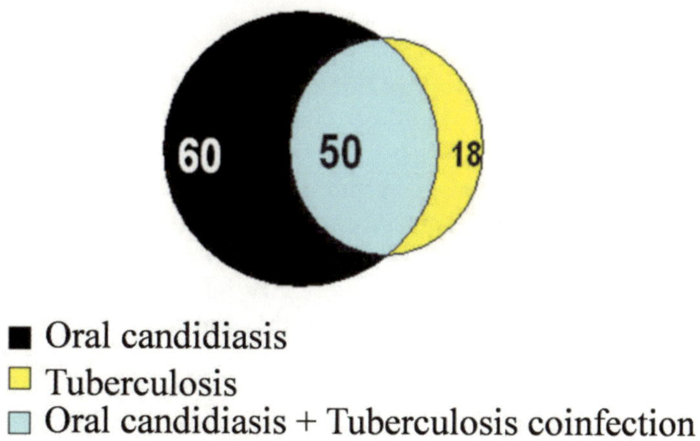

Fig. 3. Co-infection of Oral candidiasis with E coli

Oral candidiasis was found to be prevalent amongst 110 of the 125 HIV/AIDS infected patients as mentioned previously. TB infection was found to be prevalent amongst 68 of the AIDS/HIV infected patients. Amongst them, 50 developed co-infection of these two OIs. Thus, only 18of the 58 patients infected with TB did not develop any infection from Oral candidiasis.

From our study, it again becomes very prominent that HIV/AIDS patients suffering from TB develop high possibility of developing infection from Oral candidiasis.

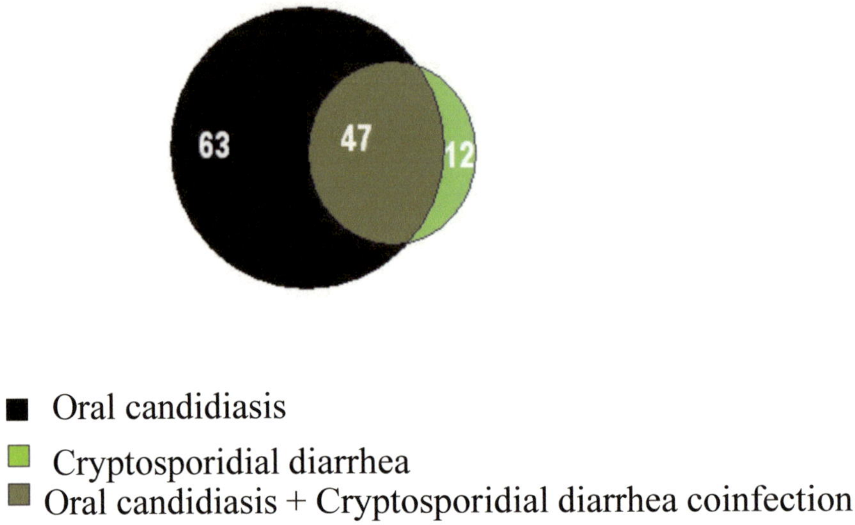

Fig. 4. Co-infection of Oral candidiasis with Cryptosporal diahorrhea

Oral candidiasis was found to be prevalent amongst 110 of the 125 HIV/AIDS infected patients as mentioned previously. Cryptosporal diahorrheal infection was found to be prevalent amongst 59 of the AIDS/HIV infected patients. Amongst them, 47 developed co-infection of these two OIs. Thus, only 12 of the 59 patients infected with TB did not develop any infection from Oral candidiasis.

From our study, it again becomes very prominent that HIV/AIDS patients suffering from Cryptosporal diahorrhea develop high possibility of developing infection from Oral candidiasis.

In another different study undertaken by our research group, (published as *Incidence of multiple herpesvirus infection in HIV seropositive patients, a big concern for Eastern Indian scenario* published in Virology Journal 2010, **7**:147) we were also eager to study the spread of the different *betaherpes* virus infection amongst these HIV infected patients. All herpes viruses share a characteristic ability to remain latent within the body over long periods. These herpes viruses play a very important role in further worsening the scenario in case of the HIV infected patients. For this purpose, in order to investigate the incidence of the different herpes viruses amongst the HIV/AIDS patients, we reviewed 200 HIV/AIDS patients, admitted between January 2006 to November 2008 at Calcutta Medical College Hospital, Kolkata, West Bengal, Apex Clinic, Calcutta Medical College Hospital- and ART Center, School of Tropical Medicine, for the detection of viral opportunistic infections. Their HIV status was confirmed as before by three ERS (Enzyme Linked Immunosorbent Assay [ELISA], Rapid, Simple) as before, an ELISA (HIV ELISA, Rapid test)and Western Blot as recommended by the National Aids Control Organization (NACO), Ministry of Health and Family Welfare, Government of India. The admitted patients were referred to us because they presented symptoms related to HIV infection or symptoms of unknown origin such as prolonged fever. The study group comprised of 140 (70%) males and 60 (30%) females, with

mean ages of 36 ± 16 and 35 ± 12 years respectively. The patients included in the study were from different states of Eastern India.
The viral OIs were primarily diagnosed by the common clinical manifestations as diagnosed by the clinicians.

2.1.3 Primary clinical symptoms for CMV infection (As confirmed by the clinicians)

For the diagnosis of active CMV infection, the primary clinical symptoms were retinitis (an infection of the eyes), pneumonia, blindness and gastrointestinal disease. The common clinical feature of CMV disease is retinitis. Retinitis is charecterised by painless, gradual loss of vision, floaters etc. Often, retinitis begins in one eye, but then progresses gradually to the other eye. If kept without treatment, progressive damage to the retina can lead to blindness in 4-6 months or less. Even with regular treatment, the disease can worsen to blindness. This may be because CMV may become resistant to the drugs so the drugs can no longer kill the virus, or because the patient's immune system has deteriorated further. Patients with CMV retinitis also have a chance of developing retinal detachment, in which the retina detaches from the nerves of the eye, causing blindness.
Other symptoms following active CMV infection include oesophagitis. Cytomegalovirus (CMV) esophagitis is a viral infection of the esophagus, which is the muscular tube through which food travels from the mouth to the stomach. It is charecterised by dysphagia - difficulty in swallowing or Odynophagia - painful swallowing,low grade fever, mouth sores.
Colitis is another clinical symptom due to active CMV infection. The clinical presentation ae as follows: pain abdomen, bloody diarrhea, fever, anorexia, malaise,dehydeation, weight loss, chronic watery diahorrea. HIV infected patients suffering from CMV colitis usually benefit from antiviral treatment.
CMV Pneumonitis is charecterised by cough, breathlessness. Pneumonitis is a common manifestation of CMV infection. It is highily associated with immunocompromised patients with fever and dyspnea.
Encephalitis caused by CMV is characterized by altered mental status, convulsion and headache.
Radiculoneuropathy is characterized by weakness/paralysis of lower limbs, pain lower back, urinary retention etc.

2.1.4 Primary clinical symptoms for HSV infection (As confirmed by the clinicians)

Among HIV-1 infected individuals, HSV-1 and HSV-2 infections are common, with prevalences that approximate or exceed those in the general population. Primary symptoms of HSV included persistent vesicular and ulcerative lesions of the oral and anogenital areas, often with extensive or deep ulcerations and blisters on or around the genitals or rectum. The blisters left tender ulcers (sores) that took two to four weeks to heal the first time they occurred. Other symptoms included tender tonsils covered with a whitish substance that made swallowing difficult or blisters present in the mouth.

2.1.5 Primary clinical symptoms for EBV infection

EBV+ and HIVincreases by many fold the risk of non-Hodgkins lymphoma (NHL) over general population, though overall risk remains small. In HIV, EBV most highly associated with Lymphoma, Primary CNS (PCNSL). Primary diagnosis of EBV was based on the clinical symptoms of fever, sore throat and swollen lymph glands. The commonestclinical presentation of EBV disease in HIV positives is Oral hairy Leukoplakia (OHL).

2.1.6 Primary clinical symptoms for HSV infection

Patients with HIV disease are at risk for developing severe illness from either varicella or zoster. Progressive primary varicella, a syndrome with persistent new lesion formation and visceral dissemination, may occur in HIV-infected patients and may be life-threatening. Zoster eruptions in HIV-infected patients can be extensive and locally destructive, and can become secondarily infected. Zoster may also disseminate cutaneously, and has been reported as the cause of encephalitis in patients with HIV disease (Quinnan et al. 1984;
Cone & Schiffman, 1984 ;Sandor *et al.* 1984 ;Ryder *et al.*1986; Friedman-Kien *et al.*1986; Cohen *et al.*1988; Colebunders *et al.*1988; Cohen, & Grossman, 1989 ; Gilson *et al.* 1989; Eidelberg *et al.*1986) was primarily diagnosed based on the clinical manifestations of severe headaches, backache, general malaise and fever accompanied by the typical exanthem (rash) of chickenpox. Other symptoms of VZV included painful oral lesions, vesicular rash, facial numbness and loss of hearing/ ear pain.

All the clinical manifestations were confirmed by ELISA test. The following diagnostic test kits were used for the assay of the opportunistic viruses:

Anti- CMV

Serum anti-CMV was determined by a commercially available test kit, CMV IgM, IgG ELISA Test kit was used to detect antibodies against the CMV.

Anti - EBV 1

Serum anti-EBV was determined by a commercially available test kit, EBV IgG, IgM ELISA Test kit was used to detect antibodies against the EBV 1.

Anti- HSV 2

Serum anti- HSVwas determined by a commercially available test kit, HSV type1 IgM ELISA Test kit supplied was used to detect antibodies against the affinity chromatographically purified recombinant antigen HSV-2.

Anti - VZV

Serum anti-VZV was determined by a commercially available test kit, VZV IgM, IgG, IgA Was used to detect antibodies against the Ellen Strain antigen (ATCC).

Of these herpes viruses studied, our study within the studied population suggests that, the occurrence of CMV is the highest. It accounts to 49% of the total population studied across the range of CD4+.

From the different tests performed, the results were as follows:

The following table (3) represents the cases of viral OIs in these HIV infected patients:

Study population= 200

We were also interested to study the trend of co-infection with CMV amongst these HIV patients.

Type of Viral infection	No. of positive cases	%
CMV	98	49
HSV	94	47
VZV	52	26
EBV	65	32.5

Table 3. Represents the cases of viral OIs in these HIV infected patients.

CMV was found to be associated predominantly with HSV followed by EBV and VZV.
Presence of CMV associated viral OIs in HIV infected population
The following table (4) represents the cases of dual infection with CMV in these HIV infected patients:
Study population= 200

Viral Co-infections	No. of positive cases	%
CMV+HSV	71	35.5
CMV+VZV	32	16
CMV+EBV	41	20.5

Table 4. Represents the cases of dual infection with CMV in these HIV infected patient

The Venn diagrams below to demonstrate the actual distribution of these viral infections amongst the immunocompromised patients under our study:

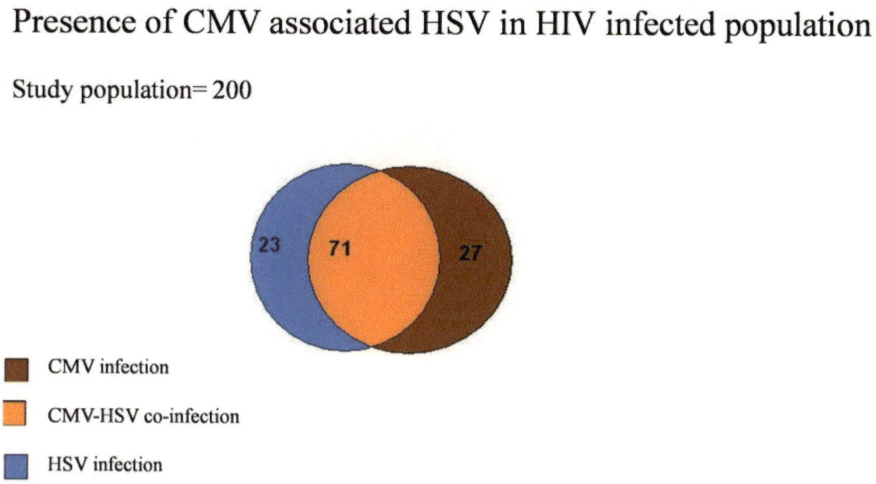

Fig. 5. Co-infection of CMV with HSV

CMV was found to be prevalent amongst 98 of the 200 HIV/AIDS infected patients as mentioned previously. HSV infection was found to be prevalent amongst 94 of the AIDS/HIV infected patients. Amongst them, 71 developed co-infection of these two OIs.

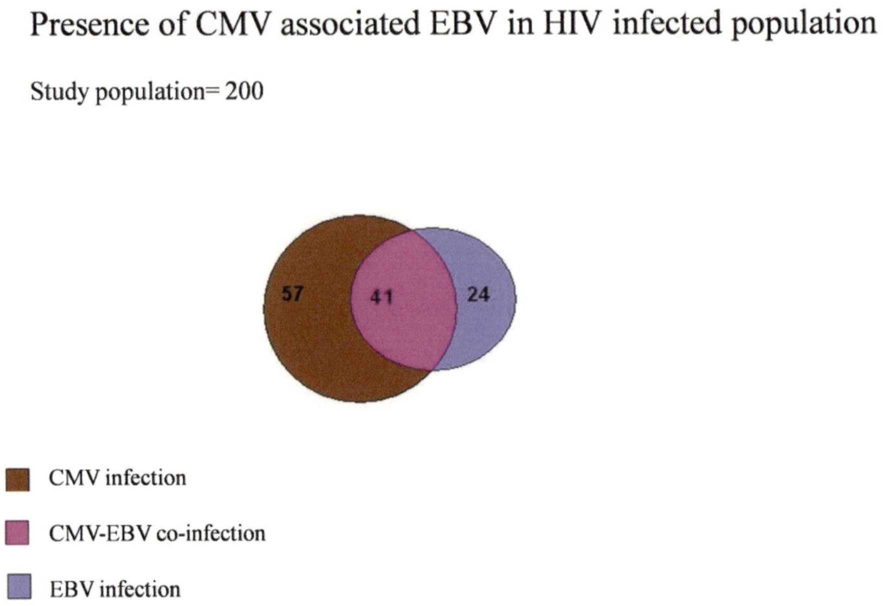

Fig. 6. Co-infection of CMV with EBV

CMV was found to be prevalent amongst 98 of the 200 HIV/AIDS infected patients as mentioned previously. HSV infection was found to be prevalent amongst 65 of the AIDS/HIV infected patients. Amongst them, 41 developed co-infection of these two OIs.

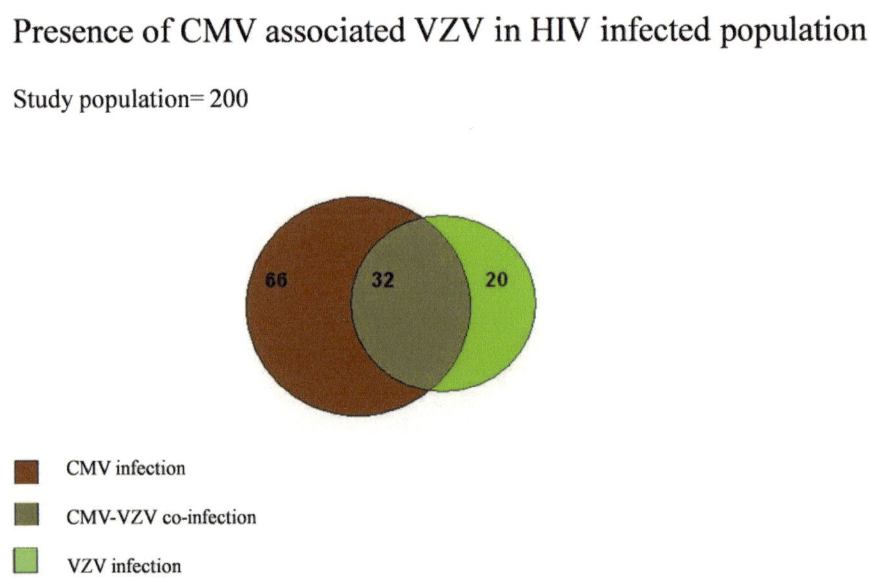

Fig. 7. Co-infection of CMV with EBV

CMV was found to be prevalent amongst 98 of the 200 HIV/AIDS infected patients as mentioned previously. VZV infection was found to be prevalent amongst 52 of the AIDS/HIV infected patients. Amongst them, 45 developed co-infection of these two OIs.

The incidence of CMV was higher among males than females 59/39. HSV was also found to be more predominant in the males 63/ 31. The incidence of VZV and EBV was also found to be dominant in the male population, the dominancy being 46/19 and 31/21 respectively.
HSV infection is found to be dominating in the heterosexual individuals among the study group. There are no significant variations among the homophiles, the drug users and the blood transfusion patients.The incidence of the different viral OIs was also assessed with respect to the CD4+ cell count/µl of blood and patients with mean CD4+ cell count of 51-100 showed the highest prevalence of opportunistic viral antibodies. This was followed by the group with CD4+ count of 101-150, 51-100, 151-200 and >200.
Age related prevalence of opportunistic viral antibodies in the serum of 200 HIV infected patient cohorts was assessed and results showed that individuals in the age group of 21- 40 years had the highest incidence of viral opportunistic infections as evident from the Table below.
The following table (5) represents the HIV-seropositive patient groups in various risk factors:

Risk Behavior	**Male**	**Female**
Blood transfusion	13	6
IVD abuse	25	3
Heterosexual	82	39
Homophiles	20	12
Occupation		
Unemployed	12	46
Government Service	13	-
Non Government Service	115	14
Deaths	3	2

Table 5. Represents the HIV-seropositive patient groups in various risk factors.

Viral opportunistic infections and HIV/AIDS having become so intertwined have constituted a major public health problem in the country. The opportunistic infections, Therefore, play a major role in clinical presentations and remain one of the most frequent causes of death in these patients. The Table below shows the association of the different OIs with the different modes of transmission of HIV amongst the different sexes amongst patients suffering from HIV/AIDS.
The following table (6) represents the different opportunistic viruses which infects HIV/AIDS patients of different age groups

	Risk Factors of HIV transmission							
	Heterosexual		Homophile		IDU		Blood transfusion	
Opportunistic Viruses	Male	Female	Male	Female	Male	Female	Male	Female
CMV	27	19	13	8	13	2	9	3
EBV	23	13	5	2	7	-	2	-
HSV	43	12	11	6	9	3	7	3
VZV	19	9	13	5	11	-	6	2

Table 6. Represents the different opportunistic viruses which infects HIV/AIDS patients of different age groups

From our study, as mentioned previously, CMV was obtained as the most prevalent amongst the different viral OIs amongst the patients suffering from HIV/AIDS. Infection by cytomegalovirus (CMV) is the major cause of morbidity and mortality in individuals with depressed cell mediated immunity of congenital origin, iatrogenic origin and that associated with acquired immunodeficiency syndrome (AIDS). The clinical diagnosis of AIDS with CMV infection can be difficult in the absence of CMV retinitis, polyradiculopathy and the classical CMV syndrome (Wiley & Nelson ,1988; Santosh *et al.*1998). The diagnosis poses difficulties because a 2-3 week period is mandatory for virus isolation. While IgM antibodies as detected by ELISA correlate poorly with the clinical status of CMV infection and facilities for culture are usually not available in most centers (Lanjewar *et al.* 1996). There are a few reports available of CMV infection in Indian patients with HIV/AIDS, which are based primarily on clinical or autopsy evaluation (Lanjewar *et al.* 1988; Becker *et al.* 1996; Nebuloni *et al.* 1998). We found CMV as the most incidental co infection in HIV/ AIDS patient with the overall incidence of 49%. Human immunodeficiency virus (HIV) infection is associated with an increased risk for human herpesviruses (HHVs) and their related diseases. The incidence of HSV in human immunodeficiency virus (HIV)-seropositive patients has not been focused, with reports generally focusing on individual infection (Mcclain *et al.* 1995). In this report, the serum prevalence of HSV is found to be higher in HIV seropositive patients; the overall incidence is around 47%. VZV infection, the overall incidence being 32.5% is the third most incidental coinfection in HIV seropositive patients. VZV is one of the common aetiological agents of viral retinitis. Neurological complications of the reactivation of VZV occur most frequently in elderly persons and immunocompromised patients (Sixbey *et al.* 1989). Gray *et al.*(1994) reported VZV infection of the CNS in more than 4% of patients with AIDS examined at autopsy. In AIDS patients, VZV tends to reactivate from multiple dorsal root ganglia levels, and the disease is often disseminated.

EBV is the least prevalent among the four HHVs studied in our work which is 26% of the total. EBV has been identified as a co-factor in the pathogenesis of a significant proportion of HIV related lymphoproliferative disorders and in oral hairy leukoplakia (Sculley *et al.* 1988). However, only limited information exists on the status of EBV in the course of HIV infection and the extent of its interaction with HIV. There is also growing interest in the biological properties and pathogenic potential of the different EBV subtypes, EBV-1 and EBV-2. Serological findings and studies in saliva and blood have indicated a high incidence of EBV-

2 infection in the course of HIV disease, but there is limited information regarding its significance (Sixbey *et al.* 1989; Sculley *et al.* 1988).

The analysis of the association of immunological status and the presence of viral OIs revealed that the CD4 count was significantly associated with the presence of viral OIs. An increasing CD4 count significantly protected patients from expressing HHVs in our patient cohorts as indicated by the correlation as in Figure 2. It has been detected clinically that more frequently virus infections are associated with the compromised immunity in HIVinfected patients (Kyaw et al.1992). We found that, HIV-infected patients with CD4+ cell counts of around 200 cells/mm3 are less likely to be infected with any virus examined here suggesting that a higherCD4+ cell count does play a role in immunity against virus infection. This clinical outcome is consistent with our finding of significantly lower CD4 cell count in HIV patients with viral OIs, indicating that the diagnosis of viral opportunistic

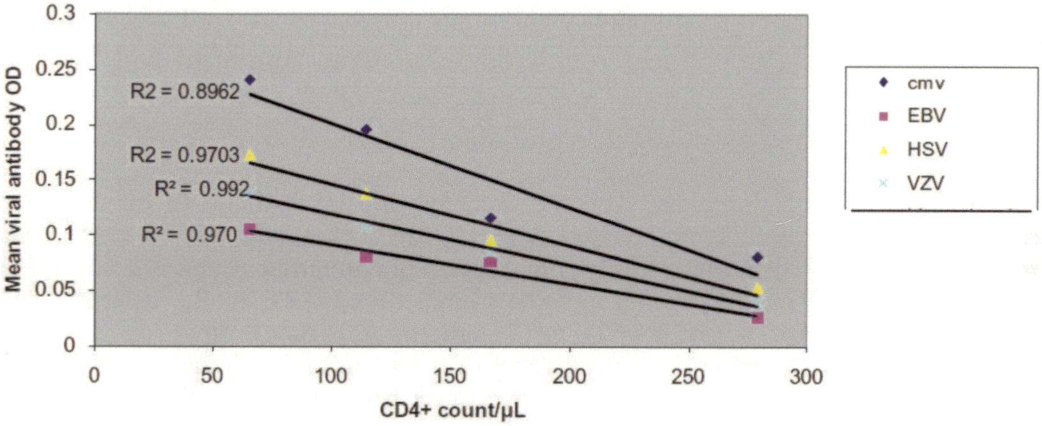

Fig. 8. CD4+ counts/µL of blood versus the antibody titres against the different opportunistic viruses in the patients. The CD4+ count ranges between 50/µL to 300/µL and the antibody titres showing the mean OD of the triplicate ELISA reading.

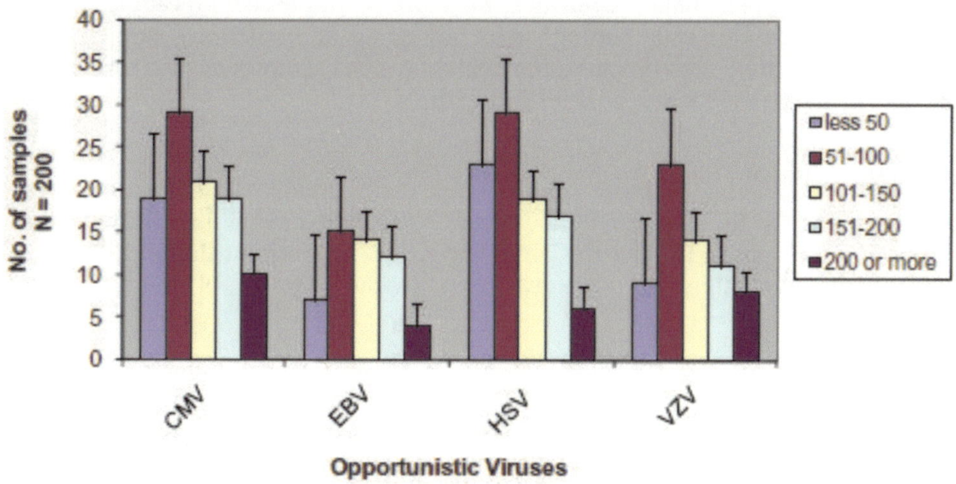

Fig. 9. Antibody prevalence of the corresponding viruses in different age groups of our patients samples.

infections can indeed be correlated with the clinical manifestation and thus is helpful in predicting disease progression. Figure 3 clearly shows that the patient group with CD4+ counts between 51 and 100 cells/µl is most susceptible to viral OI in HIV/AIDS patient.
The groups with CD4+ count less than 50 cells/µl are showing least opportunistic viruses which could be due to the advanced HAART treatment. This study is aimed at providing baseline data on viral opportunistic infections in HIV seropositive population as part of the preliminary investigation on the dynamics of viral opportunistic infections in immunocompromised population of India. One of the major problems is the lack of specific investigations that can provide rapid and reliable confirmation of a clinical diagnosis. A high level of alertness is needed at both clinical and laboratory level and routine surveillance studies need to be undertaken. Institutions in India and other developing countries need to be equipped to face the emerging challenge, in the form of updating the present knowledge, by way of education and training of the personnel, acquisition of skills of improved procedures, and their implementation in appropriate settings with adequate administrative support.

3. Conclusion

This study is aimed at providing baseline data for different pathogenic opportunistic infections in HIV seropositive population as part of the preliminary investigation on the dynamics of viral opportunistic infections in immunocompromised population of Eastern India. As many HIV/AIDS patients in India cannot afford ART, so the detection and awareness towards OIs related to HIV is of immense importance especially in Indian perspective or with respect to other developing countries also. These data may also be of immense importance especially to those countries of the tropical region as the spread of OIs might be comparable to that of our study. A high level of alertness is needed at both laboratory and clinical level and routine surveillance studies need to be undertaken. Institutions in India and other developing countries need to be equipped to face the emerging challenge, in the form of updating the present knowledge, by way of education and training of the personnel, acquisition of skills of improved procedures, and their implementation in appropriate settings with adequate administrative support. Further investigations have to be undertaken with matched control samples as case control analysis with respect to all OIs in HIV seropositive individuals.

4. Acknowledgment

The authors thank the technical staffs Mr. Probal Kanti Ray and Mr Tapan Chakrabarti for their laboratory help and Mr. Avirup Chakraborty, PhD student for doing desk work. The work was supported by fund received from Indian Council of Medical Research, Government of India.

5. References

A Talib, V.H., Khurana, S.K., Pandey, J., et al. (1993): Current concepts: tuberculosis and HIV infection. Indian J. Pathol. Microbiol., 36, 503-511.

Becker TM, Lee F, Daling JR, Nahmias AJ: Seroprevalence of and risk factors for antibodies to herpes simplex viruses, hepatitis B, and hepatitis C among southwestern

Hispanic and non-Hispanic white women. Sexually Transmitted Diseases 1996, 23(2):138.

Centers for Disease and Control (1982): Update on acquired immune deficiency syndrome (AIDS)-United States. Morb. Mortal. Wkly. Rep., 31, 507-514.

Centers for Disease Control (1992): 1993 revised classification system for HIV infection and expanded surveillance case definition for AIDS among adolescents and adults. Morbid. Mortal. Wkly. Rec., 41, RR-17.

Cohen PR, Beltrani VP, Grossman ME.Disseminated herpes zoster in patients with human immunodeficiency virus infection. Am J Med. 1988 Jun;84(6):1076-80

Cohen PR, Grossman ME. Clinical features of human immunodeficiency virus-associated disseminated herpes zoster virus infection--a review of the literature. Clin Exp Dermatol. 1989 Jul;14(4):273-6 [PubMed ID: 2686873]

Colebunders R, Mann JM, Francis H, Bila K, Izaley L, Ilwaya M, Kakonde N, Quinn TC, Curran JW, Piot P. Herpes zoster in African patients: a clinical predictor of human immunodeficiency virus infection. J Infect Dis. 1988 Feb;157(2):314-8

Cone LA, Schiffman MA. Herpes zoster and the acquired immunodeficiency syndrome. Ann Intern Med. 1984 Mar;100(3):462 [PubMed ID: 6696374]

da Silva, A. and Pieniazek, N. (2003): Latest advances and trends in PCR-based diagnostic methods. p. 397-412. In Dionisio, D. (ed.),Textbook-Atlas of Intestinal Infections in AIDS. Springer

Eidelberg D, Sotrel A, Vogel H, Walker P, Kleefield J, Crumpacker CS: Progressive polyradiculopathy in acquired immunedeficiency syndrome. Neurology 1986, 36:912-6.

Finkelstein, D.M., Williams, P.I., Molenbergs, G., et al. (1996): Patterns of opportunistic infections in patients with HIV-infection. J. Acquir. Immune Defic. Syndr. Hum. Retrovirol., 12, 38-45.

Friedman-Kien AE, Lafleur FL, Gendler E, Hennessey NP, Montagna R, Halbert S, Rubinstein P, Krasinski K, Zang E, Poiesz B. Herpes zoster: a possible early clinical sign for development of acquired immunodeficiency syndrome in high-risk individuals. J Am Acad Dermatol. 1986 Jun;14(6):1023-8

Gilson IH, Barnett JH, Conant MA, Laskin OL, Williams J, Jones PG. Disseminated ecthymatous herpes varicella-zoster virus infection in patients with acquired immunodeficiency syndrome. J Am Acad Dermatol. 1989 Apr;20(4):637-42

Gray F, Belec L, Lescs M, Chretien F, Ciardi A, Hassine D, Flament-Saillour M, Truchis P, Clair B, Scaravilli F: Varicella-zoster virus infection of the central nervous system in the acquired immune deficiency syndrome. Brain 1994, 117(5):987.

Kolmer, J.A., Spaulding, E.H. and Robinson, H.W. (1969): Approved Laboratory Technic, Appleton-Century-Crofts, Inc. p. 627-630.

Kyaw MT, Hurren L, Evans L, Moss DJ, Cooper DA, Benson E, Esmore D, Sculley TB: Expression of B-type Epstein-Barr virus in HIV-infected patients and cardiac transplant recipients. AIDS Research and Human Retroviruses 1992, 8:1869-1874.

Lanjewar D, Anand B, Genta R, Maheshwari M, Ansari M, Hira S, Dupont H: Major differences in the spectrum of gastrointestinal infections associated with AIDS in India versus the west: an autopsy study. Clinical Infectious Diseases 1996, 23(3):482-485.

Lanjewar DN, Shetty CR, Catdare G: Profile of AIDS pathology in India. An autopsy study. In Recent advance in pathology New Delhi: Jaypee Brothers Medical Publishers; 1988:183-9.

Luft, B.J. and Remington, J.S. (1992): Toxoplasmic encephalitis in AIDS. Clin. Infect. Dis., 15, 211-222.
Luft, B.J. and Remington, J.S. (1992): Toxoplasmic encephalitis in AIDS. Clin. Infect. Dis., 15, 211-222.
Mcclain KL, Leach CT, Jenson HB, Joshi VV, Pollock BH, Parmley RT, Dicarlo FJ, Chadwick EG, Murphy SB: Association of Epstein-Barr virus with leiomyosarcomas in young people with AIDS. The New England Journal of Medicine 1995, 332(1):12.

Moore, R.D. and Chassion, R.E. (1996): Natural history of opportunistic disease in an HIV-infected urban clinical cohort. Ann. Intern. Med., 124, 633-642.

National AIDS Control Organization, Ministry of Health and Family Welfare, Government of India (2000): Surveillance for HIV Infections/AIDS Case in India (1986 - 1999). New Delhi, India.

Nebuloni M, Vago L, Boldorini R, Bonetto S, Costanzi G: VZV fulminant necrotizing encephalitis with concomitant EBV-related lymphoma and CMV ventriculitis: report of an AIDS case. Journal of Neurovirology 1998,4(4):457-460.

Pitche, P., Mouzou, T., Padonou, C., et al. (2005): Stevens-Johnson syndrome and toxic epidermal necrolysis after intake of rifampicin isoniazid: report of 8 cases in HIV-infected patients in Togo. Med. Trop.(Mars), 65, 359-362.

Progressive encephalitis three months after resolution of cutaneous zoster in a patient with AIDS. Ann Neurol. 1986 Feb;19(2):182-8

Quinn TC: Global burden of the HIV pandemic. Lancet 1996, 348:99-105.

Quinnan GV, Masur H, Rook AH, Armstrong G, Frederick WR, Epstein J, Manischewitz JF, Macher AM, Jackson L, Ames J. Herpesvirus infections in the acquired immune deficiency syndrome. JAMA. 1984 Jul;252(1):72-7 [PubMed ID: 6328055]

Ran K, Hemalatha R: Oral lesions in HIV infection in developing countries: an overview. Advances in Dental Research 2006, 19:63.

Ryder JW, Croen K, Kleinschmidt-DeMasters BK, Ostrove JM, Straus SE, Cohn DL.

Sandor E, Croxson TS, Millman A, Mildvan D. Herpes zoster ophthalmicus in patients at risk for AIDS. N Engl J Med. 1984 Apr;310(17):1118-9 [PubMed ID: 6608691]

Santosh Vani T, Yasha C, Panda KM, Das S, Satishchandra P, Gourie-Devi M, Ravi V, Desai A, Khanna N, Chandramuki A, Swamy HS, Nagaraja D, Kolluri V, Sastry R, Shankar SK: Pathology of AIDS--Study from a Neuropsychiatric Centre from South India. Annual Indian Academical Neurology 1998, 1:71-82.

Sculley T, Cros S, Borrow P, Cooper D: Prevalence of antibodies to Epstein-Barr virus nuclear antigen 2B in persons infected with the human immunodeficiency virus. Journal of Infectious Disease 1988, 158:186-192.

Selik, R.M., Haverkis, H.W. and Curren, J.W. (1984): Acquired immune deficiency syndrome (AIDS) trends in the United States. 1978-1982. Am. J. Med., 76, 493-500.

Sixbey J, Shirley P, Chesney P, Buntin D, Resnick L: Detection of a second widespread strain of Epstein-Barr virus. Lancet 1989, ii:761-765.

Solomon S, Solomon S, Ganesh A: AIDS in India. British Medical Journal 2006, 82:545.

Stein, D.S., Korvick, J.A. and Vermund, S.H. (1992): CD4+ lymphocyte cell enumeration for prediction of clinical course of human immunodeficiency virus disease: a review. J. Infect. Dis., 165, 352-363.

Wiley CA, Nelson JA: Role of human immunodeficiency virus and cytomegalovirus in AIDS encephalitis. American Journal of Pathology 1988, 133:73-81.

Part 3

Social Impact and Awareness of HIV-Infection

9

Challenges Associated with the Effective Management of HIV Infection in a Low Income Setting in Sub Saharan Africa: Case Study of Nigeria

Osaro Erhabor et al.*
Blood Sciences Department Royal Bolton Hospital Bolton
UK

1. Introduction

Nigeria's size is 923,768 sq km, slightly more than twice the size of California in the US. The terrain is mixed with southern lowlands merging into central hills and plateaus. There are mountains in the southeast, and plains in north. The climate varies with equatorial weather in south, tropical in the centre, and arid in north. The lowest point in Nigeria is the Atlantic Ocean at 0 m. The highest point is Chappal Waddi at 2,419 m. Nigeria is home to one of Africa's most important rivers, the Niger, which enters the country in the northwest and flows southward through tropical rain forests and swamps to its delta in the Gulf of Guinea. Just over 135 million people live in Nigeria, making it the most populated country in Africa.

* Oseikhuemen Adebayo Ejele[1], Chijioke Adonye Nwauche[1], Chris Akani[2], Eyindah Cosmos[2] Dennis Allagoa[2], Edward Alikor A.D.[3], Ojule Aaron C.[4], Hamilton Opurum[4], Orikomaba Obunge[5], Seye Babatunde[6], Nnenna Frank-Peterside[7], Sonny Chinenye[8], Ihekwaba E. Anele[8], Teddy Charles Adias[9], Emmanuel Uko[10], Agbonlahor Dennis E.[11], Fiekumo Buseri I.[11], Zacheus Awortu Jeremiah[11], Wachuckwu Confidence[12], Obioma Azuonwu[12], Abbey S.D.[12], Onwuka Frank[13], Etebu Ebitimi N.[14], Seleye-Fubara D.[14] and Osadolor Humphrey [15]
[1]*Department of Haematology and Immunology, University of Port Harcourt, Nigeria*
[2]*Obstetrics and Gynaecology, University of Port Harcourt, Nigeria*
[3]*Department of Paediatrics, University of Port Harcourt, Nigeria*
[4]*Department of Chemical Pathology, University of Port Harcourt, Nigeria*
[5]*Department of Medical Microbiology and Parasitology, University of Port Harcourt, Nigeria*
[6]*Department of Community Health Medicine, University of Port Harcourt, Nigeria*
[7]*Department of Microbiology, University of Port Harcourt, Nigeria*
[8]*Department of Internal Medicine, University of Port Harcourt, Nigeria*
[9]*College of Health Technology Bayelsa State, Nigeria*
[10]*Department of Haematology University of Calabar, Nigeria*
[11]*Department of Medical Laboratory Science Niger Delta University, Amassoma Bayelsa State, Nigeria*
[12]*Department of Medical Laboratory Science Rivers State University of Science and Technology Port Harcourt Nigeria, Nigeria*
[13]*Department of Biochemistry University of Port Harcourt, Nigeria*
[14]*Department of Anatomical Pathology, University of Port Harcourt Teaching Hospital, PMB 6173, Port Harcourt, Nigeria*
[15]*Department of Biochemistry, University of Benin, Nigeria*

Nigeria is made up of 36 states. Figure 1 show the map of Nigeria. Life expectancy is around 47 years. Birth rate is on average 5.45 per woman. Literacy rate is just over 68%. English is the official language. Hausa, Yoruba, Igbo (Ibo) and Fulani are commonly spoken by the major ethnic groups. Nigeria is composed of more than 250 ethnic groups. The most populous and politically influential ethnic groups includes: Hausa and Fulani 29%, Yoruba 21%, Igbo (Ibo) 18%, Ijaw 10%, Kanuri 4%, Ibibio 3.5%, and Tiv 2.5%. Nigeria is a multi-religious nation. Muslims constitute 50% of the population while Christians constitute 40% while 10% practice their indigenous beliefs. British influence and control over what became Nigeria grew through the 19th century. A series of constitutions after World War II granted Nigeria greater autonomy and eventually independence came on October 1st, 1960. Following nearly 16 years of military rule, a new constitution was adopted in 1999, and a peaceful transition to civilian government was completed. The government faces the daunting task of reforming a petroleum-based economy, whose revenues have been squandered through corruption and mismanagement. In addition, the defusing longstanding ethnic and religious tensions are a priority if Nigeria is to build a sound foundation for economic growth and political stability. Oil-rich Nigeria, long hobbled by political instability, corruption, inadequate infrastructure, high rate of unemployment and poor macroeconomic management and suboptimal health infrastructure is undertaking some reforms under a new reform-minded administration. Nigeria's former military rulers failed to diversify the economy away from its overdependence on the capital-intensive oil sector, which provides 20% of GDP and 95% of foreign exchange earnings, and about 65% of budgetary revenues. The largely subsistence agricultural sector has failed to keep up with rapid population growth. Nigeria is Africa's most populous country - and the country, once a large net exporter of food, now must import food.

Despite being the largest oil producer in Africa and the 12th largest in the world (Energy Information Administration, 2007), Nigeria is ranked 158 out of 177 on the United Nations Development Programme (UNDP) Human Poverty Index (UNDP, 2007). This poor development position has meant that Nigeria is faced with huge challenges in fighting its HIV and AIDS epidemic. In Nigeria, an estimated 3.6 percent of the populations are living with HIV and AIDS (UNGASS, 2010). Although HIV prevalence is much lower in Nigeria than in other African countries such as South Africa and Zambia, the size of Nigeria's population (around 149 million) means that by the end of 2009, there were 3.3 million people living with HIV (UNAIDS,2010). Approximately 220,000 people died from AIDS in Nigeria in 2009 (UNAIDS, 2010). With AIDS claiming so many lives, Nigeria's life expectancy has declined significantly. In 1991 the average life expectancy was 54 years for women and 53 years for men (WHO, 2008).In 2009 these figures had fallen to 48 for women and 46 for men (CIA World Fact book, 2010). The major sources of HIV infection in Nigeria include heterosexual transmission, through unsafe blood transfusion and from mother to child transmission. Approximately 80-95 percent of HIV infections in Nigeria are a result of heterosexual sex (UNGASS, 2010). Factors contributing to this include a lack of information about sexual health and HIV, sexual promiscuity, low levels of condom use, and high levels of sexually transmitted diseases. Women are particularly more vulnerable to HIV. In 2009 women accounted for 56 percent of all adults aged 15 and above living with the virus (UNGASS, 2010). HIV transmission through unsafe blood and blood products accounts for the second largest source of HIV infection in Nigeria (Federal Ministry of Health, 2009). Not all Nigerian hospitals have the technology to effectively screen blood and therefore there is a risk of using contaminated blood. Women and children are particularly at risk as a result of malaria and pregnancy-related anaemia. The Nigerian Federal Ministry of Health have responded by backing legislation that requires hospitals to only use blood from the National Blood Transfusion Service, which has far more advanced blood-screening technology (Nigeria Exchange, 2008). Each year around 57,000 babies are born with HIV (UNGASS, 2010). It is estimated that 360,000 children are living with HIV in Nigeria, most of who became infected from their mothers (UNGASS, 2010). This has increased from 220,000 in 2007 (UNAIDS, 2008). In Nigeria there is a distinct lack of HIV testing programmes. In 2007, just 3 percent of health facilities had HIV testing and counseling services (WHO, UNAIDS & UNICEF, 2008) and only 11.7 percent of women and men aged 15-49 had received an HIV test and found out the results (UNGASS, 2010). In 2009 there was only one HIV testing and counseling facility for approximately every 53,000 Nigerian adults .This is an indication of how desperately the Nigerian government needs to scale up HIV testing services.

Sex is traditionally a very private subject in Nigeria and the discussion of sex with teenagers is often seen as inappropriate. Attempts at providing sex education for young people have been hampered by religious and cultural objections (Odutolu, 2005). In 2009 only 23 percent of schools were providing life skills-based HIV education, and just 25 percent of men and women between the ages of 15 and 24 correctly identified ways to prevent sexual transmission of HIV and rejected major misconceptions about HIV transmission (UNGASS, 2010). In some regions of Nigeria girls marry relatively young, often to much older men. In North Western Nigeria around half of girls are married by age 15 and four out of five girls are married by the time they are 18 (Erulkar and Bello, 2007). Studies have found that those who are married at a younger age have less knowledge about HIV and AIDS, and are more likely to believe they are low-risk for becoming infected with HIV (Erulkar and Bello, 2007). HIV and AIDS education initiatives need to focus on young married women, especially as these women are less likely to have access to health information (Odutolu, 2005). In sub-Saharan Africa (Brenan et al., 2008) and in other parts of the world, (Barnes et al., 1991) it is estimated that there are 12 to 13 infected women for every infected man. Biological, cultural and socio-economic factors contribute to women's greater vulnerability to HIV/AIDS. Women are four times more at risk of becoming infected with HIV during unprotected vaginal intercourse than men. The vagina's large surface area of susceptible tissue and micro trauma during intercourse makes women more physiologically vulnerable (Nyobi et al., 2008). The synergy between HIV and other sexually transmitted infections (STIs) is another biological factor that makes women more vulnerable. Socio economic factors including women's lack of access to education or personal income perpetuate women's lower status. Moreover widespread poverty drives some women into commercial sex work. Cultural traditions such as forced marriage, female genital mutilation and older men's preference for younger women all risk factors prevalent in Nigeria contribute to increased female vulnerability to HIV (Pieniazek et al., 1991).

HIV pandemic is one of the most serious health crisis faced by the world today. Sub-Saharan Africa remains by far the worst affected region. In 2007, it contained an estimated 68% of people living with HIV and 76% of all Acquired Immunodeficiency Syndrome (AIDS) deaths (De Cock and Weiss, 2000). An estimated 33.4 million people were living with HIV/AIDS as at 2009 (UNAIDS, 2008). The HIV/AIDS epidemic has already devastated Nigeria, with nearly a million people dead and more than two million children orphaned. By 2003, the virus had infected approximately 5% of the adult population of about 100 million people (UNAIDS/WHO, 2005). In 2002, the National Intelligence Council identified the five countries expected to bear the heaviest burden of HIV infection in the expanding worldwide epidemic: India, China, Nigeria, Ethiopia, and Russia (Eberstadt, 2002). The

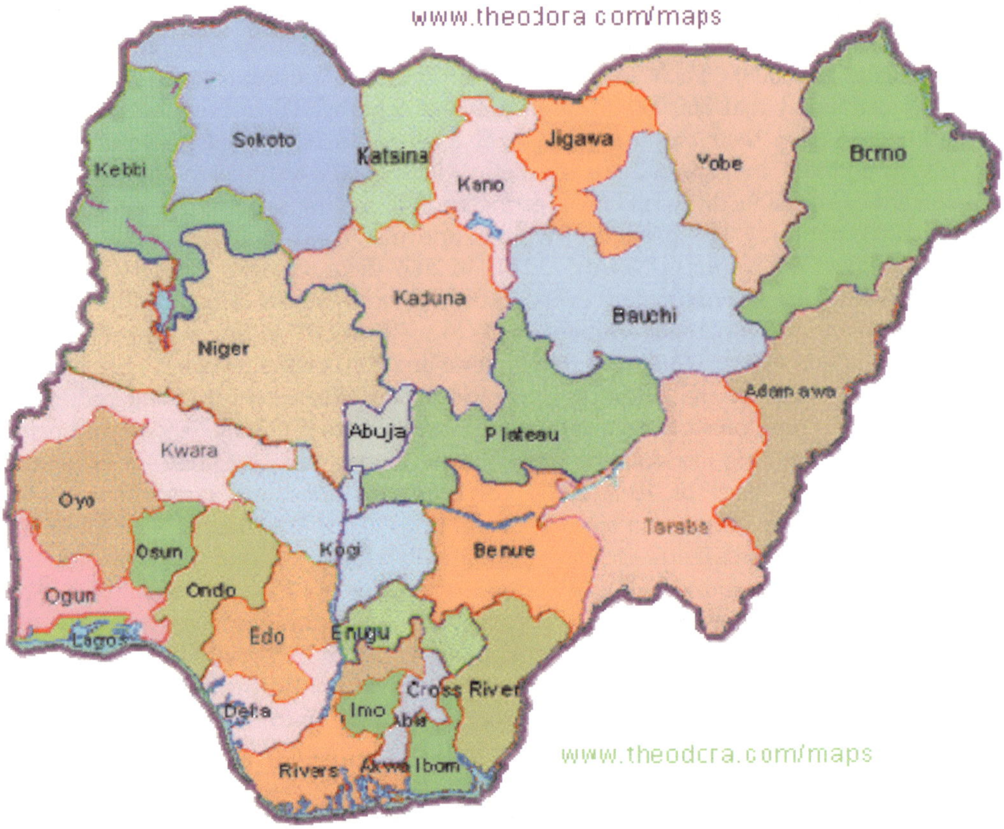

Fig. 1. Map of Nigeria showing the 36 states

council predicted that Nigeria and Ethiopia would be especially hard hit, with the number of people living with HIV/AIDS in Nigeria projected to balloon to ten to fifteen million by 2010, or as much as 26 percent of the adult population. Without effective prevention on a large scale, Nigeria will experience not only the tragedy of countless lives forever altered by the virus, but also untold adverse social and economic effects. In Nigeria the prevalence of HIV has increased from 1.8% in 1991 to 3.8% in 1993, 4.5% in 1999, 5.8%, 5.0% in 2003, 4.4% in 2005 to 4.6% in 2008 (Federal Ministry of Health Nigeria, 2009). Nigeria's population has grown rapidly in recent decades. In 1991 the total population was 88.9 million, and projections by the National Population Commission of Nigeria estimated that by 2003 the population would rise to 133 million (National Population Commission of Nigeria, 1991).The prevalence of HIV in Nigeria may not be as high as it is in most countries in Southern part of Africa. The prevalence is however significant considering the population of the country. There has been great concern in the international community as to whether Nigeria with her sub-optimal health infrastructure will be able to manage this pandemic.

Poverty is a major challenge associated with the increasing prevalence of HIV in Nigeria. With her annual income per capita below the average for other low-income countries, Nigeria is considered a "poor" nation. The country's health status indicators also are worse than average; Nigeria spends less than average on health. The United Nations Development

Programme has ranked Nigeria 152 out of 175 on the Human Development Index, a composite measure of income coupled with access to education and health services (United Nations Development Programme, 2004). By some estimates, two-thirds of Nigerians live on less than US$1 per day. Youth unemployment is a major problem, with estimates ranging between 40% and 60% (World Bank, 2004).Poverty—combined with economic vulnerability, institutional weaknesses, and socio-cultural complexity—exacerbates the difficulties inherent in tackling the Nigerian HIV epidemic and is responsible for the high HIV prevalence observed in selected groups; blood donors (commercial remunerated), unemployed, long distance truck drivers, abandoned babies, tuberculosis patient and unbooked antenatal women. The complexity of the HIV/AIDS epidemic stems from its links with all aspects of society and culture. Social and cultural factors affect not only viral transmission, but also the success of prevention strategies and the compassion with which people living with the virus are treated. A clear understanding of these factors therefore becomes a point of significance for planning the control of the epidemic. Heterosexual transmission accounts for as many as 95% of HIV infections in Nigeria, where having multiple sexual partners has been a major behavioural factor fuelling the epidemic. Non-sexual traditional practices—particularly male and female circumcision and the custom of creating facial and body markings with shared, non-sterile skin-piercing implements—expose significant numbers of people to infection as well. The aim of this chapter is to present the challenges associated with the management of HIV/AIDS pandemic in Nigeria.

2. HIV prevalence among Most At Risk Populations (MARPs)

2.1 HIV among blood donors and challenges of providing safe blood and blood products

Blood transfusions particularly in sub Saharan Africa currently face interesting challenges of accessing safe and adequate quantities of blood and blood products. The risk of transfusion -transmissible infections including HIV amongst others have provoked a greatly heightened emphasis on safety with inescapable implications on complexity and cost of providing a transfusion service (Tagny et al., 2008). Blood transfusion continues to be an important route of transmission of HIV particularly in developing countries among young children and pregnant women following transfusion for malaria associated anaemia and pregnancy-related complications (Foster and Buvé, 1995). A study undertaken to determine the seroprevalence of human immunodeficiency virus infection among 1,500 blood donors living in the Niger Delta area of Nigeria has shown a prevalence of 1.0%. The highest prevalence occurred among commercial remunerated donors (Ejele et al., 2005). Similarly a study of 33,682 and 1259 blood donors screened in two tertiary hospitals in Nigeria has indicated overall HIV seroprevalence rate of 7.66% (Fasola et al.,2008) and 0.71% (Salawu and Murainah, 2006) respectively. Studies to investigate the risk of transfusion transmissible HIV infection among Malian blood donors have indicated a prevalence of 2.6% (Diarra et al., 2009) and 4.5% (Tounkara et al., 2009). Undetectable HIV infections in blood banks pose a serious threat to public health (Zohoun et al, 2004). In Kenya, blood donations from high school students are preferred over adult samples due to lower HIV infection prevalence within this population. However a study carried out using stimmunology, an in vitro lymphocyte stimulation technique has unveiled a significant number of early, pre-seroconversion HIV carriers both among adult and teenage Kenyan populations (Mumo et al., 2009, Minga et al., 2010). A mathematical model constructed to quantify transfusion risks across 45 sub-Saharan African countries using three components: the risk of a contaminated unit entering the blood supply, the risk that the unit will be given to a susceptible patient and the risk that receipt of the unit will lead to infection in the recipient. Variables included prevalence of infection in donors, extent of blood testing, test sensitivity, and susceptibility of recipients. Data from the World Health Organization (WHO) African Region and a systematic review of the literature were used to parameterize the model. Data suggest that the median overall risks of becoming infected with HIV from a blood transfusion in SSA were 1 infection per 1000 units (Jayaraman et al., 2010). A study to determine the prevalence of HIV among adolescent donors in Zimbabwe during the period between 2002 and 2003 has revealed that the prevalence of HIV in 2002 and 2003 were 0.48% and 0.38%, respectively. Prevalence was higher among first time and female donors (Mandisodza et al., *2006).* A study to estimate the prevalence of transfusion-transmissible HIV infection in two groups of blood donors at Douala city over the period of 1995 -2004 has indicated that the prevalence of HIV ranged from 2.2% to 8.12% at the Douala University and 7.89% at the blood bank of Laquintinie Hospital (Mogtomo et al.,2009). Remunerated and family replacement donors are at more risk of being HIV positive (Batina et al., 2007). Areas with high HIV-incidence rates compared to the developed world may benefit from additional testing in blood banks and may show more favourable cost-effectiveness ratios.

2.2 HIV infection and unemployment

Youth unemployment is a major problem in Nigeria, with estimates ranging between 40% and 60% (World Bank, 2004). Poverty—combined with economic vulnerability, institutional weaknesses, and socio-cultural complexity—exacerbates the difficulties inherent in tackling the Nigerian HIV epidemic. Human immunodeficiency virus (HIV) infection is highly endemic in Nigeria, particularly with the prevalence in 2001 at 5.8%. A previous study (Ejele at al., 2005) to determine the prevalence of HIV among 868 unemployed individuals in Port Harcourt comprising of 373 males and 495 females indicated a sero-prevalence rate of (3.19%). HIV seroprevalence was relatively higher among females (3.6%) compared to males (2.4%). The highest prevalence was found in the <19 years age group (5.1%) and lowest in the 40-49 years age group (2.3%), although the difference was not statistically significant ($X^2 = 4.86$, $p = 0.09$). The highest prevalence occurred among separated subjects (7.7%) compared to singles (3.9%) and married subjects (1.8%).This study indicates a 3.1% prevalence of HIV infection among unemployed individuals studied and calls for urgent and concerted efforts aimed at promoting behavioural, cultural and social changes that will reverse the current trend in the prevalence of HIV among the unemployed.

2.3 HIV among abandoned babies in Nigeria

Paediatric HIV infection is fast assuming a serious dimension in developing countries. In addition, the early death of mothers creates a large number of orphans and vulnerable children, many of whom succumb to AIDS or complications of other infections and malnutrition. This trend is eroding gains of child survival efforts of previous decades. Disease progression in children who acquire HIV infection from their mothers is more rapid in Africa than in developed countries, probably because African children are exposed to early and multiple infections. Abandonment of newborn babies dates back to the bible days with the story of Moses. In Nigeria, it is a common observation to find babies abandoned in the hospital after birth, in gutters and hidden places possibly because the mother tested positive for HIV. The act of child abandonment is greatly influenced by socio-economic constraints. In this era of the HIV Pandemic, many of the abandoned babies are feared to be babies of HIV sero positive mothers who for fear of stigmatisation, discrimination and the burden of caring for an HIV positive child, abandon their babies. HIV infection is endemic in Nigeria and is an important cause of infant mortality and morbidity. A previous study (Akani et al.,2006) was undertaken to determine the sero-epidemiology of HIV among One hundred and forty (n = 140) consecutively recruited abandoned babies with mean age of 11.5 ± 24.1 weeks made up to 79 males and 61 females. The babies were referred to the HIV screening unit from motherless baby's homes in Port Harcourt for pre-adoption HIV screening within a five years period (1999 - 2003). Babies were screened for HIV using the WHO approved immunocomb HIV I & II kits (Organics, Israel) - an enzyme linked immunosorbent assay for the quantitative and differential diagnosis of HIV in serum or plasma. Initially reactive samples were continued using Genscreen HIV 1 & 2 (p24) antigen test (Bro Rad, France). HIV was detected in 19(13.6%) of babies tested. Sero-prevalence was highest in babies 9 - 16 weeks (25.0%). Males accounted for the highest infection burden (57.9%) compared to (42.1%) for females. Data indicated that the prevalence of HIV declined from 12.5% in 1999 to 8.3% in 2000 and increased subsequently to 20% in 2001 but declined steadily to 16.1% in 2002 and 14.3% in 2003. HIV-1 accounted for the predominant viral subtype among babies sero-positive for HIV (89.5%). Chi square analysis indicates that symptom at abandonment was an independent risk factor for HIV infection among abandoned babies ($\chi^2 = 40.97$; $p = 0.0001$). This hospital-based study has confirmed a high prevalence of HIV among abandoned babies tested and highlights the importance of HIV screening for abandoned babies before transfer to foster parents and brings to bare the challenge associated with child adoption in Nigeria. Government, non-governmental organizations and Faith Based Organizations (FBO's) should embark on care and support programmes by providing young people with knowledge, information and youth-friendly health services in a bid to address the issue of child abandonment and HIV infection. The findings emphasize the need for capacity building of personnel working in motherless babies home to enable them cope with the challenges of the increasing incidence of child abandonment and HIV. There is the need to strengthen the family planning services for sero positive mothers who do not wish to have more babies. The issue of therapeutic termination of pregnancy in HIV-infected mothers in cases of unwanted pregnancies may need to be reconsidered.

2.4 HIV infection and the Nigerian military

Epidemiologic evidence indicates that throughout the world men and women in the military are among the most susceptible subpopulations to sexually transmitted infections (STIs), including HIV. In peacetime, STI rates in the military are two to five times higher than in comparable civilian populations; during wartime the rates tend to rise (UNAIDS, 1998). Conflict situations involving troops, vulnerable populations, and humanitarian workers further promote the transmission of HIV. In many African countries, the uniformed services report HIV prevalence rates higher than the national averages. In Uganda (27% versus 8.3%) (U.S. Bureau of the Census, Population Division, 1998) in South Africa (60% to 70%, compared with 20%) (Sarin, 2003), Cameroon (6.2% compared to 2%) (Adebajo et al., 2002), Sierra Leone (11% versus 5%) (Lovgren, 2001). Similarly in Malawi, 25% to 50% of army officials are already HIV positive (UNAIDS, 2005). Interestingly HIV/ AIDS is becoming the leading cause of death in the military and police forces in many settings in sub Saharan

Africa, accounting for as much as half of in-service mortality (Noah and Fidas, 2000). These findings have serious consequence on the territorial security. HIV/AIDS has the potential to wipe out the capability and experience of military forces when prevalence rates are high and prevention and mitigation efforts are ineffective or insufficient. In sub-Saharan Africa, the number of states at war or involved in significant lethal conflicts increased from 11 in 1989 to 22 in 2000 (Bakhireva et al., 2004, Nwokoji et al., 2004). In a survey conducted in Sierra Leone recently, Physicians for Human Rights estimated that 215,000 to 257,000 internally displaced women and girls experienced rape or other forms of sexual violence in war, as well as non-combat situations. This demonstrates the potential for women to be exposed to HIV during conflicts (Lovgren, 2001). Although Nigeria has not experienced a national war in the past 37 years, limited internal, inter-ethnic, and religious skirmishes have occurred in several regions. Moreover, women and children have become victims of forced sex and other human rights abuses. Several studies have shown that HIV prevalence among soldiers in Africa is elevated, with prevalence rates as high as 60% in the militaries of Angola and the Democratic Republic of Congo (Fleming,1988).Many African military forces have infection rates as high as five times those of civilian populations (Nwokoji et al., 2004, Bakhireva et al., 2004). It is important to remember that HIV transmission does not end when conflict ceases; when infected soldiers return to their communities, they continue to spread the virus. In Nigeria, this trend was confirmed by the increased HIV seroprevalence among soldiers returning home from a peacekeeping mission (Lovgren S, 2001). Peacekeeping operations by Nigerian soldiers in Liberia, Sierra Leone, Côte d'Ivoire, the former Yugoslavia, and Somalia at various times have produced other distinct strands of net transfer of infection from these countries to Nigeria. The lifestyle of peacekeeping officers is characterized by high levels of multiple sexual partners, low condom use, and exposure to blood transfusions in the line of duty. After an initial period of secrecy surrounding the extent of the HIV/AIDS problem in the military and among returning peacekeeping forces, the Nigerian military is addressing the spread of HIV among soldiers (Raufu, 2001).The coming out of soldiers living with HIV/AIDS has raised awareness of the impact of peacekeeping expeditions on the spread of HIV. It has also helped shape the public policy on HIV in Nigeria. The privileged position of the military means that policies made for it set standards to which the public HIV/AIDS policy can aspire, such as the introduction of a free antiretroviral program for infected soldiers (Raufu, 2002). Nigerian police officers also have been involved in peacekeeping operations, mostly within Nigeria but occasionally abroad. Their sexual lifestyles are no less risky than those of soldiers (Akinnawo et al., 1995). They maintain modest levels of condom use and high rates of STIs, take advantage of modern medical treatment, and report good rates of partner notification when infected but low rates of notifying their spouses about infection episodes. A previous study by Azuonwu et al (Azuonwu et al., 2011) investigated the prevalence of HIV among a total of One hundred and fifty military personnel aged between 20 and 55 years in the Niger Delta of Nigeria and observed an overall HIV prevalence rate of 14.67%. The HIV prevalence among the male was higher than that of the female group (84% versus 16%). There was a negative correlation between the CD4 count and HIV infection ($r = -0.443$, $p < 0.01$). The military community is considered a high-risk environment for HIV transmission. There are several compelling risk factors that increase the susceptibility of military personnel to HIV infection; danger and risk taking are integral parts of the military profession, military personnel tend to be young, single, and sexually active, they are highly mobile and stay away from their families and home communities for extended periods, they are often influenced by peer pressure rather than social convention, they are inclined to feel invincible and involve in high risk sexual behaviour and they have more ready cash than other males where they are deployed and hence are surrounded by opportunities for casual and commercial sex.

2.5 HIV infection among long distance truck drivers

Truck drivers play an important role in HIV/AIDS transmission in many countries (Pandey et al., 2008, Sunmola, 2005). Previous report in Bangladesh and India found HIV prevalence of 15.9% and 17.8% respectively among long distance drivers (Gibney et al., 2003, Manjunath et al., 2002). Condom use among long distance drivers is low and /or inconsistent (Sugihantono et al., 2003). Long distance truck drivers are vulnerable to sexually transmitted diseases for several reasons; truckers are always on the move, have little or no access to sexual health services, migratory nature of their occupation often disconnect them from family and community, truck drivers rarely interact with orthodox medical practitioners and instead seek the help of quacks and home remedies to cure Sexually Transmitted infections (STIs) and many lack information about STIs and HIV/AIDS and their prevention. Previous report (Azuonwu et al., 2010) on a total of one hundred long-distance truck drivers in the Niger Delta of Nigerian aged between 21 and 60 years and mean age of 42.36 ±5.23 years that were screened for the presence of HIV antibodies indicated a prevalence of 10%. The prevalence of HIV was significantly higher in the 31-40 years. HIV 1 was the predominant viral subtype among the subjects (90%) while (10%) had HIV-2. None of the HIV-positive subjects had dual HIV 1 and 2 infections. The mean CD4 lymphocyte count for subjects positive for HIV was 380 ± 68.0 (range 312 – 448 cells/μl) while CD4 count for HIV negative subjects was 780 ± 76 cells/ μl (range 704 - 856 cells/μl. A significant negative correlation was observed between HIV positivity and CD4 count r-0.010 (p = 0.01). Authors recommended that intensive preventive measures be instituted coupled with the implementation of a vigorous enlightenment campaign targeting behavioural change from high risk culture among truckers. Efforts are urgently needed to provide access to sexual health education, treatment services and HIV testing facilities to reduce their vulnerability to HIV infection.

2.6 HIV infection among tuberculosis – infected Nigerians

Nigeria, with estimated 259,000 cases of tuberculosis, has the sixth largest population of people with tuberculosis (TB) in the world. The arrival of HIV/AIDS has caused a secondary tuberculosis epidemic in many African countries. Before the HIV epidemic, the incidence rate of new cases of tuberculosis had been estimated at 2 per 1,000. Tuberculosis (TB) and human immunodeficiency virus (HIV) have been closely linked since the emergence of acquired immunodeficiency syndrome (AIDS). HIV infection has contributed to a significant increase in the worldwide incidence of TB (Low and Eng, 2009). By producing a progressive decline in cell-mediated immunity, HIV alters the pathogenesis of TB, greatly increasing the risk of developing the disease in co-infected individuals, leading to more frequent extrapulmonary involvement and atypical radiographic manifestations. Although HIV-related TB is treatable and preventable, incidence rates continue to climb in developing nations where HIV infection and TB are endemic and resources are limited. Worldwide, TB is the most common opportunistic infection affecting HIV sero-positive individuals and it is the most common cause of death in patients with AIDS (API consensus expert committee, 2006). The prevalence of HIV infection among TB patients in several African countries ranges from 20% to 60%.1 The World Health Organization (WHO) estimates that about 8 million new cases of TB and nearly 2 million deaths from the disease occur each year and approximately 10 million people are estimated to be co-infected with TB and HIV, and over 90% of these dually infected individuals reside in developing nations. In some areas of sub-Saharan Africa, the rates of co-infection exceed 1,000 per 100,000 populations (Yusuph, 2005). Worldwide, a similar change has occurred in some developed countries. The HIV epidemic has increased the global TB burden and focused attention on the need to strengthen links between TB and HIV/AIDS program. In response to these health emergencies, the WHO has developed an expanded strategy aimed at reducing the burden of HIV-related TB infection through close collaboration between TB and HIV/AIDS programmes. Infection with HIV is the most well known risk factor for the development of TB. Because of the prevalence of TB amongst HIV-infected patients the joint statement by the American Thoracic Society, Centres for Disease Control and Prevention, and Infectious Diseases Society of America recommends that all patients with TB undergo testing for HIV infection after counselling (Blumberg et al., 2003). A recent study (Erhabor et al., 2010) investigated the prevalence of HIV infection among 120 patients diagnosed with microbiologically proven TB. Subjects were Nigerians aged 18 to 54 years with a mean age of 39.5 years (standard deviation 6.75). Of the 120 TB patients tested (25%) were positive for HIV infection. HIV-1 was the predominant viral subtype. HIV prevalence was significantly higher in subjects in the 38-47 and 28-37 years age groups. The mean CD4 lymphocyte count of the HIV-infected TB subjects was significantly lower (195 ± 40.5 cells/µL) compared to the non-HIV infected (288 ± 35.25 cells/µL $p = 0.01$). This finding is in agreement with previous reports among 59 patients with pulmonary TB studied in Kampala, Uganda (De Cock et al., 1992) in which two-thirds of the patients were HIV sero-positive. Similarly in Sagamu, Nigeria Daniel and colleagues (Daniel et al., 2004) observed a 14.9% HIV prevalence amongst their cohort of TB infected patients. Of patients with confirmed pulmonary TB in Zambia, 49% were positive for HIV (Elliott et al., 1990). Studies among TB patients in Kenya (Barnes et al., 1991) observed 40.7% prevalence while nearly 40% of the smear-positive TB patients in Tanzania were attributable to HIV (Cantwell et al 1994). However, out of 13,269 patients diagnosed with TB in the Netherlands who were then tested for HIV between 1993 to 2001, 542 were HIV positive (4.1%) (Haar et al., 2006). Among 184 newly diagnosed TB patients tested for HIV in Singapore, 15 (8.2%) was seropositive (Eriki et al., 1991).

2.7 Challenges of mother – to child transmission of HIV among unbooked antenatal patriuents

Mother-to-child transmission (MTCT) of HIV represents an especially tragic dimension of the burden of HIV/AIDS, particularly in resource-constrained settings, where fragile and poorly funded health care systems hamper care and prevention efforts. The global HIV epidemic continues to expand, with an estimated five million people becoming infected each year. Over the decades, the epidemic, once dominated by infected males, has become progressively feminized. In sub-Saharan Africa, where about two-thirds of the global disease burden resides, 57% of adults living with HIV are women (UNAIDS, 2004). As more women contract the virus, the number of children infected from their mothers has been growing. Worldwide, an estimated 640,000 children acquired HIV in 2004 alone (UNAIDS, 2004), with more than 90% of the infections occurring through mother-to-child transmission. MTCT has become a critical children's health problem in Africa, contributing to severe morbidity and significant mortality and undermining the impact of programs that had significantly reduced child mortality in previous decades. Women can transmit HIV to their babies in utero, during birth, and through breastfeeding. Without preventive interventions, approximately 25% to 40% of infants born to HIV-positive mothers will contract the virus. In the developed world with lower HIV prevalence rates, mother-to-child transmission has dropped to less than 2% with the implementation of universal Voluntary Counselling and Testing (VCT), ARV prophylaxis, elective caesarean section, and the avoidance of breastfeeding (Mofenson, 2003). Unfortunately, in Nigeria and other countries with poor health systems, particularly with poor maternal and child health programs, this transmission route continues to cause great concern. The key entry point to PMTCT programs is the VCT offered to pregnant women. The experiences of PMTCT programs in Nigeria and other African nations demonstrate that much of their success is determined by the proportion of women, who agree to be tested for HIV, return to obtain their test results, and accept the ARV prophylaxis, which is often a single dose of nevirapine. The infrastructure, capacity building, and training are required to maximize the "uptake" of VCT, as well as the development of clinically proven ARV prophylaxis protocols. ARV prophylaxis significantly reduces the rate of mother-to-child transmission of HIV. This consists of single or double ARVs during the last trimester of pregnancy or at delivery with a goal of lowering viral load to decrease the risk of transmission. Trials of various PMTCT protocols have been conducted in the developing world; yet viral drug resistance remains a problem (Mofenson et al., 1999). Although the current use of single dose nevirapine to HIV-infected pregnant women does significantly reduce mother-to-child transmission, it also leads to the development of nevirapine resistance in 12% to 40% of women (Eshleman et al., 2001). The development of drug resistance in either the mother or infant compromises ARV provision since nevirapine is often used in first-line regimens for adults and infants in developing country programs (Lallement, 2005). To date, the use of various short courses of ARVs given during the last trimester of pregnancy reduce levels of viral load and significantly lower the risk of in utero and intrapartum infection. HIV transmission through breast milk, however, continues to be a major obstacle for PMTCT efforts, particularly in Africa, where strong cultural and economic factors favour breast milk feeding rather than expensive breast milk substitutes. Furthermore, employment of safe breast milk substitutes is complicated by the fact that many HIV-infected women lack access to clean water and sanitation. Organized preventive screening programs for antenatal care were first introduced in Western Europe in the twentieth century with the hope that routine antenatal care would contribute to a reduction in maternal and infant mortality rates. Figures on maternal mortality in the developed world show that the risk of death as a result of pregnancy and child birth is approximately 1 in 7000 compared with 1 in 23 for women living in parts of Africa where antenatal care is poor or nonexistent (Carroli et al., 2001).

Most children living with HIV in Nigeria acquire the infection through mother-to-child transmission (MTCT), which can occur during pregnancy, labour, delivery, or breastfeeding. In the absence of any intervention, the risk of such transmission is 15%–30% in non-breastfeeding populations. Breastfeeding by an infected mother increases the risk by 5%–20% to a total of 20%–45% (de Cock et al., 2000). The risk of MTCT can be reduced to less than 2% by interventions that include antiretroviral prophylaxis given to women during pregnancy and labour and to the infant in the first weeks of life, during elective caesarean delivery (prior to the onset of labour and rupture of membranes), and avoidance of breastfeeding (European collaborative study, 2005). With these interventions, new HIV infections in children are becoming increasingly rare in many parts of the world, particularly in high-income countries. In many resource-constrained settings, elective caesarean delivery is seldom feasible (Stanton and Holtz 2006), and it is often neither acceptable nor safe for mothers to refrain from breastfeeding. However, recent guidelines from the World Health Organization (World Health Organization, 2010) recommend that mothers known to be HIV-infected (and whose infants are HIV-uninfected or of unknown HIV status) should exclusively breastfeed their infants for the first six months of life, introducing appropriate complementary foods after that. Breastfeeding should then be stopped only when a nutritionally adequate and safe diet without breast milk can be provided. In these settings, efforts to prevent HIV infection in infants initially focused on reducing MTCT around the time of labour and delivery. The unknown HIV status of these unbooked women presenting to clinic for the first time in the third trimester of pregnancy poses a risk not only to the patient and her baby, but also to the staff caring for them in the peripartum period. A recent study (Akani et al., 2010) was undertaken to determine the seroprevalence of HIV infection among unbooked pregnant women in the Niger Delta of Nigeria. One hundred and eighteen consecutively recruited unbooked subjects presenting to the isolation ward at the University of Port Harcourt Teaching Hospital were screened for HIV. Among the 118 subjects studied, 30 (25.4%) were positive for HIV. HIV-1 was the predominant viral strain. Gestational age of subjects at presentation was 28–40 weeks and mean age was 35.04 ± 8.06 years. The majority of subjects were primigravidas 66 (55.9%), while 52 (44.1%) were multigravidas. The prevalence of HIV was significantly higher among unbooked pregnant women with less formal education: 14 (11.9%) compared with 9 (7.6%), 5 (4.2%), and 2 (1.7%) for those with primary, secondary, and tertiary education, respectively ($P = 0.01$). Among the occupational groups, the prevalence of HIV was significantly higher among traders 14 (11.9%) than in career women 5 (4.2%, $P = 0.04$). Multigravid women were more susceptible to HIV infection 17 (14.4%) than primigravid women. Perinatal mortality and emergency caesarean section was high among unbooked pregnant women. These findings are very pertinent to health care delivery, because this pool of unbooked patients may not be benefiting from the Prevention of Maternal to Child Transmission program, thus increasing the paediatric HIV burden in our environment.

3. Challenges of HIV sero- discordance and HIV serostatus disclosure

The disclosure of HIV serostatus is a difficult emotional task creating opportunity for both support and rejection (Yashioka and Schustack, 2001). Barriers to disclosure include fear of accusation of infidelity, abandonment, discrimination and violence (Medley et al., 2004. Stigmatizing belief about AIDS and the associated fear of discrimination can influence decision to disclose ones HIV serostatus (Chesney and Smith, 1999). A considerable body of evidence has associated the act of disclosing personal trauma-related information with improved physiological health and that it can lead to support that facilitates initiation of and adherence to treatment (Chandra et al., 2003, Klitzman et al.,2004).The dilemma of choosing to disclose personal information is somewhat of a cruel paradox (Harber, 1992).Often people long to share a trauma or secret with another, yet they fear the possible rejection or alienation by the listener (Silver et al., 1990). A previous study (Akani et al., 2006) in the Niger Delta of Nigeria evaluated the rate, patterns and barriers to HIV serostatus disclosure. A pre-tested interviewer-administered questionnaire from 187 HIV infected people residing in a resource-limited setting in the Niger Delta of Nigeria was analysed. Of the 187 HIV seropositive patients studied, 144 (77.0%) had disclosed their HIV-serostatus while 43 (23.0%) had not. Results showed that the patients had disclosed their HIV-serostatus to:

parents (22.3%), siblings (9.7%), pastors (27.8%), friends (6.3%), family members (10.4%) and sexual partners (23.6%) ($p = 0.004$). Females were more likely (59.7%) to disclose their HIV serostatus compared with males (40.3%) ($p = 0.003$). Mothers were twice as likely (65.6%) to be confided in compared with fathers. Barriers to HIV serostatus disclosure included fear of stigmatization, victimization, fear of confidants spreading the news of their serostatus and fear of accusation of infidelity and abandonment ($p = 0.002$). Married respondents were more likely to disclose their status. Better-educated respondents with tertiary education were more likely to disclose their HIV-serostatus. Expectation of economic, spiritual, emotional and social support was the major reason for disclosure. The ratio of disclosure to non-disclosure among patients with non-formal education was (2.6:1.0), primary education (2.3:1.0), secondary education (3.3:1.0) and tertiary education (10.0:1.0). Disclosure of HIV serostatus can foster economic social and economic support. There is need for the re-intensification of interventional measure that combines provider, patients and community education particularly in the aspect of anti-stigma campaign, partner notification and skill building to facilitate appropriate HIV serostatus disclosure.

4. Reproductive health challenges associated with HIV – infection in Nigeria

Availability and use of antiretroviral drugs has changed the landscape of HIV/AIDS bringing about a change in the perception of HIV from an incurable deadly disease to a chronic manageable illness. As effective HIV treatments become more widespread, HIV-infected individuals are living longer and healthier lives. Many HIV-affected couples (sero-discordant and sero-concordant) are considering options for safer reproduction. A large body of evidence suggests that reproductive technologies can help HIV-affected couples to safely conceive with minimal risk of HIV transmission to their partner and baby. However, for most couples particularly in low income countries in sub Saharan Africa, such technologies are both neither geographically nor economically accessible (Matthews and Mukherjee, 2009). With HIV now considered to be a chronic manageable disease, attention is shifting to offering and improving quality of life particularly by the provision of reproductive health options/care to men and women living with HIV-1. Many HIV-infected men and women are now expressing their desire to father or mother a child. Assisted reproductive technologies, including intrauterine insemination (IUI), in vitro fertilisation (IVF) and intracytoplasmatic sperm injection (ICSI) in combination with semen washing have been used to decrease the risk of HIV -1 transmission in HIV-1-infected discordant couples with an HIV-1-infected man (van et al., *2009*) . Previous report indicates that in HIV-positive men taking HAART, seminal viral load is decreased but not eliminated and fertilization should be achieved through sperm washing to offer maximum protection for the uninfected female. Pregnant HIV-positive women on antiretroviral medication have a reduced risk of transmitting the virus, but should still be counselled about the possibility to further limit the chances of infecting their infant through elective Caesarean section (Semprini et al., 2004, Semprini et al., 2004b, Barreiro et al.,2007, Matthews et al., 2010) . HIV sero-discordant couples with strong desire for childbearing have a dilemma of risking HIV infection or infecting their spouse. Some risk transmission of HIV infection to reproduce. Over two-thirds of 104 couple wanting to procreate surveyed reported unprotected sex with their partner in the past 6 months. Most respondents, regardless of serostatus, said that viral load testing and awareness of post-exposure prevention had no effect on their condom use (van der Straten et al., 2000). A study to assess the reproductive health concerns among 195 persons living with HIV/AIDS in the Niger Delta of Nigeria Akani et al (in press) showed that 111 (56.9 %) indicated their desire to have children. Single subjects were more inclined to having children (66.6%) compared to married (53.4%) *p= .03*. Persons with no formal education are about twice as likely to have children (66.7%) compared to persons educated to tertiary education level (37, 0%) (*p=.01*). Knowledge about reproductive health options available to reduce risk of infecting their partners and or baby was poor. There is the need to support the sexual and reproductive rights of HIV-infected individuals, offer additional training to HIV counsellors on evidence-based best and affordable practices regarding reproductive health issues, develop policies that support the availability and accessibility to relevant reproductive and sexual health services.

5. Challenges of management of occupational exposure to HIV and availability of post exposure prophylaxis

HIV transmission in health care settings occurs when workers are stuck with needles or sharp instruments contaminated with HIV-infected blood or, less frequently, when workers are exposed to infected blood through an open cut or a mucous membrane, such as the eyes or nasal passages (Campbell, 2004). Patients in African settings may be more likely to be infected with HIV. This predisposes health care workers to HIV infection particularly in the absence of proper universal precautions. In developed countries, post-exposure prophylaxis is part of most health care policies. Post-exposure prophylaxis—a short course of triple-drug ART provided to prevent possible HIV infection has yet to be broadly institutionalized in Nigeria's health care facilities. It is hoped that with the increased availability of ARVs, this may be feasible in the near future. Sharp injuries and other exposure to patient's blood carry a risk of transmission of blood borne infections including HIV. Despite the long-standing recommendations in the developed world that Health Care Workers exposed to infected blood and blood product be offered post exposure prophylaxis, they remain unavailable to healthcare workers in most resource-limited settings in Sub-Saharan Africa. Also there is absence of established occupational health policy and policy for minimising the risk and management of percutaneous and mucosal exposure to high risk patient's blood and body fluids. A previous study (Erhabor et al, 2007) was carried out to demonstrate the epidemiology and risk of occupational exposure to HIV, HBV and HCV among health care workers (HCWs) and highlight areas where greater training is required. The study population included 13 health care workers; 5 males (38.5%) and 8 females (61.5%), mean age 34.15 +/- 6.8 years including 3 doctors (23.1%), 2 laboratory scientist (15.4%), 1 laboratory technician (7.7%), 6 medical students (46.2%) and 1 trainee laboratory assistant (7.7%). The care and follow-up provided to the health care workers in a 500 -bed tertiary health hospital in the Niger Delta of Nigeria who had percutaneous exposure to patient's blood between June 2002 and June 2005 were analyzed. All exposed health care workers were evaluated and offered follow up counselling. Five millilitres of blood from each of the HCWs and the source patients were screened by immmuno-enzymatic testing for HIV, HBV, and HCV. Exposures were concentrated in few areas of the hospital; paediatrics (46.2%); surgery (15.4%); obstetrics and gynaecology (7.7%) and laboratory unit (30.8%) (p = 0.05). Risk of exposure was significantly higher among females (61.5%) compared to males (38.5%) (p = 0.001). All exposed HCWs were seen and offered post exposure prophylaxis within 24 hours of exposure. All the exposed health care workers were sero-negative to HIV,

HBsAg and anti-HCV at exposure. The source patients were known in all cases. Evidence of HIV was present in 5 (38.5%); 1 (7.7%) had HBV while none had HCV infection. Of all the HCWs who completed the follow-up, only 1(7.7%) confirmed case of HBV sero-conversion occurred in a HCW who was not previously vaccinated against HBV but who received post exposure HBV vaccination. Exposure rate was significantly higher among house officers 7 (53.9%) followed by registrars 3 (23.1%) and laboratory scientist 3 (23.1) ($p = 0.01$). There is need to urgently address the issue of occupational exposure in Nigeria by the formulation of occupational health policy in Nigeria as well as provision of training on universal precaution, phlebotomy, modifying procedures that have high risk, developing institutional policy for handling of sharps and post-exposure management of healthcare workers as well as the provision of protective post exposure prophylaxis for all exposed HCWs.

6. Challenges of availability of affordable laboratory-monitoring tests and trained manpower required for the implementation of HIV therapy

Few laboratories in resource-constrained countries can afford to perform laboratory-monitoring tests required for the implementation of HIV therapy. Flow cytometric techniques are expensive and require a significant infrastructure to perform. In addition, the measurement of quantities of virus in the blood—known as viral load—is an important clinical parameter to evaluate the severity of disease and to monitor the efficacy of therapy. These expensive laboratory tests require complex technologies not previously used in much of the developing world. Scientists are devising new methodologies that they hope will be as sensitive as existing methodologies yet more cost effective. The laboratory infrastructure is the most expensive and specialized part of any institutional framework for HIV/AIDS cares (Stephenson, 2002). In Nigeria, policymakers and decision makers have tended to view laboratories in the narrow context of HIV screening. At the onset of the ART program no laboratory in the country had the full capacity needed to monitor treatment response and toxicity properly. Only a handful of institutions had the capacity to perform CD4+ counts, a necessary test for decision-making in HIV therapy. The federal government program provided the training and technical capacity for CD4+ tests to be performed in the 25 treatment centres using a manual microscopic technique. This technology is labour intensive, and one laboratory scientist cannot reliably perform more than 10 tests a day. This pace cannot accommodate the expansion of ART in these centres and in other centres that would rely on them for laboratory support. Through a generous donation from MTN Nigeria, a telecommunications company, APIN was able to equip two federal treatment centres—at University College Hospital and Jos University Teaching Hospital—with flow-cytometry-based instruments (Imade et al., 2005), which allow technicians to process more than 100 CD4+ tests daily. The instruments cut the cost of the tests four- to fivefold. All Harvard PEPFAR program sites are now equipped with these instruments. Many other programs in Nigeria, particularly the other PEPFAR programs, have opted for that investment as well. Similarly, when the ART program started in Nigeria, only one centre had the capacity to perform viral load tests routinely; these tests are used to measure the virus level in the blood of infected individuals and thereby allow clinicians to assess treatment efficacy. This centre, the Nigerian Institute of Medical Research, had been upgraded and equipped by a grant from the Ford Foundation. APIN, a project based at the Harvard School of Public Health (HSPH) and sponsored by the Bill & Melinda Gates

Foundation, has significantly affected the level of infrastructures available in its four target states of Borno, Lagos, Oyo, and Plateau. All APIN sites now routinely perform HIV viral load tests with technical assistance and/or equipment provided by HSPH. When HSPH became a PEPFAR implementation partner, it further expanded the capacity of its collaborating centres. HSPH has provided training and retraining of health professional and laboratory personnel and helped upgrade or establish six laboratories for HIV and STI services. In addition few sites have facilities to perform infant diagnostics using polymerase chain reaction (PCR), the only technique capable of diagnosing HIV infection in infants. In addition, most sites have been involved in projects in collaboration with HSPH to conduct surveillance studies of the HIV strains circulating in Nigeria and of the drug resistance levels in various patient populations. In a previous study in the Niger Delta of Nigeria (Erhabor et al., 2006) investigated the relevance of absolute lymphocyte count as a surrogate marker for CD4 lymphocyte count as a criterion for initiating HAART in HIV-infected Nigerians. A total of 100 consecutive recruited HIV-infected, previously antiretroviral naive persons and 30 HIV-negative individuals blood samples were run for absolute lymphocyte and CD4 lymphocyte counts and results were compared by a model of linear regression analysis. An overall modest correlation was observed between absolute lymphocyte count and CD4 lymphocyte (r = 0.51) and at CD4 lymphocyte threshold relevant for clinical management of HIV-infected; <200, 200-350 and >350 cells/microL (r = 0.41, 0.30 and 0.21) respectively. Mean absolute lymphocyte count of 1.60 +/- 0.77 x 10(9)/L, 1.88 +/- 1.11 x 10(9)/L and 2.04 +/- 0.54 x 10(9)/L was equivalent respectively to CD4 of <200, 200-350 and >350 cells/microL. This study indicated a modest correlation between absolute and CD4 lymphocyte counts of HIV-infected Nigerians and at CD4 lymphocyte count threshold significant for clinical management of HIV-infected. Absolute lymphocyte count can become a minimal inexpensive alternative to CD4 lymphocyte count in conjunction with WHO staging and clinical status of patient in determining the optimal time to initiate therapy particularly in resource limited settings where other expensive methods of CD4 enumeration are unavailable. The infrastructure for the diagnosis of HIV and monitoring of patients on antiretroviral therapy in Nigerians is still sub-optimal and the capacity to monitor patients on ARV therapy is inadequate. These diagnostic limitations have hindered the effective monitoring of patients on antiretroviral therapy. There is need to improve the facilities for HIV diagnosis and treatment monitoring as well as manpower development of biomedical scientist to effectively carry out these specialized diagnostic services.

7. Challenges of deciding the optimal time to start antiretroviral treatment

Highly active antiretroviral therapy (HAART) has changed the landscape of HIV- related care in the developed world with marked reduction in mortality and morbidity (Cameron et al., 1998). This possibility however is beyond the reach of a vast majority of HIV-infected in sub Saharan Africa. Following the development of HAART, many physicians were quite aggressive in treating patients at virtually any stage of this human retroviral disease. Increasing concern related to drug toxicities, pill burden, cost and ability of patients to adhere to strict and complicated regimens, have complicated the decision-making process for physicians and patients alike (Volberding, 2000). Despite promised price-reduction and increased availability of generic drugs in some countries, cost remains a major factor in deciding when to start therapy. Early intervention suggested that a higher proportion of patients achieved a viral load of < 500 cells/µl if started on HAART at a CD4+ count of >500 cells/µl and >350 cells/µl rather than at < 200 cells/µl (Meibohm et al., 2000, Moore et al., 2000). Long-term clinical outcomes data however are not available to fully endorse this approach. The British HIV association recommends that therapy be initiated once CD4+ cell count falls to 350 cells/µl (British HIV Association (BHIVA), 2000). The argument for a conservative approach in the initiation of HAART is that most regimen are difficult to tolerate, non- adherence leads to the development of resistance, thus limiting future treatment options (Molla et al., 1996, d' Arminio Monforte et al., 2000) and that considerable reconstitution of the immune system seems possible even in patients initiating HAART at a low CD4+ cell count (Miller et al., 1999). Increasing concerns related to cost, drug toxicity, pill burden, tolerability ability of patient to adhere to strict and complicated regimen and emergence of drug resistance has complicated the decision making process of the optimal time to initiate antiretroviral therapy in Nigeria. A previous study (Ejele et al.,2004) aimed at determining if there is any immunological advantage in initiating HAART at a pre-therapeutic CD4 count of > 350cells/µl rather than at 200-350 or < 200 cells/µl investigated one hundred HIV-infected previously antiretroviral- naive individuals grouped under 3 $CD4^+$ lymphocyte count thresholds; < 200, 200 - 350 and > 350 cells/µl who were randomized to take HAART of stavudine (40mg) lamivudine (150mg) and nevirapine (200mg) orally twice daily. CD4 lymphocyte count was determined serially every 8 weeks for an observation period of 48 weeks. CD4 lymphocyte count responses were compared statistically based on pre-therapeutic CD4 lymphocyte counts. The overall increase in CD4 lymphocyte count irrespective of baseline CD4 count was 122 cells/µl ($p < 0.01$). CD4 lymphocyte count response to 48 weeks HAART was significantly higher in patients initiating HAART at a pre-therapeutic CD4 count of <200 cells/µl (163 cells/µl) compared to 118 and 50 cells/µl respectively for those initiating at 200 - 350 and > 350 cells/µl respectively. HIV-related morbidity of 3% was found among subjects who initiated HAART with a pre-therapeutic CD4 count of < 200 cells/µl. Steven -Johnson syndrome was the commonest adverse clinical event observed occurring in 15% of subjects. This study indicates that there is no long-term advantage in terms of CD4+ lymphocyte response in initiating HAART at a pre-therapeutic CD4 count of > 350 cells/µl rather than at 200 - 350 cells/µl. This present study appears to support postponing the initiation of therapy in some patients until the CD4+ count approaches 200 cells/µl particularly in sub-Saharan Africa where drug accessibility and affordability constitutes a major challenge.

8. Challenges of adherence, compliance, drug resistance and universal access to antiretroviral treatment

With the widespread use of antiretrovirals particularly in the developed world, there has been a transformed perception of HIV/AIDS from a fatal incurable disease to a manageable chronic illness (Palella et al., 1998) .However access to ART remains limited, especially in developing countries where paradoxically a significant number of HIV-infected live but with only an insignificant 28% of the 7.1 million in need of treatment having access (WHO/UNAIDS/UNICEF 2007). Antiretroviral treatment (ARV) was introduced in Nigeria in the early 1990s; they were only available to those who paid for them. As the cost of the drugs was very high at this time and the overwhelming majority of Nigerians were living on less than $2 a day, only the wealthy minority were able to afford the treatment. In 2002 the

Nigerian government started an ambitious antiretroviral treatment programme, which aimed to supply 10,000 adults and 5,000 children with antiretroviral drugs within one year. An initial $3.5 million worth of ARVs were to be imported from India and delivered at a subsidized monthly cost of $7 per person (Odutolu et al., 2006). The programme was announced as Africa's largest antiretroviral treatment programme. By 2004 the programme had suffered a major setback as too many patients were being recruited without a big enough supply of drugs to hand out. This resulted in an expanding waiting list and not enough drugs to supply the high demand. The patients who had already started the treatment then had to wait for up to three months for more drugs, which can not only reverse the progress the drugs have already made, but can also increase the risk of HIV becoming resistant to the ARVs. Eventually, another $3.8 million worth of drugs were ordered and the programme resumed. Resources needed to provide sufficient treatment and care for those living with HIV in Nigeria are seriously lacking. A study of health care providers found many had not received sufficient training on HIV prevention and treatment and many of the health facilities had a shortage of medications, equipment and materials (Physicians for Human Rights, 2006). The government's National HIV/AIDS Strategic Framework for 2005 to 2009 set out to provide ARVs to 80 percent of adults and children with advanced HIV infection and to 80 percent of HIV-positive pregnant women, all by 2010 (WHO, UNAIDS, UNICEF,2007). However, only 31 percent of people who needed treatment for advanced HIV infection received it in 2009. According to the latest WHO guidelines (2010), which advise starting treatment earlier, HIV treatment coverage is only 21% (WHO, UNAIDS, UNICEF, 2010). As a result of this slow progress the treatment goals were set back to 2015 in the revised framework (2010 to 2015) (NACA, 2009). It has been estimated that the Nigerian government are contributing an insignificant 5 percent of the funds for the antiretroviral treatment programmes (HERFON, 2007). The majority of the funding comes from development partners. The main donors are PEPFAR (the President's Emergency Plan for AIDS Relief), the Global Fund and the World Bank. In 2002, the World Bank loaned US$90.3 million to Nigeria to support the 5-year HIV/AIDS Programme Development Project (HERFON, 2007). In May 2007 it was announced that the World Bank were to allocate a further US$50 million loan for the programme (World Bank, 2008). In 2008 PEPFAR provided approximately US$448 million to Nigeria for HIV/AIDS prevention, treatment and care, (PEPFAR, 2008) the third highest amount out of PEPFAR's 15 focus countries. In the same vein, the Global Fund in 2008 disbursed US$95 million in funds for Nigeria to expand treatment, prevention, and prevention of mother-to-child transmission programmes (Global fund 2009). Even the availability of financial resources has not brought the number of patients on ART to the level desired particularly in some settings in Africa.

For example the Global fund has put forward US$1.9 billion in order to scale-up access to ART (UNAIDS 2006). In some settings in Africa, the cost of antiretrovirals does not seem to be the most important constraint of access to ART, as many of the drugs are supplied free of cost to eligible patients through combined efforts by countries and bilateral and multilateral partners. Mozambique, a country with one of the highest HIV/AIDS burden, only 14% of those in need received ART by the end of 2006 (WHO/UNAIDS/UNICEF 2007). Mozambique spent less than 30% of the donor funds earmarked for the health ministry (Nemes et al., 2006).This poor absorptive capacity of the public institutions in most countries in Africa shows that there are other factors; health- systems level barriers (insufficient human resources and judicious use of donor funds) and population -level barriers (lack of information about ART, stigmatization and discrimination) may prevent or restrict access to ART.

Antiretroviral treatment causes improvement in the immunologic status and reduction in the viral load (Erb et al., 2000) thus reducing the incidence of hospitalization and mortality (Paterson et al., 2000) .Treatment effectiveness however requires a high level of adherence to medication regimens (Vanhove et al., 1996).Missing of even a few doses of antiretroviral medication can lead to drug resistant strains of HIV (Bangsberg et al., 2000).A previous study (Erhabor et al., 2009) to investigate the short-term effect of highly active antiretroviral therapy on the CD4 lymphocyte count of HIV-infected Nigerians at the Haematology Department of the University of Port Harcourt Teaching Hospital involving 70 HIV-infected subjects placed on highly active antiretroviral therapy and thirty HIV-infected yet to start therapy due to unaffordability were monitored as controls. CD4 lymphocyte count was determined at baseline for subjects and controls. Subjects were placed on HAART for 12 weeks while controls that were yet to start therapy were monitored as controls. CD4 lymphocyte count was repeated after 12 weeks and the differences compared statistically. We observed that subjects and control patients did not differ significantly in their CD4 lymphocyte count at baseline ($p > 0.05$), but after 12 weeks HAART in subjects, there was a mean increase in CD4 count of (39 cells/µl) in subjects, while untreated controls showed a mean decline of (12 cells/µl) $p < 0.05$. There was a statistically significant variation in the therapy dependent increases in CD4 count of HAART treated subjects based on pre-therapeutic baseline CD4 count ($\chi^2 = 180.39$, $p < 0.05$). The HAART dependent increase in CD4 counts was higher in younger subjects 19-28 years (31 cells/µl) compared to older subjects 49-58 years (21 cells/µl) ($p = 0.01$). Similarly CD4 response was found higher in females compared to males ($p = 0.01$). Low adherence has been associated with detectable viral load (>500 viral RNA copies/ml of plasma (Ruthbun et al., 2005) and possible cross resistance to other antiretrovirals of the same class (Tchetgen et al., 2001). A previous study (Nwauche et al., 2006) to evaluate the factors militating against adherence to antiretroviral therapy among 187 HIV-infected persons on a combination therapy of two-nucleoside analogue; stavudine and lamivudine and one non-nucleoside nevirapine in the Niger Delta of Nigeria indicated an adherence rate of 49.2%.Factors associated with non-adherence included; cost of antiretrovirals, educational status of subjects, medication adverse effects, occupational factors and high pill burden of prescribed regimen. There is need for universal access to antiretroviral treatment .Cost constraint remains a major limiting factor on adherence particularly in resource-limited settings (Muko et al., 2004). National government particularly those in sub Saharan Africa have prolonged reluctance to provide the best possible treatment citing numerous concerns ranging from cost to the ability of patients to adhere to complex life-long treatment. However South Africa a country with more than 5 million citizens living with HIV has proved the pundits wrong. The prices of antiretrovirals having precipitously plummeted by more than 95% as a result of the South African government developing the political will to take on board the challenge of universal access. This strategic and humanitarian obligation has resulted in an increase in adherence to a high level of more than 90%.The world health organization must remain resolute on the initiative of universal access to antiretroviral treatment particularly in developing countries where paradoxically the greatest HIV disease burden exist but with an insignificant number having access. There is an urgent need for universal access and sustainability of antiretroviral therapy particularly in resource-limited settings. There is need for supervised medication delivery. Efforts should be made towards simplifying the therapeutic regimen to reduce the bill burden and substitution with treatment combination and strategies that minimise negative adverse effects, coupled with the re-intensification of patient education and counselling.

9. Conclusion

Nigeria is the most populous nation in Africa Nigeria is the most populous nation in Africa and is home is home to more than 130 million people. These individuals belong to more than 350 ethnic and linguistic groups, and their country is ranked among the 25 poorest in the world. As many as six million people are already infected with the virus. HIV prevalence rates in some states are as high as 12 percent. At least two million children have been orphaned by AIDS. Health facilities in Nigeria are suboptimal. Nigeria faces many daunting challenges in dealing with its HIV/AIDS epidemic.

Public education must play a key role in the success of prevention programs and increase in the uptake of HIV testing. Behavioural change programs must encourage individuals to reduce their risk of HIV acquisition. The stigmatization and discrimination that have typified societal responses must be dealt with promptly, as they compromise the effectiveness of prevention programs. The early involvement and support of the government in the HIV/AIDS campaign can set the necessary groundwork for a continuing strong leadership that will be critical for initiating and sustaining an effective nationwide prevention program. Stigmatization and discrimination against PLWHAs are common in Nigeria. Often both Christian and Muslim religious leaders view immoral behaviour as the cause of the HIV/AIDS epidemic. PLWHAs often lose their jobs or are denied health care services because of the ignorance and fear surrounding the disease. There is need for increased national campaigns and more visible and vocal societies and support groups for people infected with or affected by HIV as well as education of the public about HIV/AIDS in a bid to dispelling myths and giving the disease a human face.

New methods to detect antibodies to HIV are needed for diagnosis, and although the simple rapid test and the enzyme-linked immunosorbent assay formats have been improved, they remain expensive for Nigerian patients. Furthermore, voluntary counselling and testing (VCT) programs are still based in urban centres, where they remain inaccessible to many Nigerians. Clinical management of HIV infection requires the regular measurement of CD4+ lymphocytes in the blood. Flow cytometric techniques are expensive and require a significant infrastructure to perform. In addition, the measurement of quantities of virus in the blood—known as viral load—is an important clinical parameter to evaluate the severity of disease and to monitor the efficacy of therapy. These expensive laboratory tests require complex technologies not previously used in much of the developing world. Scientists are devising new methodologies that they hope will be as sensitive as existing methodologies yet more cost effective. To accommodate these new and critical diagnostic clinical tools, Nigerian institutions will need ongoing training, capacity building, and infrastructure development. These requisites will grow even more acute as the country scales up its ART program.

Healthcare workers are at risk of acquiring HIV infection occupationally through percutaneous or mucosal exposure to contaminated blood and body fluids. There is need to urgently address the issue of formulation of occupational health policy in Nigeria as well as provision of training on universal precaution, phlebotomy, modifying procedures that have high risk, developing institutional policy for handling of sharps and post-exposure management of healthcare workers, provision of HIV post-exposure prophylaxis for exposed healthcare workers.

Blood transfusion continues to be an important route of transmission of HIV particularly in Nigeria among young children and pregnant women following transfusion for malaria associated anaemia and pregnancy-related complications. Nigeria faces several enduring challenges; chronic blood shortages, high prevalence of transfusion-transmissible infections, absence of functional national blood transfusion service, recruitment and retention of voluntary non –remunerated donors. Blood safety remains an issue of major concern in transfusion practice in Nigeria where national blood transfusion services and policies, appropriate infrastructure, trained personnel and financial resources are inadequate to support the running of a voluntary non-remunerated donor transfusion service. This is further aggravated by the predominance of family replacement and commercially remunerated blood donors, rather than regular benevolent, non-remunerated donors who give blood as a result of altruism. We advocate that commercial remunerated donation of blood be discouraged. There is need for unlimited supply of highly sensitive HIV test kits for the testing of donors. Political will and open-mindedness to innovative ways to improve supply and safety of blood are essential to promote more evidence-based approaches to blood transfusion practice in Nigeria.

The development and widespread use of antiretrovirals in the developed world has brought about a transformed perception of HIV/AIDS from a fatal incurable disease to a chronic manageable illness. There is an urgent need for universal access and sustainability of antiretroviral therapy particularly in Nigeria. There is need for supervised medication delivery. Efforts should be made towards simplifying the therapeutic regimens to reduce the pill burden and substitution with treatment combination and strategies that minimize negative adverse effects coupled with the re-intensification of patient's education and counselling.

There is concern in the developed world about the ability of Nigeria to effectively manage her HIV epidemic particularly in the midst of her sub-optimal health infrastructure including widespread poverty and a large and sexually active youthful population. The most effective interventions has to be multi-sectoral, with a high-level government commitment to tackle the problem, policy changes resulting from an awareness of the impact of HIV/AIDS on society, and the development of communications and media efforts, health interventions targeting high-risk populations, laboratory and field research, and scientific training. Without effective multi-sectoral intervention on a large scale, Nigeria is likely to experience not only the tragedy of countless lives forever altered by the virus, but also untold adverse social and economic effects.

10. References

[1] Adebajo SB, Mafeni J, Moreland S, et al (2002). Knowledge, Attitudes and Sexual Behaviour among Nigerian Military Concerning HIV/AIDS and STD: *Final Technical Report.* Abuja, Nigeria: Policy Project.

[2] Akani CI, Erhabor O (2006). Sero-epidemiology of HIV infection among abandoned babies in Port Harcourt, Nigeria. *Annals of African Medicine, Vol. 5(1): 6 – 9.*

[3] Akani CI, Erhabor O, Allagoa DO (2010). Human immunodeficiency virus prevalence in an unbooked obstetric population in the Niger Delta. *HIV/AIDS - Research and Palliative Care, 2:179–184.*

[4] Akinnawo EO (1995). Sexual networking, STDs, and HIV/ AIDS transmission among Nigerian police officers. *Health Transit Rev, (Suppl 5):S113–S121.*

[5] API consensus expert committee. API TB Consensus guidelines (2006). Management of pulmonary TB, extra-pulmonary TB and TB in special situations. *J Assoc Physicians India,* 54:219–234.

[6] Azuonwu O, Erhabor O, Frank-Peterside N (2010).HIV Infection in Long-Distance Truck Drivers in a Low Income Setting in the Niger Delta of Nigeria. *J Community Health.,* 36(4):583-587.

[7] Azuonwu O, Erhabor O, Obire O. HIV Seroprevalence among military personnel in the Niger Delta of Nigeria. J Community Health.2011 May 17.[Epud ahead of print].PMID:21584818.

[8] Bangsberg DR, Hetcht FM, Charlebois ED, Zolopa AR, Holodniy M, Sheiner L, Bamberger JD, Chesney MN, Moss A (2000).Adherence to protease inhibitor and development of drug resistance in an indigent population.*AIDS,14:357-366.*

[9] Bakhireva LN, Abebe Y, Brodine SK, et al (2004). Human immunodeficiency virus/acquired immunodeficiency syndrome knowledge and risk factors in Ethiopian military personnel. *Mil Med, 169(3): 221–226.*

[10] Bangsberg DR, Hetcht FM, Charlebois ED, Zolopa AR, Holodniy M, Sheiner L, Bamberger JD, Chesney MN, Moss A (2000).Adherence to protease inhibitor and development of drug resistance in an indigent population.*AIDS,14:357-366.*

[11] Barnes PF, Bloch AB, Davidson PT, Snider DE Jr (1991). TB in patients with human immunodeficiency virus infection. *N Engl J Med,* 324(23):1644–1650.

[12] Barreiro P, Castilla JA, Labarga P, Soriano V (2007). Is natural conception a valid option for HIV-serodiscordant couples? *Human Reproduction, 22(9): 2353-2358.*

[13] Batina A, Kabemba S, Malengela R (2007). Infectious markers among blood donors in Democratic Republic of Congo (DRC). *Rev Med Brux, 28(3):145-149.*

[14] Blumberg HM, Burman WJ, Chaisson RE, et al (2003). American Thoracic Society/Centres for Disease Control and Prevention/Infectious Diseases Society of America: treatment of TB. *Am J Respir Crit Care Med,* 167:603–662.

[15] Brenan CA, Bodelle P, Coffey R, et al (2008). The prevalence of diverse HIV-1 strains was stable in Cameroonian blood donors from 1996 to 2004. *J Acquir Immune Defic Syndr,*49(4):432–439.

[16] British HIV Association (BHIVA) (2000). Guidelines for the treatment of HIV-infected adults with antiretroviral therapy. *HIV Med, 1: 76 – 101.*

[17] Cameron DW, Heath- Chiozzi M, Danner S, et al (1998). Prolongation of life and prevention of AIDS complications in a randomized controlled clinical trial of ritonavir in patients with advanced HIV disease. *Lancet, 351: 543 – 549.*

[18] Cantwell MF, Snider DE Jr, Cauthen GM, Onorato IM (1994). Epidemiology of TB in the United States, 1985 through 1992. *JAMA,* 272(7):535–539.

[19] Carroli G, Rooney C, Villar J (2001). How effective is antenatal care in preventing maternal mortality and serious morbidity? An overview of the evidence. *Paediatr Perinat Epidemiol,* 15(1):1–42.

[20] Chandra PS, Deepthivarma S, Manjula V (2003). Disclosure of HIV infection in South India: patterns, reasons and reactions. *AIDS Care, 15:207-215.*

[21] d' Arminio Monforte A, Lepri AC, Rezza G, et al (2000). Insight into reason for discontinuation of the first HAART regimen in a cohort of antiretroviral naïve patients. *AIDS, 14: 499 – 507.*

[22] Daniel OJ, Salako AA, Oluwole FA, Alausa OK, Oladapo OT (2004). Human immunodeficiency virus sero-prevalence among newly diagnosed adult pulmonary TB patients in sagamu, Nigeria. *Nigeria Journal of Medicine,* 3(4):393–397.

[23] de Cock KM, Fowler MG, Mercier E, et al (2000). Prevention of mother- to- child HIV transmission in resource-poor countries: Translating research into policy and practice. *JAMA,* 283(9):1175–1182.

[24] De Cock KM, Soro B, Coulibaly IM, Lucas SB (1992). TB and HIV infection in sub-Saharan Africa. *JAMA,* 268:1581–1587.

[25] De Cock KM and Weiss HA. The global epidemiology of HIV/AIDS (2000). *Tropical Medicine International Health,* 5: 3-9.

[26] Diarra A, Kouriba B, Baby M, Murphy E, Lefrere JJ (2009). HIV, HCV, HBV and syphilis rate of positive donations among blood donations in Mali: lower rates among volunteer blood donors. *Transfus Clin Biol, 16(5-6):444-447.*

[27] Eberstadt N (2002). The future of AIDS. *Foreign Aff,* 81(6); 22-45.

[28] Ejele OA, Nwauche AC, Erhabor O (2004). Highly active antiretroviral therapy (HAART) in HIV-infected Africans: The question of the optimal time to start. *Proceedings of the World AIDS conference, Bangkok, 203 – 208.*

[29] Ejele OA, Nwauche CA, Erhabor O (2005). Seroprevalence of HIV among unemployed individuals undergoing pre-employment medical examination in Port Harcourt. *Niger J Med, 14(4):419-421.*

[30] Ejele OA, Nwauche CA, Erhabor O (2005). Seroprevalence of HIV infection among blood donors in Port Harcourt, Nigeria. *Niger J Med; 14(3):287-289.*

[31] Elliott AM, Lout N, Tembo G, et al (1990). Impact of Human immunodeficiency virus on TB patients in Zambia, a cross-sectional study. *BMJ,* 301(6749):412–415.

[32] Erb P, Battegay M, Zimmerli W, Rickenbach M, Egger M (2000). Effect of antiretroviral therapy on viral load, CD4 cell count and progression of acquired immunodeficiency syndrome in a community of human immunodeficiency virus-infected cohort study. *Arch Intern Med, 160: 1134-1140.*

[33] Energy Information Administration (2007).Official energy statistics from the U.S government. Nigerian energy profile.

[34] Erhabor O, Akani CI, Eyindah CE. Reproductive Health Options among HIV-Infected Persons in a Low Income Setting in the Niger Delta of Nigeria. In press

[35] Erhabor O, Uko EK, Adias T (2006). Absolute lymphocyte count as a marker for CD4 T-lymphocyte count: criterion for initiating antiretroviral therapy in HIV infected Nigerians. Niger J Med,15(1):56-59.

[36] Erhabor O, Ejele OA, Nwauche CA (2007). Epidemiology and management of occupational exposure to blood borne viral infections in a resource poor setting: the case for availability of post exposure prophylaxis. *Niger J Clin Pract, 10(2):100-104.*

[37] Erhabor O, Jeremiah ZA, Adias TC, Okere CE (2010). The prevalence of human immunodeficiency virus infection among TB patients in Port Harcourt Nigeria. *HIV/AIDS - Research and Palliative Care: 2 1–5.*

[38] Eriki PP, Okwere A, Aisu T (1991). The Influence of human immunodeficiency virus infection of TB in Kampala, Uganda. *Annual Review of Respiratory Diseases.* , 40:128–132.
[39] Erulkar AS, Bello M (2007).The experience of married adolescent girls in northern Nigeria. The Population Council,1-19.
[40] Eshleman SH, Mracna M, Guay L, et al (2001). Selection and fading of resistance mutations in women and infants receiving nevirapine to prevent HIV-1 vertical transmission (HIVNET 012). AIDS. 2001 Oct 19; 15(15):1951-1957.
[41] European collaborative study (2005). Mother-to-child transmission of HIV infection in the era of highly active antiretroviral therapy. *Clin Infect Dis,* 40(3):458–457.
[42] Fasola FA, Kotila TR, Akinyemi JO (2008). Trends in transfusion-transmitted viral infections from 2001 to 2006 in Ibadan, Nigeria. *Intervirology; 51(6):427-431).*
[43] Federal Ministry of Health, Nigeria (2009).National Blood Transfusion Service- About us.
[44] Federal Ministry of Health, Nigeria (2009). Report of the 2008 National HIV seroprevalence sentinel survey among pregnant women attending antenatal clinic in Nigeria: 1-46.
[45] Fleming AF (1988). Sero epidemiology of human immunodeficiency viruses in Africa. *Biomed Pharmacother,* 42(5):309–320.
[46] Foster S, Buvé A (1995). Benefits of HIV screening of blood transfusions in Zambia. *Lancet, 22; 346(8969):225-227.*
[47] Gibney L, Saquib N, Matzger J (2003). Behavioural risk factors for STD/HIV transmission in Bangladesh trucking industry. *Social Science and Medicine, 56:1411-1424.*
[48] Harber KD, Pennebaker J (1992). Overcoming traumatic memories. In: Christianson SA, ed. The handbook of emotion and memory. Hillsdale (NJ): Erlbanin, 359-387.
[49] Imade GE, Badung B, Pam S, et al (2005). Comparison of a new, affordable flow cytometric method and the manual magnetic bead technique for CD4 T-lymphocyte counting in a northern Nigerian setting. *Clin Diagn Lab Immunol,* 12(1):224–227.
[50] Jayaraman S, Chalabi Z, Perel P, Guerriero C, Roberts I (2010). The risk of transfusion-transmitted infections in sub-Saharan Africa. *Transfusion; 50(2):433-442.*
[51] Klitzman RL, Kirshenbaum SB, Dodge B, et al 92004). Intricacies and inter-relationships between HIV disclosure and HAART: a qualitative study. *AIDS Care, 16:628-640.*
[52] Lallement M (005). Response to the therapy after prior exposure to nevirapine. *3rd IAS Conference on HIV Pathogenesis and Treatment, Rio de Janeiro, Brazil, July 24–27. (Abstract TuFo0205).*
[53] Lovgren S (2001). African Army hastening HIV/AIDS spread. *Jenda: A Journal of Culture and African Women Studies;* 1, 2.
[54] Low SY, Eng P (2009). Human immunodeficiency virus testing in patients with newly-diagnosed TB in Singapore. *Singapore Med Journal,* 50(5):479–481.
[55] Mandisodza AR, Charuma H, Masoha A, Musekiwa Z, Mvere D, Abayomi A. (2006). Prevalence of HIV infection in school based and other young donors during the 2002 and 2003 period. *Afr J Med Med Sci; 35(1):69-72.*

[56] Manjunath JV, Thappa DM, Jaisankar TJ (2002). Sexually transmitted diseases and sexual lifestyles of long –distance truck drivers: A clinic-epidemiologic study in South India .*International Journal of STD and AIDS, 13:612-617.*

[57] Matthews, L. T., Mukherjee, J. S. (2009). Strategies for harm reduction among HIV-affected couples who want to conceive. *AIDS Behaviour, 13(1), 5-11.*

[58] Matthews, L. T., Baeten, J. M., Celum, C., Bangsberg, D. R. (2010). Periconception pre-exposure prophylaxis to prevent HIV transmission: benefits, risks, and challenges to implementation. *AIDS, 24(13): 1975-1982.*

[59] Meibohm A, Alexander JR J, Robertson M (2000). Early versus late initiation of indinavir (IDV) in combination with zidovudine (ZDV) and lamivudine (3TC) in HIV-infected individuals. *Seventh conference on retroviruses and opportunistic infections. San Francisco, January – February 2000.*

[60] Miller V, Staszewski S, Nisius G, Lepri AC, Sabin C, Phillips AN (1999). Risk of new AIDS disease in people on triple therapy. *Lancet, 353 – 343.*

[61] Mofenson LM, Lambert JS, Stiehm ER, et al (1999). Risk factors for perinatal transmission of human immunodeficiency virus type 1 in women treated with zidovudine. *N Engl J Med,* 341:385–393.

[62] Mofenson LM (2003). Advances in the prevention of vertical transmission of human immunodeficiency virus. *Semin Pediatr Infect Dis,* 4(4):295–308.

[63] Molla A, Korneveva M, Gao Q, et al (1996). Ordered accumulation of mutation in HIV confers resistance to ritonavir. *Nat Med, 2: 760 – 766.*

[64] Moore R, Kemly J, Barlet J, Chiasson R (2000). Start HAART early (CD4 < 350 cells/µl) or later? Evidence for greater effectiveness if started early. *Seventh conference on retroviruses and opportunistic infections. San Francisco, January – February 2000.*

[65] Muko KN, Ngwa VC, Chingan LC, Ngwa IG, Shu EN, Meiberg A (2004). Adherence to highly active antiretroviral therapy (HAART). A selection of reported case study from a rural area of Cameroon. *Medical Journal, 7:119-124.*

[66] National Agency for the Control of AIDS (NACA) (2009). National HIV/AIDS strategic framework (NSF) 2010-15.

[67] National Population Commission of Nigeria (1991). *Population Census of the Federal Republic of Nigeria: Analytic Report at the National Level.* Abuja: National Population Commission of Nigeria.

[68] Nemes MIB, Beaudoin J, Conway S, Kivumbi GW, Skjelmerud A, Vogel U (2006).Evaluation of WHO's contributions to 3'by 5':Annex 5:Regional Office and Country Visit Notes. WHO, Geneva.

[69] Nigerian exchange (2008). Ministry of Health alerts Nigerians to the transfusion of unsafe blood in hospitals.

[70] Noah D, Fidas G (2000). *The Global Infectious Disease Threat and Its Implications for the United States.* Washington, DC: National Intelligence Council, 2000.

[71] Nwauche CA, Erhabor O, Ejele OA, Akani CI (2006). Adherence to antiretroviral therapy among HIV-infected subjects in a resource-limited setting in the Niger Delta of Nigeria. African Journal of Health Sciences, 13 (3-4):13-17.

[72] Nwokoji UA, Ajuwon AJ (2004). Knowledge of AIDS and HIV risk-related sexual behaviour among Nigerian naval personnel. *BMC Public Health,* 2004; 4:24.

[73] Nyobi BM, Kristiansen KI, Bjune G, Muller F, Holm-Hansen C (2008). Diversity of human immunodeficiency type 1 subtype in Kegera and Kilimanjaro regions, Tanzania. *AIDS Res Hum Retroviruses,* 24(6):761–769.

[74] Odutolu O (2005). Convergence of behaviour change models for AIDS risk reduction in sub-Saharan Africa. *Int J Health Plann Manage, 20(3):239-52.*

[75] Odutolu O, Ahonsi BA, Gboun M, Jolayemi OM (2006). AIDS in Nigeria: A nation on the threshold. The National Response to HIV/AIDS. Harvard Center for Population and Development Studies.

[76] Palella FJ, Delaney KM, Moorman AC, Loveless MO, Fuhrer J, Satten GA, Aschman DJ, Holmberg SD (1998).Declining morbidity among patients with advanced human immunodeficiency virus infection.HIV outpatients study investigation. N Engl J Med, 338: 853-860.

[77] Pandey A, Benara SK, Roy N, Sahu D, Gayle H, et al (2008). Risk behaviour, sexually transmitted infections and HIV among long-distance drivers: a cross-sectional survey along national highways in India. AIDS, 22(5):S81-90.

[78] Physicians for Human Rights (2006) 'Nigeria: Access to Health Care for People Living with HIV and AIDS.

[79] Paterson DL, Swindell S, Mohr J, Bester M, Vergis EN, Squier C, Wagener MM, Singh N (2000).Adherence to protease inhibitor therapy and outcomes in patients with HIV infection. Ann Intern Med, 133:21-30.

[80] PEPFAR (2008). FY2008 Country profile: Nigeria. Annual report to congress.

[81] Pieniazek D, Ellenberger D, Janini LM, et al (1991). Predominance of human immunodeficiency virus type 2 subtype in Abidjan, Ivory Coast. *AIDS Res Hum Retroviruses,* 15(6):603–608.

[82] Raufu A (2001). AIDS scare hits Nigerian military. *AIDS Anal Afr; 11*(5):14.

[83] Raufu A (2002). Nigeria promises free antiretroviral drugs to HIV positive soldiers. *Br Med J*; 13; 324(7342):870.

[84] Ruthbun RC, Farmer KC, Stephens JR, Lockhard SM (2005). Impact of an adherence clinic on behavioural outcomes and virologic response in treatment of HIV infection: a prospective randomized controlled pilot study. Clinical Therapy, 25:199-209.

[85] Salawu L, Murainah HA (2006). Pre-donation screening of intending blood donors for antibodies to infectious agents in a Nigerian tertiary health institution: a pilot study. *Afr J Med Sci; 35(4):453-456.*

[86] Sarin R (2003). *A New Security Threat: HIV/AIDS in the Military.* Washington, DC: World Watch Institute.

[87] Semprini A E, Vucetich A, Hollander L (2004). Sperm washing, use of HAART and role of elective Caesarean section. *Current Opinion in Obstetrics and Gynaecology, 16(6): 465-470.*

[88] Semprini, A. E., Fiore, S. (2004) b. HIV and reproduction. *Current Opinion in Obstetrics and Gynaecology, 16(3): 257-262.*

[89] Silver RL, Wortman CB, Crofton C (1990). The role of coping in support provision: the self-presentation dilemma of victims of life Crisis.In: Sarason BR, Sarason IG, Piece GR, eds. Social Support: An International view. New York: John Wiley and Sons: 379-426.

[90] Stanton CK, Holtz SA (2006). Levels and trends in caesarean birth in the developing world. *Stud Fam Plann,* 37(1):41–48.

[91] Stephenson J (2002). Cheaper HIV drugs for poor nations bring a new challenge: monitoring treatment. *JAMA,* 288(2):151–153.

[92] Sugihantono A, Slidell M, Syaifudin A, Pratjojo H, Utami IM, Sadjimin T, et al (2003). Syphilis and HIV prevalence among commercial sex workers in central Java, Indonesia: Risk-taking behaviour and attitude that may potentiate a wider epidemic. AIDS Patient Care and STDs, 17:595-600.

[93] Sunmola AM (2005). Sexual practices, barriers to condom use and its consistent use among long distance truck drivers in Nigeria. AIDS Care, 17:208-211.

[94] Tagny CT, Mbanya D, Tapko JB, Lefrère JJ (2008). Blood safety in Sub-Saharan Africa: a multi-factorial problem. Transfusion; 48(6):1256-261.

[95] Tchetgen E, Kaplan EH, Friendland GH (2001).Public health consequences of screening patients for adherence to highly active antiretroviral therapy. Journals of AIDS, 26: 118-129.

[96] The Global Fund (2009). Nigeria and the Global Fund.

[97] The World Bank (2008). Nigeria receives US million additional funding for HIV/AIDS project program.

[98] Thorne, CN and Patel, D and Fiore, S and Peckham, C and Newell, ML (2005) Mother-to-child transmission of HIV-1 in the era of highly active antiretroviral therapy. Clinical Infectious Diseases, 40 (3), 458 – 465).

[99] Tounkara A, Sarro YS, Kristensen S, Dao S, Diallo H, Diarra B, Noumsi TG, Guindo O (2009). Seroprevalence of HIV/HBV co-infection in Malian blood donors. *J Int Assoc Physicians AIDS Care (Chic Ill) ; 8(1):47-51.*

[100] UNAIDS (1998). *AIDS and the Military*. Best Practice Collection. Geneva.

[101] UNAIDS (2004). *AIDS Epidemic Update.* Geneva: UNAIDS, December 2004.

[102] UNAIDS (2005). Engaging Uniformed Services in the Fight Against HIV/AIDS. Accessed at https://uniformed services.unaids.org on July 8.

[103] UNAIDS/WHO (2005). *AIDS Epidemic Update: December 2005.* Geneva: UNAIDS.

[104] UNAIDS (2006).Report on the Global AIDS epidemic: May 2006.Joint United Nations Programme on HIV/AIDS.UNAIDS, Geneva.

[105] UNAIDS (2008). Uniting the World against AIDS Report on the global AIDS epidemic. Available t:http://www.unaids/en/KnowledgeCentre/HIVData/ Global Report /2008/2008_Global_report.asp. Accessed Aug 11, 2010.

[106] UNAIDS (2010). UNAIDS reporton the global AIDS epidemic.

[107] UNGASS (2010).UNGASS country progress report, Nigeria.

[108] United Nations Development Programme (2004). *Human Development Report.* New York: United Nations Development Programme: 141.

[109] U.S. Bureau of the Census, Population Division (1998). *International Programs Centre HIV/AIDS Surveillance Data.* Washington, DC: U.S. Bureau of the Census.

[110] UNDP 92007/2008). Human and income poverty: developing countries. In 2007/2008 human development report.

[111] Vanhove GF, Schapiro JM, Winters MA, Iversen A, Merigan TC (1996). Patient's compliance and drug failure in protease inhibitor monotherapy.JAMA, 276:1955-1956.

[112] van Leeuwen E, Repping S, Prins J M, Reiss P, van der Veen F. (2009). Assisted reproductive technologies to establish pregnancies in couples with an HIV-1-infected man. *Netherland Journal of Medicine, 67(8), 322-327.*
[113] Volberding P (2010). When and where to start: guidelines for the initiation of antiretroviral therapy. AIDS Reader, 10: 150 - 155.
[114] WHO (2008).WHO African region: Nigeria.
[115] WHO/UNAIDS/UNICEF (2007). Towards Universal Access: Scaling up Priority HIV/AIDS Interventions in the Health Sector. Progress Report, April 2007.WHO, Geneva.
[116] WHO/UNAIDS/UNICEF (2008). Towards Universal Access: Scaling up Priority HIV/AIDS Interventions in the Health Sector. Progress Report, WHO, Geneva.
[117] WHO/UNAIDS/UNICEF (2010). Towards Universal Access: Scaling up Priority HIV/AIDS Interventions in the Health Sector. Progress Report, WHO, Geneva.
[118] World Bank (2004). Memorandum of the President of the International Development Association and the International Finance Corporation to the Executive Directors on a World Bank Group Second Joint Interim Strategy Progress Report for the Federal Republic of Nigeria.
[119] World Health Organization (2010). Rapid advice: Revised WHO principles and recommendations on infant feeding in the context of HIV.2009.Available at: http://whqlibdoc.who.int/publications/2009/9789241598873_eng.pdf.Accessed Aug 11, 2010.
[120] Yashioka MR, Schustack A (2001). Disclosure of HIV status: cultural issues of Asian patients. *AIDS Care STDs, 15:77-82.*
[121] Yusuph H (2005). Prevalence of HIV infection, in TB patient in Nguru, North Eastern Nigeria. *Sahel Medical Journal,* 8(3):65–67.
[122] Zohoun A, Lafia E, Houinato D, Anagonou S (2004). Risk of HIV-1 or 2 infections associated with transfusion in Benin. *Bull Soc Pathol Exot; 97(4):261-264.*

10

Prevention Strategies for HIV Infection Risk Reduction Among Hispanic/Latino Adolescents

Diana M. Fernández-Santos, Wanda Figueroa-Cosme,
Christine Miranda, Johanna Maysonet,
Angel Mayor-Becerra and Robert Hunter-Mellado
Universidad Central del Caribe, School of Medicine
Puerto Rico

1. Introduction

Adolescence is defined as a "period of development characterized by biological, cognitive, emotional and social reorganization with the ultimate goal of adapting to the cultural expectations of becoming an adult" (Lerner & Steinberg, 2004, p. 16). It is also a developmental period associated with sexual debut as well as risk taking practices. Adolescents are in a stage of experimentation and exploration, and in a search of their sexual identity. The use of alcohol and other drugs enhances sexual arousal and performance, increments impulsive risk decision making, and may function as a stimulus for sensation seeking. These factors may synergistically increase the probability of unsafe sexual practices and illicit drug use (*National Institute on Alcohol Abuse and Alcoholism* [Robles 2004). Despite HIV prevention efforts during the past decade, teenagers represent one of the fastest growing groups of newly HIV-infected persons. Sexual transmission accounts for most cases of HIV during adolescence.

The physiological, psychological, and social–cultural changes that take place during the adolescence period places this group of young individuals at higher levels of risk to get infected with HIV. These factors contribute to the increment of the newly acquired HIV infection seen among adolescents in developing and developed countries.

Hispanic/Latino adolescents have presented a high incidence of HIV infection for many years. Several research studies have examined the risk factors and scenarios among this group and have developed HIV prevention strategies to lessen HIV infections. Most of these studies have been evaluated within Hispanic/Latino populations residing in the United States. It is relevant to validate and confirm these observations in other countries around the world. However, it is important to develop and test interventions that are directed to address HIV infections among other Hispanic/Latino countries.

This chapter describes and analyzes the HIV epidemiology, HIV-related risk factors, and prevention strategies for Hispanic/Latino adolescents based on a literature review and our experience with "A Supportive Model for HIV Risk Reduction in Early Adolescent" (ASUMA Project). We will also discuss future implications for the development of strategies to address HIV prevention for Hispanic/Latino adolescents.

2. Epidemiology of HIV infection among Hispanic/Latino adolescents

The Human Immunodeficiency Virus (HIV) is a retrovirus transmitted by contact with blood and other body fluids usually via risky behavioral practices incurred during sexual activities, intravenous drugs use, and in the past with the administration of blood products. In 2008, an estimate of 33.4 million people, in which 2.1 million were children under 15 years old, were living with HIV worldwide (Joint United Nations Programme on HIV/AIDS [UNAIDS] & World Health Organization [WHO] 2009).

Teenagers represent one of the fastest growing groups of newly HIV-infected persons. In 2008, a global estimate of 430,000 new HIV infections occurred among children under the age of 15 (UNAIDS & WHO, 2009). Despite the number and extent of HIV preventive strategies, young people accounted for about 40% of all new adult HIV infections worldwide. (UNAIDS & WHO, 2009). For the vast majority of individuals, sexual relations begin in adolescence, in which the use of illicit drugs and alcohol function as mediators in the adolescents' engagement in sexual risky behaviors.

Until 2008, Latin America occupied the third position in HIV prevalence, accounting for 2 million persons living with HIV/AIDS (UNAIDS & WHO, 2009). UNAIDS and WHO (2009) reported an increase in the number of newly infected children from 6,200 children in 2001 to 6,900 children in 2008. The modes of HIV transmission varied according to the geographic location and the individual's social and cultural backgrounds. Men who have sex with men (MSM) is the predominant transmission mode in North and Latin America, Central and Western Europe, and Oceania; while heterosexual transmission is the highest transmission mode in Africa, Guyana, and in some countries in Central America and the Caribbean (Wilson, Wright, Safrit, & Rudy, 2010).

The Centers for Disease Control and Prevention (CDC, 2008) estimated that 1,106,400 adults and adolescents were living with HIV in the United States at the end of 2006. As of 2009, an approximate of 4.8% (551,455 cases) of the 1,108,611 AIDS cases in the U.S. were adolescents between the ages of 13 and 24 years (CDC, 2009). From 2006 to 2009, an increase in the number of HIV infections among adolescents and young adults living in the U.S. was reported (Centers for Disease Control and Prevention [CDC], 2009). In 2009, most HIV infections and the highest HIV infection rate (36.9 per 100,000 persons) were among persons aged 20 to 24 years (CDC, 2009). For the same year, the incidence rate of HIV infection in the group between 15 and 19 years in the U.S. increased from 9.6 per 100,000 in 2006 to 12.0 per 100,000 (CDC, 2009). Similarly, the incidence rates in the group between 20 and 24 years increased from 28.2 per 100,000 in 2006 to 36.9 per 100,000 in 2009 (CDC, 2009). On the other hand, the rates of adolescents and young adults with AIDS diagnosis increased from 1.9 to 2.2 per 100,000 in the age group between 15 and 19 and from 7.7 to 9.7 per 100,000 in the group 20 to 24 between the years 2006 and 2009 (CDC, 2009).

The CDC Youth Risk Behavior Surveillance System (YRBSS) conducted a survey among junior and high school students from public and private schools in the U.S. mainland and its territories. The 2009 survey results reported that 46.0% of U.S. junior and high school students had sexual intercourse; and among those, 34.2% reported being sexually active during the three months prior to the survey (CDC, 2009). The survey also revealed that twenty-one percent of sexually active students drank alcohol or used illegal drugs before their last sexual intercourse (CDC, 2009).

Furthermore, the number of Hispanic/Latino living with an AIDS diagnosis in the United States and its territories (including PR) increased since 1996 and continued over years until

2008 (CDC, 2008). Hispanic/Latino living in the U.S. had the second highest HIV infection rate in 2008 (CDC, 2008). Specifically, Puerto Rican born females and male adults held the second and third positions of HIV infections in the U.S. respectively. According to the 2009 YRBSS, Hispanic/Latino students, had the second highest prevalence of having sexual intercourse (49.1%), of which 14.2% reported having four or more partners during their lifetime, only preceded by African American students (CDC, 2009).

Until March 2011, the Puerto Rico HIV/AIDS Surveillance Office reported 43,100 cumulative HIV/AIDS cases in Puerto Rico where 50 cases were among adolescents aged 13 to 14 years old and 19,549 (45%) were among adolescents and young adults aged 15-34 years old. This fact indicates that many of these young adults were infected during adolescence since the median incubation between the HIV infection and AIDS diagnosis ranges between 4 to 10 years. In PR, the highest HIV modes of transmission are intravenous drug use (IDU) (46%) followed by heterosexual contact (27%) and men who have sex with men (MSM) (23%) (Puerto Rico HIV/AIDS Surveillance, 2011). Robles et al. (2007) reported an early age of sexual initiation among Puerto Rican adolescents at age 15 (26.8%), where the proportion of sexually active adolescents nearly doubled from elementary to intermediate school and from intermediate to high school.

In general, the adolescent population is a growing vulnerable age group at risk of acquiring the HIV virus. For this reason, future studies with special emphasis on prevention to reduce the HIV/AIDS morbidity and mortality should be conducted.

3. Factors related to HIV infection among Hispanic/Latino adolescents

Several factors related to HIV infection among adolescents have been studied using an ecological approach. In Hispanic/Latino adolescents, few studies had been performed involving the nature of the interplay between individual, family, and social factors in a synergistic manner to decrease HIV infection among them.

3.1 Individual factors

Papalia and Wendkos (1997) define adolescence as a transition period of development between childhood and adulthood. This developmental stage fluctuates between ages 12 and 19 years. Biologically, adolescent's immature reproductive and immune systems make them more vulnerable to infection by various STI pathogens (Cates, & McPheeters, 1997; as cited in Sales, & DiClemente, 2010, p. 2). Offer and Offer (1974) found that one third of adolescents had difficulty facing unexpected events and frequently came back to immature behaviors and were displeased during difficult times. Adolescents frequently use alcohol, cannabis, or tobacco. Recently a new drug known as ecstasy has emerged. Drugs provoke un-inhibited effects in human behavior. Some of the published explanations for the high transmission rates of STI in adolescents include the use of oral contraceptives. That results in unprotected sex, a feeling of invulnerability towards STI, the presence of a non-susceptible belief, and the desire for sensation seeking.

3.2 Sensation seeking

Sensation seeking is a personality factor that could have an important role in HIV risk behavior. Sensation seeking focuses on the need for new and varied experiences through un-inhibited behavior, these include dangerous activities, a non-conventional lifestyle, and a rejection of monotony (Zuckerman, 1979; Zuckerman 1971). Few studies have demonstrated the relationship between high-risk behavior and sensation seeking among adolescents. Romer & Hennessy (2007) reported that sensation seeking increases adolescent risky behaviors such as the use of alcohol, tobacco, or other drugs. Martin (2002) found that sensation seeking mediates the relationship between pubertal development and drug use in adolescent's males and females. Arnett (1990) found a significant relationship between high sensation seeking scores and sexual relationships without contraception among 145 adolescents in Atlanta. Also, some studies have found a relationship between sensation seeking and alcohol consumption among high school students (Clapper et al., 1994) and first year college students (Johnson & Cropsey, 2010). Erikson (1968) presented a way to understand young people needs in relation to their society. He developed the psychosocial developmental theory, defining seven developmental stages. Adolescence is the stage of identity versus confusion. The most important question in this developmental stage is who am I? Having an identity involves making deliberate decisions related to occupation, sexual orientation, and life philosophy.

Adolescents with high sensation seeking are more receptive to intense or novel stimuli, which make them more likely to engage in HIV risk behaviors (Donohew, Palmgreen, Zimmerman, Harrington, & Lane, 2003; Zucherman, 2007). Zuckerman (2003) affirmed that imparting information alone or using scare tactics are not effective for preventing risky behavior in adolescents with high sensation seeking. Also, Donohew et al. (2003) and Zuckerman (2003) recommended incorporating strategies that enhance self-esteem through cognitive and behavioral interventions to help mediate impulsive decision-making and sensation seeking. These strategies teach adolescents skills to resist peer pressure and to exert self-control (e.g. critical thinking and positive decision making). According to Donohew et al. (2003) and Zuckerman (2003) using sensational messages are effective to capture the attention of adolescents with high sensation seeking; such as messages that are "novel, creative, unusual, complex, emotional, graphic, unconventional, fast paced, and suspenseful, with intense sound, hard-edged music and visual effects" (Zucherman, 2006, p. 216).

3.3 Self-esteem

Self-esteem has proven to be a predictor of risk behaviors (e.g. smoking initiation and alcohol use) in adolescents and adults, which predispose them to poor physical health (Birndorf, Ryan, Auinger, & Aten, 2005 as cited in Figueroa, Miranda, Fernandez, Maysonet, & Ramon, 2010, p. 37). Researchers found that Puerto Rican boys were more likely than girls to report high self-esteem in all grades (8th, 10th and 12th) ($p < 0.001$) (Figueroa, et al., 2010). In grade eigth, 39.2% of boys versus 27.4% of girls reported high self-esteem. Factors common to both - boys and girls- included positive family communication at baseline self-esteem measurement (Figueroa, et al., 2010). An adolescent with low self-esteem can be more exposed to peer pressure than an adolescent with adequate self-esteem. A longitudinal study followed over two years was conducted with seventh grade students, revealed that boys with higher self-esteem were 2.4 times more likely to initiate intercourse, while girls with higher self-esteem were more likely to remain virgin than those with lower self-esteem who were 3 times more likely to initiate intercourse (Sumter, Bokhorst, Steinberg, Westernberg as cited in Figueroa et al., 2010). Low self-esteem, psychological distress, sexual abuse, and depression also place many adolescents at risk to engage in STI/HIV associated sexual behaviors (DiClemente et al., 2001; Shrier, Harris, Sternberg, & Beardslee, 2001; Shrier, Harris, & Beardslee, 2002; Spencer, Zimet, Aalsma, & Orr, 2002; Parrillo, Freeman, Collier, & Young, 2001; as cited in DiClemente et al., 2008, p. 598).

3.4 Invulnerability

Adolescents believe that they are invincible from disease, accidents, and death (Hochhauster, 1988). Also, adolescents rely more on peer networks and are more concerned with immediate risks than with long term risks. Mason, Olson, and Parish (1988) indicated that adolescent's attitudes towards risk behaviors often include the denial of any chance of contamination and the adoption of the belief that they are invulnerable. Peltzer (2001) found that the behavioral factors that influence HIV risk among high school seniors in South Africa were attitudes towards the use of condom as well as feeling invulnerable to HIV/AIDS. Since many adolescents do not perceive themselves at risk for HIV infection, they engage in sexual and drug use behaviors that put them at risk not only for HIV infection, but also for unwanted pregnancies, and sexually transmitted infections (Kipke et al., 1990). Hingson et al. (1990) consistently found that even though most adolescents have some information about HIV/AIDS; they still engage in risky sexual behavior. Although adolescents typically perceive HIV as a severe disease, a great deal of variability exists regarding individual perception of susceptibility (DiClemente et al., 2008). Studies have suggested that adolescents who perceive that they are at risk for STIs/HIV tend to engage in less risky sexual behavior than those who do not have these perceptions (Boyer, Shafer, Wibbelsman, Seeberg, Teitle, Lovell, 2000; Sieving, Resnick, Bearinger, Remafedi, Taylor, Harmon, 1997; Zimet, Bunch, Anglin, Lazebnik, Williams, Krowchuck, 1992; as cited in DiClemente, Crittenden, Rose, Sales, Wingood, Crosby, Salazar, 2008, p. 598).

3.5 Risky behaviors

Alcohol and drug use have been identified as the most important predictors for STDs and HIV infection among high school students; both have strong effects in the age of sexual debut (Schafer et al., 1991). According to a study by the American Federation of AIDS Research (2001), sexual behavior of young people is highly influenced by the use of alcohol and drugs, which in turn negatively affects their decision-making skills and ultimately their behavior. As previously cited, the CDC (2010) reported that 21.6% of adolescents had drunk alcohol or had used drugs before their last sexual intercourse (YRBS, 2010). Kraft and Rise (1999) found a relationship between alcohol consumption and sexual behavior among adolescents. A recent study showed that young people with substance abuse problems are more likely to engage in risky sexual behaviors during adolescence and continue in risky sexual behaviors while substance problems persist (Tapert et al., 2001). Among adolescents surveyed in New Zealand, alcohol misuse was significantly associated with unprotected intercourse and sexual activity before age 16 (Fergusson & Lynnskey, 1996). Forty-four percent of sexually active teenagers in Massachusetts said they were more likely to have sexual intercourse if they had been drinking and 17 percent said they were less likely to use condoms after drinking (Strunin & Hingson, 1992). Similar results have been found among Hispanic/Latino adolescents. As previously published, HIV risk behavior (e.g. alcohol use, drugs use, and/or sexual intercourse) was measured among Puerto Rican early-adolescents enrolled in the ASUMA project at baseline. Researchers found that none of them reported illicit drug use, 26.3% and 1.2% reported alcohol use and sexual intercourse at some point in their lives, respectively (Fernandez et al., 2008). Latinas are 2.8 times more exposed than non-Latina whites to give birth at ages 15-19. Overall, Latinas have the highest pregnancy rate and birthrate among all ethnic groups in the U.S.. Although Latina women initiate sexual intercourse at later ages than non-Latinas, they are less likely to use contraceptives once they start having sex (Stoneas cited in Deardorff, Tschann, Flores, & Ozer, 2010, p. 23). Female virginity was positively associated with women's nonuse of condoms, rather than consistent use, during the first month of their current relationship" (Deardorff et al., 2010). In males, "the importance of satisfying sexual needs increased with the numbers of lifetime and recent sexual partners and with inconsistent condom use in the first month of their relationship" (Deardorff et al., 2010).

3.6 Lack of HIV/AIDS knowledge

A lack of HIV/AIDS knowledge and inaccurate information are factors that lead to infection with HIV (Alpabio, Asuzu, Fajemilehin, & Ofi, 2008 as cited in Figueroa et al., 2010). A study among Puerto Rican high school students found low HIV/AIDS knowledge and HIV risk behaviors (Mojorele, Brook, & Kachienga as cited in Figueroa et al., 2010). Another study performed in a sample of 7th grade students from Puerto Rico, found that they did not have enough knowledge about transmission modes and preventive behaviors (Morrison et al., 2007 as cited in Figueroa et al, 2010).

3.7 Family factors

Lescano et al. (2009) identified a set of family cultural factors that have been linked to adolescent risk behavior, these are: acculturation, religiosity, HIV knowledge and sexual communication, gender role and sexual socialization, and parental monitoring practices.

3.8 Communication

Some studies have demonstrated inadequate HIV/AIDS communication between parents and adolescents. In a study conducted in a neighborhood with high HIV seroprevalence, researchers found that parents overestimate how much they talk about HIV with their children (Krauss et al., 1997). Latino youth that talks with their parents about sex, engage in less sexual activity and are less likely to become pregnant (Adolph, Ramos, Linton, & Grimes, 1995; Gilliam et al., 2007). Parent-adolescent communication with adolescent females reduces sexual risk behavior (DiClemente et al., 2001). Open discussion with parents can help postpone sexual activity, protect them from engaging in risky behaviors, and support the healthy sexual socialization of youth (Leland & Barth, 1993). These findings demonstrate the importance of involving parents in HIV prevention efforts directed to adolescents.

As cited by Dancy et al. (2006), mothers often do not have the correct information to assist their daughters in developing risk-reduction behaviors. The same was reported in the qualitative study with African American females performed by Aronowitz et al. (2007) were mothers admitted that it is uncomfortable to talk about sex with their daughters. In another study by Meneses et al. (2006), Latino and Asian mothers demonstrated the highest levels of discomfort and infrequent communication about sex. Lefkowitz (2007) exposed that conversations between parents and adolescents about sexuality are often difficult for both.

This represents a barrier to communicate openly about sexuality and consequently their daughters may receive less prevention information.
DiClemente et al. (as cited in Figueroa et al., 2010) suggested that adolescents that perceived positive family support, family closeness, parental monitoring and parent-adolescent communication are less likely to perform risky sexual behaviors (as cited in Figueroa et al., 2010). Moreover, a study conducted in Puerto Rico by Robles (2007) found that adolescents whose parents reported poor or little communication, monitoring, or control over their children were almost three times more likely to engage in early sexual activity (Robles et al., 2007 as cited in Figueroa et al., 2010).

3.9 Social factors

The trend towards peer linkage is high at this stage. Many adolescents start using drugs by curiosity or by peer pressure. The peer group is critical to an adolescent's emotional development and teenagers prefer each other's company to that of their parents. Risk-taking is seen as a way of coping with normal developmental tasks such as exploration, achieving autonomy (Lavery, Siegel, Cousins, & Rusovits, 1993; Millstein & Igra, 1995) and those difficulties that adolescents face when making decisions (Furby & Beyth-Marom, 1992). Peer pressure can be a negative force in the lives of adolescents, often resulting in their experimentation with tobacco, alcohol, illegal drugs and sexual relations. An adolescent with low self-esteem could be more exposed to negative peer pressure than an adolescent with adequate levels of self-esteem. Peer pressure affects the early onset and prevalence of sexual behaviors (Romer et al., 1994). A national representative phone survey among 510 teens between the ages of 12 to 17 found that 83% of males and 89% of females reported that their peers felt an element of extrinsic pressure when asked on sex and relationships; and 41% of males and 31% of females reported that they personally face pressure when it comes to sex and relationships (SIECUS, 2000).

4. HIV prevention among adolescents

Many studies have identified several risk factors associated with multiple problem behaviors (Biglan, Brennan, Foster & Holder, 2004). Various HIV risk reduction strategies for adolescents have been performed in the United States to mediate biological, cognitive, social, and emotional factors (Biglan et al., 2004). Biglan et al. (2004) stated that effective interventions should address multiple problem behaviors according to the following factors: (1) individual level factors such as mood disorders, anxiety, impulsivity, hyperactivity, attention problems, and early aggression; (2) family level factors such as: absence parental problem solving skills, inconsistent discipline and monitoring, and barriers of parent-adolescents communication; and (3) social level factors such as violence, drug and alcohol use and smoking, social stigma, discrimination, lack of health services and public policy to enhance HIV risk reduction strategies and programs.

4.1 Evidence-based interventions

HIV evidence-based interventions are "behavioral, social, and structural interventions that are relevant to HIV risk reduction have been tested using a methodologically rigorous design, and have been shown to be effective in a research setting" (CDC, 2003). Evidence-based interventions employ several cognitive, social, behavioral, motivational, humanistic and/or existential psychodynamic theoretical models to address the core components of each intervention. Evidence-based interventions have to be implemented exactly as intended and within a context similar to the original intervention. If they are to be adapted and tailored to a different target population the core elements of the intervention need to be maintained. (Dworkin et al., 2008; McKleory et al., 2006; Rebchook et al., 2006; Rohrbach et al., 2006; Stanton et al., 2005 as cited in Rotheram-Borus et al., 2009). However, some community interventionists reject the replication with fidelity of an evidence-based program because they tend to customize their programs based on the community needs (Rotheram-Borus et al., 2009).

Kim et al. (1997) and Rotheram-Borus et al. (2009) evaluated and recommended a set of common factors that should be included in the design of effective HIV prevention programs for adolescents: (1) using a theoretical framework to address behavioral change; (2) focusing on the community and/or cultural aspects and issues of target population; (3) including coping skills (e.g., cognitive, affective an behavioral skills) training; (4) addressing environmental barriers; (5) providing skills and tools to support positive community healthy actions. Advocates for Youth (2003, 2006) identified several evidence based programs; known as "Programs that Works." These programs can be accessed through the CDC and the Diffusion of Effective Behavioral Interventions websites (CDC, 2010). Rotheram-Borus et al. (2009, p. 391-394) identified common principles which should be included for effective adolescent HIV prevention interventions program's goals. These include the following:

1. Develop adolescent positive self-esteem. Positive self-esteem and emotion can enhance the adolescent's ability to resist negative peer pressure and to promote self-care.
2. Provide accurate facts. Accurate information can increase HIV/AIDS knowledge and helps them understand common myths and faulty assumptions.
3. Evaluate options and consequences. Develop adolescent's skills by providing them with strategies to make informed decisions.
4. Commitment to change. Reinforce vulnerability recognition by reinforcing personal commitment for acting safely through community active participation.
5. Plan ahead and be prepared. Prepare adolescents with coping skills and avoidance of risky situations by enhancing critical thinking and communication skills.
6. Practice self-control. Enhance self-control skills that will allow the control of self-emotional states and increment the recognition of situations that might trigger the lack of control.
7. Teach exciting alternatives to avoid high-risk sexual activity.
8. Teach them how to negotiate. Provide them with guidance to enhance verbal and non-verbal negotiation skills and express their desires by enhancing self-care, self-esteem, and positive relationships.
9. Focus on their freedom to choose. Interventions should focus on the development of each adolescent's freedom to choose for themselves, thus providing them with skills to set voluntary limits that will help them protect their health.
10. Act to help others protect themselves. Enhance their responsibility to value and protect their peers.

Several evidence-based interventions were designed and tested among Hispanic/Latino adolescents by using multiple educational strategies (e.g., role play, demonstration, workshops, video/music, projects, simulation, practice, scientific research, assignment, small groups discussion) and were delivered in school (Villaruel, Jemmott, & Jemmott, 2006) or community settings (McGraw et al., 2002). The majority of these interventions focused on enhancing adolescents HIV knowledge, self-esteem, emotion and motivational factors, problem solving and decision making skills, autonomy, impulse control and self-control, critical thinking, effective communication and negotiation, social responsibility, values and norms (McGraw et al., 2002; Rotheram-Borus et al., 2009; Villaruel et al., 2006). Some of these theoretical constructs were used to design interventions for reducing HIV risk related behavior among Hispanic/Latino adolescents (e.g., risky sexual behaviors) such as intentions: subjective norms, and control beliefs. These interventions resulted in a reduction of sexual activity, a reduction in the number of sex partners, a reduction of unprotected sex, and an increase in condom use s (Gallegos, Villarruel, Loveland-Cherry, Ronis, & Zhou, 2004; Villarruel et al., 2006). Other interventions have constructed its core components on the socioecological theoretical model, which can be used to address individual, family, community, organizational, and societal determinants of HIV risk infection among Hispanic/Latino adolescents (Biglan et al., 2004). The eco-developmental model along with other social and behavioral models was used to design a Hispanic/Latino adolescent's intervention in Mexico (Gallegos et al., 2006). The outcome of the intervention showed a significant intention of condom use among adolescents in the experimental group (Gallegos et al., 2006). Some effective interventions have incorporated and evaluated the effectiveness of parental involvement as a mean to improve HIV risk practices among their children. Recent research has found high intervention attendance and retention rates among parents involved in HIV prevention programs with their children (Wyckoff et al., 2003). Also, Wyckoff et al. (2003) affirmed that parents are interested and willing to participate in activities directed to improve adolescent communication. Perrino et al. (2000) highlighted the significant contribution of families in the prevention of HIV risk behaviors among adolescents. In recent studies among Hispanic/Latino adolescents in the United States and Mexico, parent-adolescent communication was found to reduce sexual risk behaviors among adolescents (Gallegos et al., 2004; Villaruel, et al., 2006). These findings demonstrate the importance of involving parents in HIV prevention efforts directed to this group. However, many viable organizations and programs are not embracing the inclusion of parents in their HIV prevention efforts because they perceive a degree of difficulty to reach parental involvement. Adolescents recognized the importance of parental advice however they need to feel freedom to choose for themselves. Furthermore, adolescents tend to reject the imposition of adults.

According to DiClemente and Crittenden (2008) successful programs are based on theoretical or conceptual frameworks and are specifically tailored to a particular subgroup of a population. DiClemente and Crittenden (2008) affirmed that interventions that focus on the development of self-concept, self-esteem, and social competency skills are also effective to reduce risky sexual behaviors among adolescents. Addressing risky behaviors at earlier ages must be proven to be effective in modifying these behaviors and ultimately in preventing diseases (DiClemente & Crittenden, 2008). The development and implementation of culturally appropriate instruments and interventions are key elements in the prevention of disease for a specific population. Rios-Ellis et al. (2008, p.456) affirmed that designing culturally and linguistically appropriate interventions to reduce HIV/AIDS in Hispanic/Latino adolescent "requires an understanding of the many different perceptions, attitudes, and behaviors that deeply influence the Latino culture and values." Effective

Latino HIV interventions must employ culturally appropriate methods such as the story-based "fotonovelas" and "radionovelas" (Rios-Ellis et al., 2008). Spanish speaking trainers should conduct interventions at schools, community health centers, and community-based organizations in order to positively improve adolescent's HIV knowledge, which in turn lessens HIV/AIDS risk behaviors among Hispanic/Latino adolescents (Rios-Ellis et al., 2008). Also, program developers must address Hispanic/Latino cultural values such as familialism, "machismo", "marianismo", allocentrism, fatalism, power distance, personal space, time orientation, and gender roles" to design interventions that promote Hispanic/Latino parent-adolescent communication as a mean for HIV/AIDS risk reduction strategy among adolescents (Benavides, Bonazzo, & Torres, 2006, p. 92). Villarruel et al. (2006) designed and implemented the "Cuídate!" intervention which addresses Hispanic/Latino cultural factors including familialism and "machismo" to enhance abstinence and condom use in this ethnic group living in United States.

Herbst et al. (2007) examined the overall efficacy of HIV behavioral interventions to reduce HIV/AIDS or STI's risk behaviors among Hispanics in United States and Puerto Rico. Herbst et al. (2007) meta-analysis documented several effective HIV interventions which increase the likelihood of preventive HIV measures such as increasing condom use, reducing unprotected sex, reducing multiple sex partners, and reducing infection of STI. Table 1 shows a list of evidence-based interventions directed for Hispanic/Latino adolescents. Interventions are gender specific since significant differences were seen when targeted interventions for male or females were done as compared to interventions with both genders. (Herbst et al., 2007). According to Gómez and Marín (1996), Marín (2003), and Marín and Gómez (1997), Hispanic females and males might experience discomfort when discussing sexual matters in the presence of persons of the opposite gender.

4.2 A Supportive Model for HIV Risk Reduction in Early Adolescent (ASUMA): A HIV prevention model for Puerto Rican/Hispanic adolescents

In Puerto Rico we developed, implemented and evaluated an HIV prevention intervention for early adolescents known as "A Supportive Model for HIV Risk Reduction in Early Adolescent" (ASUMA) after a need assessment was performed. ASUMA followed a cohort of 135 Puerto Rican early-adolescents in public and private middle schools (7th to 9th grade). The schools were randomly divided into two groups; interventional and control groups. We developed a theoretical framework that focused on the adolescent's developmental factors and parental support as a mean to reduce HIV risk behaviors. ASUMA's theoretical framework is shown in Figure 1. We theorize that an increase in parental support and adolescent's self-efficacy will lessen HIV risky sexual behaviors. On the other hand, the intervention also focuses on decreasing adolescent's sensation seeking, on increasing HIV/AIDS knowledge and positive attitudes towards HIV/AIDS; which results from a decrease in the sense of invulnerability. Self-esteem among early-adolescents will increase by a decrease in negative peer pressure" (Fernandez et al., 2008).

The ASUMA curriculum design used pragmatic strategies to facilitate the process of active learning including group discussion, audiovisual aids, debates, brainstorming, patient testimony, reflection, and critical thinking (Fernandez et al., 2009). The intervention was centered on the cultural aspects of the target population and in the development of coping skills strategies. We conducted a total of eight workshops that provided information regarding the developmental and HIV risk related factors. The curriculum also included reinforcement of the knowledge and skills gained (Fernandez et al., 2009; Fernandez et al.,

Program	Middle School	Senior high	Gender	Delay Initiation of Sex	frequency of sex	No. of sex partners	monogamy	Incidence of unprotected sex	use of condoms	use of contraception	used of sexual health care/ treat compliance	incidence of STIs	No. or rate of teen pregnancy/ birth
1.AIDS prevention[a]		X	Both			X	X		X			X	
2.Get Real about AIDS[b]		X	Both			X			X				
3.Postponing sexual Involvement[c]	X		F	X						X			
4.Reach for Health Community[d]	X		Both	X	X				X	X			
5.Reducing the risk[e]		X	Both	X				X		X			
6.Safer Choices[f]		X	Both	X				X	X	X	X		
7.Teen Outreach Program[g]		X	Both										X
8.Adolescents Living Safely[h]	X	X	Both		X	X			X				
9.California's Project[i]	X	X	Both	X						X			X
10.Carrera Program[j]	X	X	F	X					X	X	X		X
11.¡Cuidate![k]		X	Both		X	X		X	X				
12.Poder Latino[l]		X	Both	X		X							
13.HIV Risk Reduction[m]	X	X	F			X		X				X	
14.Project Save[n]		X	F			X	X	X			X	X	
15.TLC[o]	X	X	Both			X		X			X		

Source: Adapted from Advocates for Youth (2008).
[a]AIDS Prevention for Adolescents in School; [b]Get Real about AIDS; [c]Postponing Sexual Involvement: Human Sexuality & Health Screening; [d]Reach for Health Community Youth Services; [e]Reducing the Risk; [f]Safer Choices; [g]Teen Outreach Program; [h]Adolescents Living Safely: AIDS Awareness Attitudes & Action; [i]California's Adolescent Sibling Prevention Project; [j]Children's Aid Society-Carrera Program; [k]¡Cuidate!; [l]Poder Latino: A Community AIDS Prevention Program for Inner-City Latino Youth; [m]HIV Risk Reduction for African American and Latina Adolescent Women ; [n]Project Save- Sexual Awareness for everyone; [o]TLC: Together Learning Choices

☐ School-Based Program ☐ Community –Based Program ☐ Clinic-Based Program

Table 1. Effective programs for Hispanic/Latinos in USA: Impact on Adolescents' Risk for Pregnancy, HIV & STI Programs

2008). We also, conducted a workshop for parents of early adolescents from the intervention group. This workshop was adapted from Cornell University's program "Talking with Kids about AIDS: A Program for Parents and Other Adults Who Care" (Fernandez et al., 2009; Fernandez et al., 2008). The parent's workshop focused on developing effective communication skills with kids and to increase parents HIV knowledge and attitudes. The early adolescents from the control group only received written educational materials about HIV/AIDS prevention (Fernandez et al., 2009; Fernandez et al., 2008). ASUMA was found to decrease HIV risk behaviors among early adolescents at the Puerto Rico school setting (Fernandez et al., 2008).

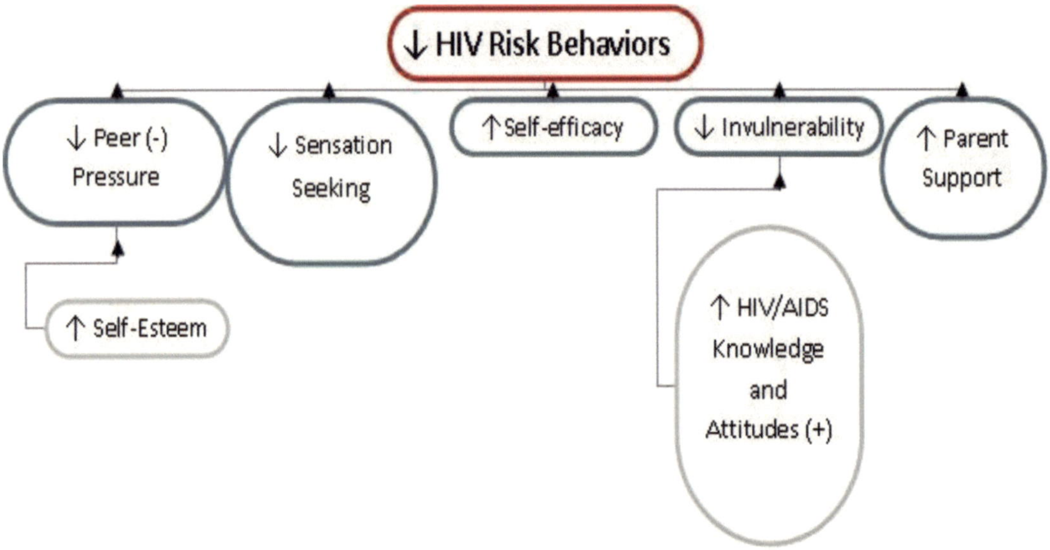

Fig. 1. ASUMA theoretical framework.

5. Barriers for HIV prevention among Latino adolescents

Researchers have identified several barriers that hinder adolescent's modification of HIV/AIDS risk behaviors among Hispanic/Latino adolescents. These barriers have been classified as individual, cultural, and environmental factors.

5.1 Individual factors

Lack of knowledge is the principal individual barrier (Paniagua, O'Boyle, & Wagner, 1997; Sheadlin, Decena, Oliver-Velez, 2005; as cited in CDC, 2010). Many Hispanic/Latino adolescents' risky behaviors are due to the lack of adequate sexual information when making health decisions. Adolescent's misconceptions of HIV/AIDS information hinder their ability to protect themselves (The Henry J. Kaiser Family Foundation, 2002). It is well known that parent-adolescent communication about sexuality correlates with sexual risk taking. Adolescents who receive more sexual information from their parents are less likely to engage in early risky sexual behavior (Benavides, Bonazzo, & Torres, 2006). Hispanic/Latino adolescents feel invulnerable from getting pregnant or getting infected with STIs or HIV (Guttmacher et al., as cited in Benavides et al., 2006). On the other hand, Hispanic mothers do not talk about sex, HIV, or condoms frequently with their children because they considered these topics disrespectful, distasteful, or indicative of promiscuity (Tinsey et al., 2004 as cited in Gomez and Marin, 1996). Other individual factors that should be considered are the invulnerability, the seeking of sensations, self-esteem, and peer pressure. Vulnerable groups are at risk for HIV infection (Henry J. Kaiser Foundation, 2002). Adolescent girls and young women are prone to have unprotected sex. On the other hand, young men who have sex with men (MSM) perceived stigma and discrimination from others. The intravenous drug users present high invulnerability and sensation seeking. Furthermore, orphaned children of HIV/AIDS parents are at higher risk of abuse and school dropout. Lastly, homeless or sexually exploited children are at risk of prostitution, trafficking, and child pornography (Henry J. Kaiser Foundation, 2002).

5.2 Cultural factors

Other important factors to be considered are cultural barriers such as poverty, values, norms and beliefs, and native tongue. According to the U.S. Census Bureau (2010) most of the Hispanic/Latino in the U.S. and Puerto Rico live in poverty. In U.S. limited literacy in English language and acculturation among immigrants represents a barrier to obtaining HIV prevention information (Organista, Carrillo, & Ayala, 2004; as cited in CDC, 2010, p. 1299).

5.3 Environmental factors

Often adolescents face multiple barriers for seeking and receiving STI and HIV testing and treatment due to lack of health insurance, money to pay, transportation, discomfort with facilities and services designed for adults, and concerns about their confidentiality (CDC, 2004; as cited in Sales, & DiClemente, 2010).

6. HIV prevention strategies for Latino/Hispanic adolescents

By strategies we refer to intended actions for enhancing health behaviors (CDC, 2003, as cited in McKenzie, Neiger, Thackeray, 2009). Interventions directed to adolescents' individual factors should focus on addressing this stressful period, which is characterized by hormonal, physical, emotional, psychological, and cognitive changes (Alloy, Zhu, & Abramson, 2003, p. 171). Alloy, Zhu, and Abramson (2003, p. 171) emphasized the need to discuss identity, self-image, independence, and intimacy issues among adolescents. Another major issue with adolescents is depression. Depression is associated with impairment in school behavior, academic performance, and family and social relationships (Gotlib, Lewinsohn, & Seeley, 1995; as cited in Alloy, Zhu, & Abramson, 2003). Adolescents with depression may display antisocial, histrionic, dependent, and passive-aggressive personality disorders that could increase HIV risk behaviors in early adulthood (Alloy et al., 2003, p.172). The Cognitive Behavioral Therapy is used to prevent depression in a school setting, by using workshops for teaching effective problem solving and encourage positive activity, to reduce stressful environmental skills among adolescents (Alloy et al., 2003). Furthermore, Alloy et al. (2003) explain that the incorporation of parents in this process can provide greater benefits for the adolescents.

6.1 Strategies to address social level factors

Achieving culturally and linguistically appropriate interventions to reduce HIV/AIDS in Hispanic/Latino adolescent requires comprehending many different perceptions, attitudes and behaviors that are deeply influenced by Latino cultures and values (Rios-Ellis, 2008, p.

456). Herbst et al. (2007) recommended that effective interventions to reduce the likelihood of the sexual risk behaviors among Hispanics should include "non-peer deliverers", should avoid peer outreach method, be at least 4 sessions, address barriers to condom use or sexual abstinence, attempt to change peer norms, include condom use practice skills, and improve problem solving skills.

7. The future of HIV prevention among Hispanic/Latino adolescents

Teenagers represent one of the fastest growing groups of newly HIV-infected persons. Despite HIV prevention efforts during the past decade, the number of HIV-positive persons has increased consistently around the world. Many of these HIV infections occur during adolescence. This developmental stage is often associated with sexual debut as well as risk taking. Adolescents are a high-risk group because: (1) they are in an age of sexual identity exploration; (2) are impulsive and might be influenced by peer group; and (3) do not feel vulnerable and are unable to foresee long-term consequences (McCormic, 1989). In the process of seeking independence, they frequently reject their parent's authority. They want to know their parents opinion, but insist in making their own decisions. The trend towards peer relationship is higher at this stage. Often they seek peer support due to a lack of parental support, which might lead to risky situations like having sex and/or using alcohol or drugs. Parental support will improve their HIV knowledge and positive attitudes, self-efficacy, and self-esteem while decreasing invulnerability, sensation seeking, and negative peer pressure. Moreover it is highly recommended to study individual, family, and social factors that put adolescents in HIV risk situations according to their cultural scenarios.

Effective programs should include the following aspects: (1) a theoretical/conceptual framework; (2) cultural aspect of the target population; (3) training in coping skills; (4) multiple strategies to impact the diversity of different types of intelligence (5) pragmatic activities to capture adolescents attention; (6) parental participation; (7) the duration of the intervention; (8) principles of community based participatory research methods; (9) the facilitator role; (10) individual or small group sections; (11) measurements of multiple factors based on the theoretical/conceptual framework; (12) an evaluation plan; and (13) a results dissemination plan. On the other hand, successful school based programs should involve pragmatic/experiential classroom and homework activities, such as small group discussions, games or simulations, brainstorming, role-playing, written exercises, verbal feedback and coaching and parental involvement (Kirby, 2002; Fernandez, 2009). Health professionals, parents, teachers, and other relatives could assume the role of facilitators to enhance the adolescent's interest in inquiring about healthier lifestyles. They should also assist in providing techniques to cope with normal developmental situations.

Programs that provide knowledge and coping skills to avoid negative behaviors should focus on abstinence, condom use, avoidance of alcohol use and illicit drug use in the specific stage of adolescence development. Program evaluation should be performed at all phases of the intervention. This action will advance the development of culturally HIV prevention efforts directed to Hispanic/Latino adolescents. Promoting collaborative efforts between government, private and community-based organizations will maximize the resources directed to enhance individual, family, and community HIV prevention services. These efforts will support the development of public health policies.

8. Acknowledgement

We want to acknowledgement Mr. Aitor González, Mr. Raul O. Ramón, Mr. Eduardo Santiago, Mrs. Magaly Torres and Mr. Gerónimo Maldonado for their support in the completion of this chapter. This manuscript was sponsored by the NIH Grant Number G12RR-03035 (UCC-RCMI Program) from the National Center for Research Resources and the Puerto Rico Clinical and Translational Research Consortium (PRCTRC) Grant Number U54RR026139-01A1. Its contents are solely the responsibility of the authors and do not necessarily represent the official views of the NIH.

9. References

Advocates for Youth. (2008). Sex Education and Other Programs that Work to Prevent Teen Pregnancy, HIV & Sexually Transmitted Infections, In: *Science and Success, Second Edition*, April 29, 2011, Available from: http://www.advocatesforyouth.org/publications/ScienceSuccess.pdf

Advocates for Youth. (2006). Additional Sex Education and Other Programs that Work to Prevent Teen Pregnancy, HIV & Sexually Transmitted Infections, In: *Science and success, Supplement 1*, April 29, 2011, Available from: http:www.advocatesforyouth.org/publications/sciencesuccess_supplement.pdf.

Akpabio, I., Asuzu, M., Fajemilehin, B., & Ofi A. (2009). Effects of School Health Nursing Education Interventions on HIV/AIDS-Related Attitudes of Students in Akwa Ibom State, Nigeria. *Journal of Adolescent Health*, Vol.44, No.2, (February 2009), pp. 118-123

Benavides, R., Bonazzo, C., & Torres, R. (2006). Parent-Child Communication: A Model for Hispanics on HIV Prevention. *Journal of Community Health Nursing*, Vol.23, No.2, (Summer 2006), pp. 81-94

Biglan, A., Brennan, P., Foster, S., & Holder, H. (2004). Helping Adolescents at Risk: Prevention of Multiple Problem Behaviors. New York: The Guilford Press.

Center for Disease Control, & AED Center on AIDS & Community Health. (October 2010). Diffusion of Effective Behavioral Interventions Project. 05.05.2011, Available from: http://www.effectiveinterventions.org/Libraries/General_Docs/10-1022_DEBI_overview_factsheet.sflb.ashx.

Centers for Disease Control and Prevention. (February 2011). HIV Surveillance Report, 2009,. 04.05.2011, Available from: http://www.cdc.gov/hiv/surveillance/resources/reports/2009report/pdf/2009SurveillanceReport.pdf

Dancy, B., Crittenden, K., & Talashek, M. (2006). Mother's Effectiveness as HIV Risk Reduction Educators for Adolescent Daughters. *Journal of Health Care for the Poor and Undeserved*, Vol.17, No.1, (February 2006), pp. 218-239

DeNavas-Walt, C., Proctor, B., Smith, J., & U. S. Census Bureau. (2010). Income, Poverty, and Health Insurance Coverage in the United States: 2009. Report P60-238. Washington, D. C.: U. S. Government Printing Office.

DiClemente, R., Crittenden, C., Rose, E., Sales, J., Wingood, G., Crosby, R., & Salazar, L. (2008). Psychological Predictors of HIV-Associated Sexual Behaviors and the Efficacy of Prevention Interventions in Adolescents at Risk for HIV Infection: What Works and What Doesn't Work? *Psychosomatic Medicine*, Vol.70, No.5, pp. 598–605

Fernandez, D., Figueroa, W., Gomez, M., Maysonet, J., Rios-Olivares, E., & Hunter, R. (2008). Changes among HIV/AIDS knowledge among early adolescents in Puerto Rico. *Ethnicity and Disease*, Vol.18, No.2, (Spring 2008), pp.146-150

Fernandez, D. (2006) Predictores de riesgo hacia la infección por VIH en estudiantes de escuela superior en Puerto Rico. Unpublished doctoral dissertation, Interamerican University of Puerto Rico, Rio Piedras, 2006

Fernandez-Santos, D., Figueroa-Cosme, W., Gomez, M., Maysonet-Cruz, J., Miranda-Diaz., C., Sepulveda, M., Rios-Olivares, E., & Hunter-Mellado, R. (2010). Changes in Developmental Factors and HIV Risk Behaviors Among Early Adolescents in Puerto Rico. *Ethnicity and Disease*, Vol.20, No.1, (Winter 2010), pp.122-126

Figueroa-Cosme, W., Fernandez-Santos, D., Miranda-Diaz, C., Maysonet-Cruz, J., & Ramon, R. (2010). Gender Differences in Social and Developmental Factors Affecting Puerto Rican Early-Adolescents. *Boletin Asociacion Medica de Puerto Rico*, Vol.102, No.3, pp. 35-44

Ford, K., & Norris, A. (1991). Urban African-American and Hispanic Adolescents and Young Adults: Who Do They Talk to About AIDS and Condoms? What Are They Learning? *AIDS Education and Prevention*, Vol.3, No.3, (Fall 1991), pp. 197–206

Gallegos, E., Villarruel, A., Gomez, M., Onofre, D., & Zhou, Y. (2007). Research Brief: Sexual Communication and Knowledge Among Mexican Parents and Their Adolescent Children. *Journal of the Association of Nurses in AIDS Care*, Vol.18, No.2, (March-April 2007), pp. 28-34

Herbst, J., Kay, L., Warren, F., Lyles, C., Crepaz, N., & Marin, B. (2007). A Systematic Review and Meta-analysis of Behavioral Interventions to Reduce HIV Risk Behaviors of Hispanics in the United States and Puerto Rico. *AIDS Behaviors*, Vol.11, No.1, (January 2007), pp. 25-47

Joint United Nations Programme on HIV/AIDS (UNAIDS). (2010). UNAIDS Report on the Global AIDS Epidemic, In: *Global Report*, April 29, 2011, Available from: http://www.unaids.org/documents/20101123_GlobalReport_em.pdf

Kim, N., Stanton, B., Li, X., Dickersin, K, & Glabraith, J. (1997). Effectiveness of the 40 Adolescent AIDS-Risk Reduction Interventions: A Quantitative Review. *Journal of Adolescent Health*, Vol.20, No.3, (March 1997), pp. 204-215

Kirby, D. (December 2002). HIV Transmission and Prevention in Adolescents, In: *HIV InSite Knowledge Base Chapter*, April 29, 2011, Available from: http://hivinsite.ucsf.edu/InSite?page=kb-07-04-03#S6X)

Lefkowitz, E., Sigman, M., & Au, T. (2000). Helping Mothers Discuss Sexuality and AIDS with Adolescents. *Child Development*, Vol.71, No.5, (September-October 2000), pp. 1383-1394

Lescano, C.M., Brown, L.K., Raffaelli, M., & Lima, L (2009). Cultural Factors and Family-Based HIV Prevention Intervention for Latino Youth. *Journal of Pediatric Psychology.* pp. 1-12.

McCormic, K. (1989). *Reducing the Risk: A School Leader's Guide to AIDS Education* (Vol.2), National School Boards Association, ISBN 10: 0883641704, Alexandria, Virginia

McGraw, S., Smith, K., Crawford, S., Costa, L., McKinlay, J., & Bullock, K. (2002). The Effectiveness of Poder Latino: A Community-Based HIV Prevention Program for Inner-City Latino Youth (Unplished manuscript).

McKenzie, J., Neiger, B., & Thackeray, R. (2009). *Planning, Implementing, and Evaluating Health Promotion Programs: A Primer.* (5th ed.), Pearson Education, Inc., ISBN-10: 032149511X, San Francisco, California

Meneses, L., Orrell-Valente, J., Guendelman, S., Oman, D., & Irwin, C. (2006). Racial/Ethnic Differences in Mother-Daughter Communication About Sex. *Journal of Adolescent Health,* Vol.39, No.1, (July 2006), pp.128-131

Miller, K., Levin, M., Whitaker, D., & Xu, X. (1998). Patterns of Condom Use Among Adolescents: The Impact of Mother-Adolescent Communication. *American Journal of Public Health,* Vol.88, No.10, (October 1998), pp. 1542-1544

Miller, K., & Whitaker, D. (2001). Predictors of Mother-Adolescent Discussions About Condoms: Implications for Providers Who Serve Youth. *Pediatrics,* Vol. 108, No.2:E28

Morojele, N., Brook, J., & Kachieng'a, M. (2006). Perceptions of Sexual Risk Behaviours and Substance Abuse Among Adolescents in South Africa: A Qualitative Investigation. *AIDS Care,* Vol.18, No.3, (April 2006), pp. 215-219

Papalia, D., & Wendkos, S. (1997). *Psicología del desarrollo. De la infancia a la adolescencia,* pp. 564-568, McGraw-Hill, México

Perrino, T., Gonzalez-Soldevilla, A., Pantin, H., & Szapocznik, J. (2000). The Role of Families in Adolescent HIV Prevention: A Review. *Clinical Child Family Psychology,* Vol.3, No.2, (June 2010), pp. 81-96

Rios-Ellis, B., Frates, J., Hoyt, L., Dwyer, M., Lopez-Zetina, J., & Ugarte, C. (2008). Addressing the Needs for Access to Culturally and Linguistically Appropriate HIV/AIDS Prevention for Latinos. *Journal of Immigrant Minority Health,* Vol.10, No.5, (October 2008), pp. 445-460

Robles, R., Matos, T., Reyes, J., Colon, H., Negron, J., Calderon, J., & Shepard, E. (2007). Correlates of Early Sexual Activity Among Hispanic Children in Middle Adolescence. *Puerto Rico Health and Sciences Journal,* Vol.26, No.2, (June 2007), pp.119-126

Rotheram-Borus, M., Ingram, B., Swendeman, D., & Flannery, D. (2009). Common Principles Embedded in Effective Adolescent HIV Prevention Programs. *AIDS Behaviors,* Vol.13, No.3, (June 2009), pp.387-398

Spencer, J., Zimet, G., Aalsma, M., & Orr, D. (2002). Self-Esteem as a Predictor of Initiation of Coitus in Early Adolesdcents. *Pediatrics,* Vol.109, No.4, (April 2002), pp. 581-584

Sumter, S., Bokhorst, C., Steinberg, L., & Westenberg, P. (2009). The Developmental Pattern of Resistance to Peer Influence in Adolescence: Will the Teenager Ever Be Able to Resist? *Journal of Adolescence,* Vol.32, No.4, (August 2009), pp. 1009-1021

The Henry J. Kaiser Family Foundation. (May 2002). The Global Impact of HIV/AIDS and Youth. *HIV AIDS Policy Fact Sheets.*

Vanoss-Marin, B., & Gomez, C. (1997). Latino Culture and Sex: Implications for HIV Prevention. In J. Garcia & M. Zea (Eds.), Psychological interventions and research with Latino populations (pp. 73–93). Boston: Allyn & Bacon.

Villaruel, A., Jemmott, J., & Jemmott, L. (2006). A Randomized Controlled Trial Testing and HIV Prevention Intervention for Latino Youth. *Archives of Pediatrics and Adolescent Medicine,* Vol.160, No.8, (August 2006), pp. 772-777

Wilson, C., Wright, P., Safrit, J., & Rudy, B. (2010). Epidemiology of HIV Infection and Risk in Adolescents and Youth. *Journal of Acquired Immune Deficiency Syndromes*, Vol.54, Suppl.1, (July 2010), pp. S5-6, ISSN 1525-4135

Wyckoff, S., Miller, K., Bush, T., Forehand, R., & Arnistead, L. (2003). Myths and Misconceptions Surrounding HIV Prevention Interventions Targeting Parents, *Proceedings of 2003 National HIV Prevention Conference*, Atlanta, Georgia, USA, July 27-30, 2003.

Youth Risk Behavior Surveillance System. (2007). Trends in the Prevalence of the Sexual Behaviors, April 29, 2011, Available from: http://www.cdc.gov/1HealthyYouth/yrbs/pdf/yrbs07_us_sexual_behaviors_trend.pdf

Zuckerman M. (1994). *Behavioral expression and biosocial bases of sensation seeking,* Cambridge University Press, ISBN 0521432006, Massachusetts, USA

11

Missed Opportunities for HIV Infection Prevention in HIV Sero-Discordant and X-Negative Concordant Couples

Netsanet Fetene[1] and Dessie Ayalew[2]
[1]*IMA World Health SuddHealth MDTF-BPHS Project*
[2]*IFHP-Pathfinder Amhara Project*
[1]*South Sudan*
[2]*Ethiopia*

1. Introduction

Most HIV-1 transmission in Africa occurs among HIV-1-discordant couples (in which one partner is HIV-infected while the other one is not) who are unaware of their discordant HIV-1 serostatus (1). HIV-negative individuals living in stable HIV-discordant partnerships are twice as likely to get infected with HIV as those living in concordant HIV-negative relationships (2). The percentages of couples in HIV sero-discordant relationships range from 5 to 31% in the various countries of Africa (3). In a study conducted at five sub-Saharan HIV affected countries, at least two thirds of the infected couples are discordant couples. Between 30 and 40 percent of the infected couples are couples where the female partner only is infected (4). The risk of HIV transmission through sexual intercourse from an HIV-positive male to an HIV-negative female was estimated as being around 1 in 10 for less than 10 unprotected contacts and around 1 in 4 after 2,000 contacts(5). What accounts for high rates of HIV-1 discordance and why some individuals remain uninfected despite repeated sexual exposure to HIV-1 is unknown. StudyingHIV-1-discordant couples may contribute to understanding correlates of HIV-1 immunity and acute infection. Additionally, HIV-1-discordant couples are an important population for prevention efforts. Consequently, HIV-1-discordant couples are increasingly viewed as a valuable source of participants for HIV vaccine and prevention trials(6).

Misconceptions about discordance are widespread among clients and counselors. Common explanations includes: the concept of a hidden infection not detectable by HIV tests, belief in immunity, the thought that gentle sex protected HIV-negative partners. Such explanations for discordance reinforce denial of HIV risk for the negative partner within discordant couples and potentially increases transmission risk. Couples identify negotiation of sexual relations as their most formidable challenge. Discordant couples represent a critical risk group and improved counseling protocols that clearly explain discordance, emphasize high risk of transmission, and support risk reduction are need(7)

The need for conception seems to lead couples to HIV infection. HIV sero-discordant couples with strong desire for childbearing have a dilemma of risking HIV infection or infecting their spouse. The main reasons for wanting a child include: ensuring lineage continuity and posterity, securing relationships and pressure from relatives to reproduce. However the challenges include: risk of HIV transmission to partner and child, lack of negotiating power for safer sex, failure of health systems to offer safe methods of reproduction(8).Natural conception could now be considered a possible alternative for HIV sero-discordant couples, as long as complete suppression of viremia with HAART is achieved in the infected partner (9). Overall, it would appear that unprotected sex for the purposes of conception in couples with the HIV-infected man not taking HAART carries a risk of HIV transmission to the female of no more than 8%(10).Given that both sexual and perinatal transmission of HIV is directly correlated with the level of viral replication, being almost negligible in patients with undetectable viremia, HAART should be given to the infected sero discordant partner to minimize the risk of transmission (11). For ethical issues raised by (assisted) reproduction for HIV positive men and women, recommendations are made concerning methods avoiding HIV transmission in the couple and to their offspring. It is concluded that, if certain precautions are taken, medical assistance to reproduction of HIV positive people is ethically acceptable. For the time being, only cases of serodiscordant couples should be considered (12).

Provision of HCT to family members of people in HIV care and treatment programs is an important intervention for case finding and prevention of HIV transmission, especially among discordant couples (13). Interventions targeting sero-discordant couples should explore contraceptive choices, the cultural importance of children, and partner communication (3). Family planning and HIV prevention programs should integrate counseling on "dual method use", combining condoms for HIV-STI prevention with a long-acting contraceptive for added protection against unplanned pregnancy (14).

In a study conducted on 535 African American HIV serodiscordant, 72% of couples reported that one or both had child sexual abuse histories. These findings underscore the heightened emotional vulnerability, and STI and HIV transmission risk taking practices, associated with sexual abuse. Adult and child sexual abuse histories among couples should be assessed to better understand how these histories may contribute to couples dynamics and risk-taking practices(15).A Study on women from three AIDS information Centres in Uganda showed alcohol abuse by the male partners was an important factor in the experience of sexual violence among the women. Their experiences evoke different reactions and feelings, including concern over the need to have children, fear of infection, desire to separate from their spouses/partners, helplessness, anger and suicidal tendencies. HIV counseling and testing centers should be supported with the capacity to address issues related to sexual violence for couples who are HIV discordant (16). Male-focused and couple-focused testing and counseling programs appear to be effective in reducing risky sexual behaviors in heterosexual couples, even if one or both partners have received testing and counseling services previously (17).

New developments in therapy, counseling, testing technology, and new trends in the HIV epidemic have increased the value of partner notification. In general, between 50 and 100% of notified partners will accept counseling about their HIV exposure, and will agree to have an HIV test (18).Such partner referral for HIV testing through partner notification reduces the missed opportunities for HIV infection prevention.

Missing the ways to prevent factors contributing for HIV infection in negative concordant and sero-discordant couples gradually lead to a new infection to the partner as well as to the other family members. The primary aim of this study is to identify factors contributing to missed opportunities for HIV infection prevention in HIV discordant and x-negative concordant partners before they become concordant HIV positive couples.This study is designed to uncover the degree and the reason why missed opportunities in HIV infection prevention occur in sero-discordant, concordant and x-sero negative concordant (who was HIV negative concordant and later became sero-discordant or positive concordant) couples.

2. Methods

A qualitative study methodology was applied both on HIV discordant (including x-negative concordants) and HIV positive concordants living together. Confidential in-depth interview

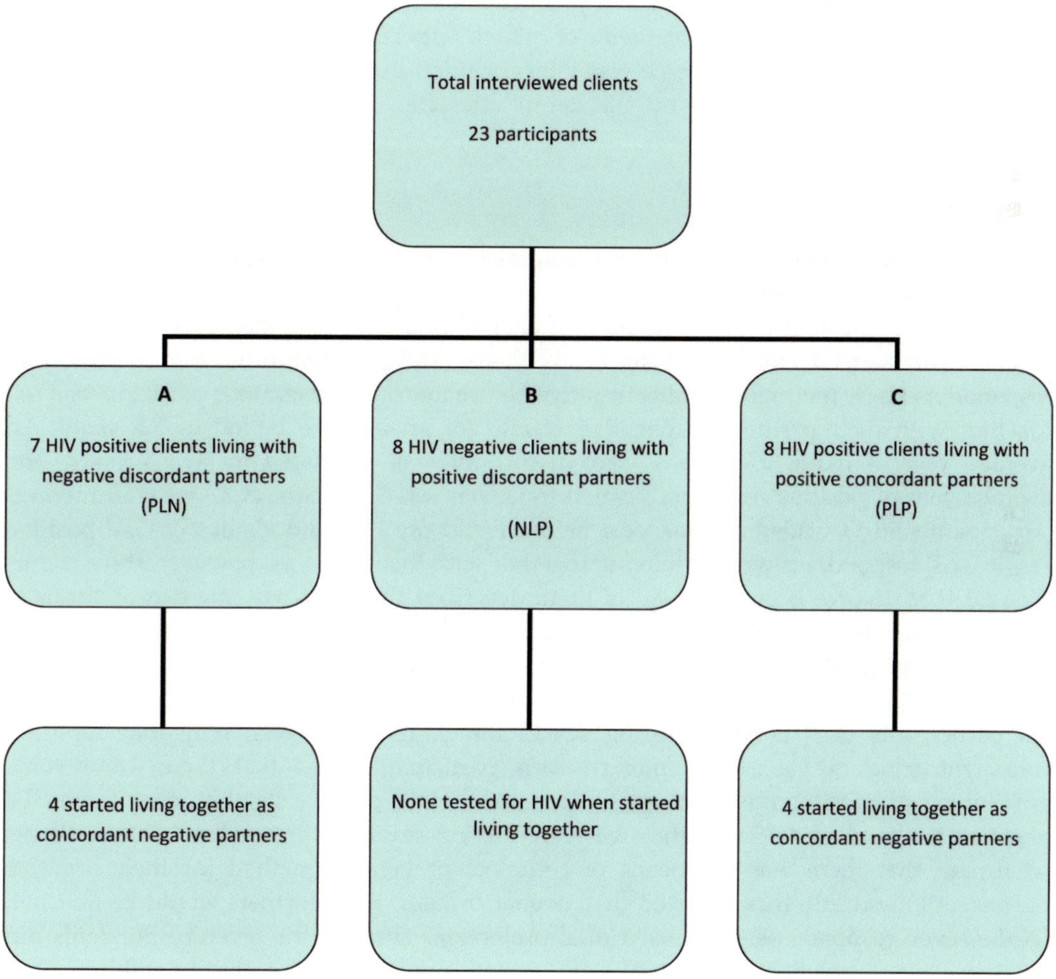

Fig. 1. Schematic representation of participants involved in the study

of HIV positive concordant and HIV discordant living clients was conducted till saturation reached. Data was collected at Mekdim clinic (a local NGO clinic mainly devoted to treating clients living with HIV), Bahirdar office, Ethiopia. Twenty three interviewed clients were categorized to three cohorts to exhaustively exploit the views from different perspectives. Category 1: Positive clients living with negative partner (PLN). Seven clients involved in the interview of this category.Catagory2: Negative clients living with positive partner (NLP). Eight clients involved in this group. Category 3: Positive clients living with positive clients(PLP) .Eight clients participated in this group. Data collection was conducted by three health professionals who were trained on VCT and ART to ensure the data quality. To maintain clients' privacy and confidentiality, clients were interviewed in separate room and clients name were not included during the tape recorded in-depth interview.
The collected data was transcribed and categorized in to the five themes. Initially four themes were identified for the analysis of the findings: the theme of timing in HIV test result awareness, the theme of knowledge and practice of clients in HIV prevention, the theme of reasons for seroconversion and the theme of missed opportunities in preventing exposure to HIV infection. One emergent theme was later included during the analysis of the finding: the theme of future intention on marital relationship. The data was analyzed using qualitative(STATA) software

3. Result

3.1 HIV positive clients living with negative discordant partners (PLN)

Seven HIV positive clients who were living with negative sero discordant partners were interviewed in the first group. The time of clients' knowledge of their HIV test result as positive was ranged from one year to six years. The majority (four out of seven) of respondents knew their blood status negative before marriage. These four participants lived together with their partners as negative couple for an average period of 3.5 years. An average year of living together as sero-discordant was calculated to be 2.4 years. The average year of positive result notification to clients was 3.28 years. A 38 years old female participant said "I waited for one year before I told my husband about my HIV positive result ".All respondents were still living together with their partners; however, three clients thought that divorce is eminent. All of them described that they had one extra partner in their life. Three participants did not satisfy with their sexual relationship because the sexual relationship is usually occurred infrequently; sometimes once in every month. The duration may be much longer due to severe illness like tuberculosis.
Six participants used condom during sexual intercourse. However, only four reported consistent condom use. Five among seven participants said that there were some possibilities of infecting their partners. A 35 years old HIV positive client living with an HIV negative husband said "Sometimes we were having sex without condom". Three clients confirmed that there was no means of complete prevention method for their negative partner. As the result, they believed that, sooner or later, their partners would be infected. Of the seven respondents, three used dual protection. Three of the seven respondents did not know the prevention methods of HIV transmission from the mother to children. Two participants had already given birth of two children (one HIV positive and one HIV negative children). Four out of seven participants wanted to have children in future but

feared that their babies might be infected. A 42 years old male participant said "We wanted to have children but we feared the virus transmission to them". The majority of patients (five) had started ART drugs with an average duration of one year and six months.

3.2 HIV negative clients living with positive discordant partners (NLP)

Eight HIV negative clients who were living with positive sero discordant partner were interviewed in another group. These HIV negative clients had been living together with their HIV positive partners for an average of five years. All of the interviewed clients didn't know their blood status until they tested together. As the result, none of the participants were able to describe if they were both negatively lived together. Similarly, sero status check up was done once in their life with an average time of five years. All negative partner who lives with positive partner preferred not to be tested any more. A 38 old man said "Once I tested negative, I did not want to be tested again for fear the result might affect my life". Three participants partner have shared their positive result immediately while four participants partner talked lately after duration ranged from 2 months to two years. Six said that they had one or more partners before their marriage. Six participants said that they were satisfied with their sexual relationships with their partner. However, three of the eight HIV negative discordant who had been living with positive partners were decided to divorce a moment later. The five participants also said that they had interested to discontinue the marriage.

Half of the eight HIV negative participants living with positive partner did not know how to prevent HIV infection. Only one participant responded the couple used condom consistently during their sexual intercourse. Three participants didn't know the availability of the reduction of HIV infection transmission from mother to child. Half of the participants wanted to have children. However, fear of positive children was their challenge. Three participants believed that their blood status would never turn out to be positive .A 34 years old male HIV negative respondent living with discordant wife said "How can I become positive?, my blood remains negative".

3.3 HIV positive clients living with positive partners (PLP)

Eight HIV positive clients living with HIV positive partner as concordant were interviewed in separate group. The average year of knowing sero status as positive for both couple was calculated to be 4.1 year. Four out of eight participants had a negative test results by the time of marriage. However, all study participants knew their positive result at the same time with their partner during the couple counselling. Five participants lived together with their partner as HIV negative couple for period ranged from one year to 20 years. A 37 years old man said " I had lived with my wife for about 20 years as HIV negative". However, as most interviewed clients were not tested while living together, they did not know if they lived as discordant couple for sometimes. For couples who tested together and proofed they were both positive, the sequence of seroconversion among the couple was difficult to sorted out putting the couples in dilemma. A 35 years old female said "We had similar results of living with HIV on the same day; therefore, it was difficult for us to say who was infected first". Three participants were not satisfied in their marital sexual relationship. Two participants had already thought of divorce because they believed that "it was difficult to live together persecuting each other all the time"

Three participants delayed the disclosure of their positive status to other family members by about one to two years of duration. Seven of HIV positive participants believed that their HIV infection easily could had been prevented if they took precautions and they condemned their past negligence. Five HIV positive clients living in concordance relationship said that they had other sexual partners out of their marriage. All of the study participants reported they were using male condom all the time they had sex with their positive partners. Two participants said that they used male condom and injectables as dual protection. Six participants knew the method of prevention from mother to child transmission.

Serial No.	Description		Positive Living with Negative partner(PLN)	Negative Living with Positive partner(NLP)	Negative Living with Positive partner(PLP)
1.	**Participant HIV status**		**Positive**	**Negative**	**Positive**
2.	**Total number interviewed**		**7**	**8**	**8**
3.	**Average age of participants**		**32.2**	**33**	**35.7**
4.	**Sex**	**Male**	**3**	**4**	**4**
		Female	**4**	**4**	**4**
5.	**Total average years of living together in marriage**		**5.75**	**5**	**6.5**
6.	**Time of HIV result seroconversion awareness(years)**		**3.3**	**4**	**4**
7.	**HIV serostatus of both couple before marriage as negative**		**4**	**unknown**	**5**
8.	**Participants who lack basic knowledge in HIV infection prevention**		**5**	**4**	**7**
9.	**Current regular and consistent condom use**		**4**	**1**	**8**
10.	**Use of dual protection**		**3**	**1**	**2**
11.	**Client/partner use of ART**		**5**	**6**	**7**
12.	**Belief in self/partner HIV infection while living as serodiscordant**		**5**	**5**	**NA**
13.	**Need of participants for children**		**4**	**4**	**2**

Table 1. Summary of result on missed opportunities in HIV sero discordant, positive concordant and x-concordant at Bahirdar Mekdim HIV/AIDS clinic, Ethiopia, Feb/2011

The majority of participants (six) did not want to have children. Two participants had already two children with both HIV positive result. Seven participants of HIV positive clients living with HIV positive partner had been taking ART. The average time since ART started was 3.5 years.

4. Discussion

4.1 The theme of timing in HIV test result awareness

The timing of HIV test result awareness of the participants' and/or the partners' positive result for all groups was less than five years (PLN=3.3yrs, NLP=5yrs, PLP=4yrs).This time was the duration since the couple became living either as discordant or concordant positive couple. Large proportion of interviewed participants knew their sero status as negative before they were married. Four out of seven HIV positive sero discordants lived sometimes as HIV negative concordants after their marriage with their recent partners (PLN=4/7).Five out of eight positive concordants Participants were both negative concordant at the time of their marriage (PLP=5/8).The important timing of living together as negative before becoming discordant positive was fairly long duration (PLN=3.3 years).

For HIV negative patients who were living together with HIV positive partners, they all knew their serodiscordance at the time of couple counselling. They were never tested before. This highly substantiates the importance of couple counselling in tracing such kind of serodiscordant married couples who has never tested before. However, failure of these clients to have their premarital HIV test result raises the concern of whether serodiscordancy was before or after the marriage. These group of clients were also not checked again once they were tested negative (average duration since tested was 5 years).The major reason for their not being tested then after and frequently was the fear of receiving positive result.

For HIV positive concordant clients who tested together as positive, the timing and origin of infection among the couples paused dilemma. Though the majority (five out of seven) started marriage tested as negative, the focus of infection among the couples remained unknown. This is highly linked with infrequent testing among the couples which negatively contributed for the inability to address the prevention methods within the available short sero discordance period among such couples (on average tested every 4.3 years). However, the majority of same couple had frequent HIV viral load test check-ups(every three to six months) after their HIV infection.

Three of the seven HIV positive interviewed sero discordant were women while four of the eight HIV negative living in serodiscordant were women. This shows proportion of male to female positive proportion among serodiscordant couples is almost similar which supports the finding stating women are as likely as men to be the index partner in a discordant couple (19).

4.2 The theme of clients HIV prevention knowledge and practice

The majority of the interviewed sero discordant participants in each groups lack the basic HIV prevention knowledge (PLN=5/7,NLP=4/8).The majority of participants living as positive concordant(PLP=7/8) said they lacked the basic HIV prevention knowledge by the time of their infection and regretted back of those occasions. The majority of respondents were not consistently and regularly using condoms (PLN=4/7,NLP=1/7,PLP=8/8).The consistent use of condom was low among the serodiscordant than concordant positive which risked the negative partners infection. Dual protection was universally low among all groups (PLN=3/7,NLP=1/7,PLP=2/8). The majority of the participants or their partners (for negative clients) were already on ART which may contributes positively for the clients living in discordance ((PLN=5/7,NLP=6/7,PLP=7/8). The majority of clients living in serodiscordant relationship believed that they would either infect their partner or be infected some time in future(PLN=5/7,NLP=5/8).

4.3 The theme of reasons for seroconversion

Large proportion of clients living in sero discordant relationship wanted to have children (PLN=4/7, NLP=4/8). This supports the study which showed 59% of the sero discordant participants desired to have children. The same study showed that the belief that serodiscordant partners wanted children was a major determinant of the desire to have children, irrespective of the HIV sero-status (20).The interest to have children was lower in HIV positive sero concordant clients; only two out of eight HIV positive concordant couple wanted children.

The fear associated with the risk of HIV infection to the negative partner as well as to the child was mentioned frequently for their desire not have children. Moreover, the majority from all groups lacked how to prevent the transmission of HIV from mother to child. Two HIV positive participants who were living with negative partner had already given birth of two children (one positive and one negative sero- status children).One negative male participant living with positive partner took the risk and had one HIV negative child. This type of occasion seems to support the idea which goes 'natural conception could now be considered a possible alternative for HIV sero discordant couples, as long as complete suppression of viremia with HAART is achieved in the infected partner' (11).

Multiple partner sexual relationship was common both in sero discordant and sero positive concordant before the seroconversion. All of the three groups, the majority described they have had extra marriage relationship before or after current marriage (PLN=5/7, NLP=6/8,PLP=5/8).Some participants were not satisfied with their sexual relationship because it was usually occurred infrequently, due to fear of infection and sometimes due to severe illness like tuberculosis. The majority of participants with HIV positive result reported that they enjoyed their sexual relationship and they usually practiced one to twice in a week. The infrequent use of condom predisposed the sero discordant couples with negative partner in further risk of infection. This result is consistent with the finding which stated that fear of transmitting the HIV to the sero negative partner is constant. Besides the fear, there are the difficulties to talk about the problem, to plan the future and to keep a satisfactory sexual life. Condom use does not seem to be an easily adopted practice (21).

HIV positive result disclosure remained a challenge to sero discordant partners. Four out of seven positive partners did not disclose their result immediately to their negative partner. They waited until 6 months to one year duration. Four HIV negative participants' partner were shared their partner positive results lately(duration ranged from two months to two years). Some participants from concordant positive partners delayed the disclosure of their positive status to other family members by about one to two years of duration. Such delay in HIV positive result disclosure has a negative impact in the prevention of the disease. Subsequently, a further missing of opportunities for HIV infection prevention occur.

4.4 The theme of missed opportunities in preventing exposure to HIV infection

From the total interviewed twenty three participants, fifteen were sero discordant clients and were lived for an average duration of 3.8 years with their partner in serodiscordant relationship. Discordant couples were living together for long period of time without using HIV infection prevention techniques. With few knowledge of HIV prevention and practices, discordant couples were missing the opportunities of preventing themselves as well as their partners from HIV infection. This result goes with the finding which showed partners in a negative serodiscordant relationship are at higher risk of HIV infection by not taking appropriate HIV transmission preventions techniques. (22).

A total fifteen HIV positive clients were interviewed. Nine of these HIV clients were married as negative. Their results became positive after lived for more than four years as negative partners. Had prevention of HIV infection intervention been made, these clients with their partners could have been saved from HIV infection. Such loss of opportunity is related to the finding which states HIV negative participants in sero concordant relationships view themselves at relatively low risk for HIV transmission and they make infrequent HIV test (22).Partner notification and referral for HIV test was delayed in most of the occasions of all group might have led to an increase in missed opportunity for prevention of further new infection. But, a study conducted to assess the outcome of partner notification showed that there is a high degree of compliance suggesting that at-risk groups are interested in obtaining information about their exposure and the options available for management provided that positive partners disclose their result (18).

The gap found in knowledge and practices of interviewed clients on HIV prevention was mainly linked to the missed opportunities by health professionals in addressing the issues while clients were in the health facilities.HIV transmission may be reduced among HIV discordant couples after initiation of ART due to reductions in HIV viral load and increased consistent condom us (11).Five of the 23(self or partner positive) clients were not on ART which increases the risk of infection.

4.5 The theme of future marital relationship

The majority of HIV positive client living together with a negative partner didn't want to think and discuss issues on future marital relationship or divorce. However, a good number of this group(three out of seven) think that divorce is inevitable. Almost all negative clients living with positive partner prefer divorce (three decided to recently divorce and five interested to discontinue the relationship).The future plan of living together in marital relationship looked stable among concordant HIV positive clients(six out of eight want to live together). However, some participants (two) mentioned their relationship would not continue because of continuous accusation of one another. A 38 years old male HIV positive client living with HIV positive partner said "it is difficult to live together persecuting each other all the time".

5. Conclusion

A large number of HIV sero discordant and x-sero negative concordant couples were living together for long period of time without using HIV prevention precautions. As the result, married or cohabiting couples started living together as HIV negative concordant have lost the opportunities of preventing HIV infection and became HIV serodiscordant and then HIV positive concordant. Factors contributing for missed opportunities for HIV infection prevention among sero discordant and x-sero negative concordant couples were found to be related to infrequent HIV testing, delayed HIV result notification to partner, lack of knowledge and practice onHIV prevention, the need for children and dissatisfaction in sexual and marital relationship.

6. Acknowledgment

We are highly grateful for the dedicated data collectors and all staffs of Mekdim Ethiopia, Bahirdar clinic, for their full collaboration while we conducted the study in the clinic. Without their assistance and group effort this study would have not been realized. Our sincere thanks goes to Mr.Menberu Getachew for reviewing and commenting on the semi-structured interview questionnaire and commenting throughout the study process. Finally, we highly acknowledge the contribution of Dr Belete Tafesse for his constructive comment till we completed the work of this study.

7. References

[1] Lingappa JR, Lambdin B, Bukusi EA, Ngure K, Kavuma L, et al (2008). Regional Differences in Prevalence of HIV-1 Discordance in Africa and Enrollment of HIV-1 Discordant Couples into an HIV-1 Prevention Trial. Plos ONE 3(1): e1411. Doi:10.1371/journal.pone.0001411

[2] Joseph K.B. Matovu Preventing HIV Transmission in Married and Cohabiting HIV-Discordant Couples in Sub-Saharan Africa through Combination Prevention. Current HIV Research, Volume 8 Issue 6 ; ISSN: 1570-162X

[3] Jolly B, Anna M, Frank K, Florence M, et al. My partner wants a child: A cross-sectional study of the determinants of the desire for children among mutually disclosed sero-discordant couples receiving care in Uganda. BMC Public Health. 2010; 10: 247.

[4] Damien de Walque. Discordant couples HIV infection among couples in Burkina Faso, Cameroon, Ghana, Kenya and Tanzania. Development Research Group, The World Bank: May 2006.

[5] Downs AM, De Vincenzi I. Probability of heterosexual transmission of HIV. Journal of Acquired Immune Deficiency Syndromes and Human Retro virology 1996; 11: 388-395.

[6] Guthrie BL, de Bruyn G, Farquhar C.HIV-1-discordant couples in sub-Saharan Africa: explanations and implications for high rates of discordancy. Curr HIV Res. 2007 Jul;5(4):416-29.

[7] Bunnell RE, Nassozi J, Marum E,etal. Living with discordance: knowledge, challenges, and prevention strategies of HIV-discordant couples in Uganda. AIDS Care. 2005 Nov;17(8):999-1012.

[8] Jolly B, Anna M, Frank K, Florence M, et al. The dilemma of safe sex and having children: challenges facing HIV sero-discordant couples in Uganda.

[9] Barreiro P, Castilla JA, Labarga P, Soriano V. Is natural conception a valid option for HIV-sero discordant couples? Hum Reprod. 2007 Sep; 22(9):2353-8. Epub 2007 Jul 19.

[10] J. T. Wilde. Conception in HIV-Discordant couples; Second Edition. Treatment of Hemophilia. April 2008 .NO 26.

[11] Pablo B, Jose Antonio C, Pablo L and Vincent S.Is natural conception a valid option for HIV-serodiscordant couples?.Human Reproduction Vol.22, No.9 pp. 2353–2358, 2007

[12] F.Shenfield , G.Pennings, J.Cohen,P.Devroey, B.Tarlatzis and C.Sureau.Taskforce 8: Ethics of medically assisted fertility treatment for HIV positive men and women. Human Reproduction Vol.19, No.11 pp. 2454–2456, 2004

[13] Were WA, Mermin JH, Wamai N, Awor AC, Bechange S, Moss S, Solberg P, Downing RG, Coutinho A, Bunnell RE. Undiagnosed HIV Infection and Couple HIV Discordance Among Household Members of HIV-Infected People Receiving Antiretroviral Therapy in Uganda. J Acquire Immune Defic Syndr. 2006 Sep; 43(1):91-5.

[14] Kristina G,Rob S,Yusuf A,etal Knowledge, Use, and Concerns about Contraceptive Methods among Sero-Discordant Couples in Rwanda and Zambia.Journal of women's health Volume 18, Number 9, 2009.

[15] The NIMH Multisite HIV/STD Prevention Trial for African American Couples Group.Prevalence of Child and Adult Sexual Abuse and Risk Taking Practices Among HIV Serodiscordant African-American Couples.AIDS Behav (2010) 14:1032–1044

[16] Donath E, Nataliya L, Pauline J , etal. Experience of sexual violence among women in HIV discordant unions after voluntary HIV counselling and testing: AIDS Care. 2009 November ; 21(11): 1363–1370.

[17] Roth DL, Stewart KE, Clay OJ,etal. Sexual practices of HIV discordant and concordant couples in Rwanda: effects of a testing and counselling programme for men. Int J STD AIDS. 2001 Mar;12(3):181-8.

[18] Kevin A. Fenton and Thomas A. HIV partner notification: taking a new look.AIDS 1997, 11:1535–1546

[19] Eyawo O, de Walque D, Ford N, Gakii G, Lester RT, Mills EJ.HIV status in discordant couples in sub-Saharan Africa: a systematic review and meta-analysis. Lancet Infect Dis. 2010 Nov;10(11):770-7.

[20] Jolly B, Anna M, Frank K ,et al my partner wants a child: A cross-sectional study of the determinants of the desire for children among mutually disclosed sero-discordant couples receiving care in Uganda.Beyeza-Kashesya et al. BMC Public Health 2010, 10:247.

[21] Camila M, Ana M.Analyzing the risk problem in couples with serodiscordance.Ciência & Saúde Coletiva, 13(6):1859-1868, 2008

[22] Lisa A. Eaton, Tessa V. West, David A. Kenny, and Seth C. Kalichman.HIV Transmission Risk among HIV Seroconcordant and Serodiscordant Couples: Dyadic Processes of Partner Selection. AIDS Behav. 2009 April ; 13(2): 185–195. Doi:10.1007/s10461-008-9480-3.

[23] Steven J, Makumbi, Frederick, et al. HIV-1 transmission among HIV-1 discordant couples before and after the introduction of antiretroviral therapy

12

Community Participation in HIV/AIDS Programs

Lawrence Mbuagbaw[1] and Elizabeth Shurik[2]
Centre for the Development of Best Practices in Health,
[1]Yaoundé
[2]Miami
[1]Cameroon
[2]USA

1. Introduction

The advent of the human immunodeficiency virus (HIV) in the last few decades has presented considerable challenges to health systems throughout the world. Many countries developed measures to combat the spread of the virus and the trends are improving, mostly due to the introduction of potent new combinations of medications, the development of effective prevention strategies and increased community awareness. These improvements would not have been possible without the mobilisation of communities around the world, who, recognising their vulnerability, have taken collective action to curb the propagation of HIV. The subsequent pages discuss the origins, development and components of community participation with respect to HIV, including examples of strong community participation initiatives.

2. What is community participation?

In order to achieve the ambitious goal of Health for All, in1978, World Health Organisation (WHO) and the United Nations Children's Fund (UNICEF) funded the International Conference on Primary Health Care (PHC) in Alma Atta, Kazakhstan. They pledged to provide basic health care for the entire world through the ingenious and comprehensive approach referred to as Primary Health Care (Werner & Sanders, 1997). The Alma Atta declaration emphasized the right and duty of communities to participate in the planning and implementation of their own health care. Apparently, strong community participation was a key element of the successful programs that led to the development of PHC principles. The previously existing but poorly recognised concept of community participation was recognised as the way forward for equitable health care.

The community participation model of health care is in many cases likened to "bottom-up" approaches and "grassroots" community action, in which the community is perceived as a third sector with the capacity to manage the more complex aspects of health care delivery historically handled poorly by the government (Botterill & Fisher, 2002). Most often, community initiatives precede the official national response to a problem.

Community participation in health can be defined along two fairly contrasting lines. It can be perceived as a movement in which the government and/or donors use community resources (i.e. land, labour, money) to meet the costs of providing health care. However, it can also be defined as a form of empowerment in which the community takes part in the decision-making process (Morgan, 1993).

The idea of community participation in health - also referred to as 'community involvement' or 'community mobilisation' - has inherited various meanings from different stakeholders who often use it for conflicting ends (Morgan, 1993; Olico-Okui, 2004). For the purposes of this book, community participation will be defined as all community contributions to prevent the spread of HIV and to improve the health care and quality of life of people living with HIV (PLHIV). The Joint United Nations Programme on HIV/AIDS (UNAIDS) recognises the following components as integral parts of community participation: raising awareness, prevention, policy and legal changes, alleviating impact, advocacy, care and support (UNAIDS, 1997).

3. Defining community participation in relation to HIV?

UNAIDS uses an all-encompassing definition of community, namely "a group of people who have something in common and will act together in their common interest" (UNAIDS, 1997). People who live together, work together or worship together belong to the same community. However, to better comprehend the need for a community to act together for their common good, it is imperative to consider exactly what the individuals have in common. In relation to HIV, it is the potential risk-factors affecting a community that determine its key characteristics. For example: people living in a village on a highway may be at higher risk for HIV due to unsafe sexual contact with truck drivers passing through. Sex workers are at a higher risk of contracting HIV by virtue of their profession. The practice of polygamy involves having multiple sexual partners, a known risk factor for HIV. Additionally, all these factors may be combined in one community, thus generating a complex situation for community medicine.

Under these circumstances, members of the community are affected, whether directly or indirectly, by the disease and should take part in deriving a solution. The way the community reacts to the disease is an important step toward developing prevention programs. Communities with high levels of stigma and discrimination create a challenging environment for initiating volunteer testing and counselling, care and support. On the other hand, in less judgmental communities it is easier to educate and empower community members and PLHIV. In other words, the community is the key to solving its own problems. A mobilized community is therefore one in which the members are aware of their vulnerability to HIV, are motivated to take action, have practical knowledge of their options to reduce their vulnerability, take action using personal resources, participate in decision-making and evaluation, all while assuming responsibility for successes and failures. Most importantly the community seeks external support when needed (UNAIDS, 1997).

4. HIV as a community illness

PLHIV are not islands off to themselves. They come from a community in which specific factors have exposed them to the virus. Children born to HIV-positive mothers represent but a link in a long chain of people who have carried and passed on the illness. The presence of an HIV-positive child usually implies that either his/her parents have HIV and/or a third party from whom the infection was contracted. Upon the demise of the parents, family members normally step in to take care of the child.

Thus, reducing vulnerability to HIV requires not only medical measures, but also social measures. For example, poor socio-economic status may reduce access to knowledge and barrier methods. Some cultural practices may limit women's ability to negotiate safer sex practices. The decimation of teachers in a community by HIV will affect the performance of students in that community. Lower levels of education will adversely affect the community. Likewise the loss of health workers to HIV or an increased burden of work due to care provided to PLHIV.

In some instances, PLHIV themselves are considered a community, and HIV activism usually stems from such communities. The control of HIV may require adapted methodologies to specific communities like commercial sex workers, men who have sex with men, medical personnel, etc.

It is becoming increasingly clear that HIV must be considered as a community problem, which needs to be solved using community-based solutions.

5. Community participation and HIV

Historically, health care projects with strong community involvement have been more successful, considering such bottom-up approaches often gain more acceptance by local populations than top-down, government-imposed solutions (Werner & Sanders, 1997). Generally speaking, and specifically in the case of HIV, countries most affected by the disease lack the financial and human resources needed to combat it. Not only did HIV decimate entire communities, creating a huge burden on the health system, it also wiped out health workers. Moreover, the spread of HIV is often linked to socio-cultural and behavioural factors that are particular to specific communities. The result is a problem that, in reality, can only be addressed within that community, by that community. Additionally, geo-political factors often slow the government response to HIV public health emergencies. The development and experimentation of new treatments and vaccines for HIV require community participation and, in many cases, community consent for necessary research.

Community participation in the response to HIV has been accepted as an essential element within health services and programs for a variety of reasons. First, HIV services have a much greater reach when stakeholder communities are involved in their design. Community contributions - in terms of money, material and manpower - can be mobilised to improve the lives of people both infected and affected by HIV. Reductions in vulnerability to HIV are achieved primarily through actions people take to protect themselves. Finally, the community has a right to be involved in decisions that affect their every-day lives (Morgan, 1993).

Community participation has played a central role in the fight against HIV since the onset of the epidemic. It has a positive effect on safer sex practices, social integration and identity (Ramirez-Valles, 2002).

6. Components of community participation in HIV

In this section, we will describe the various ways in which communities can participate in HIV programs. There are no hard lines between these components: communities of PLHIV can be involved in providing care, while also being at the forefront of activism and peer education.

6.1 Care

The already thin-stretched human resources for health in the countries most affected by HIV have been further taxed by the influx of critically and terminally ill patients into hospitals. As a result, additional hands-on-deck are required to take care of HIV patients. In-hospital care is often provided by family members and consists mostly of providing food, ensuring basic hygiene, waste disposal, bed making and the purchase of necessary medicines. Such arrangements carry their own risks, serving as another means of spreading HIV as lay people are not typically trained in the management and disposal of biological waste. However, if trained by health personnel, their efforts are invaluable.

One of the key pillars of HIV management is home-based care. This approach began as an initiative to take medication to patients who were too sick to come to the hospital themselves. It quickly spread beyond the provision of medications to cover activities such as counselling and training of family members. This activity is carried out by trained lay people often called community relay agents or community health workers. Over the years, their scope of work has become broader, including within its mandate HIV prevention and counselling for community members; educating the community on the need for testing; distribution of condoms; and social mobilisation. These community health workers operate under the supervision of regional health personnel. As the need to integrate tuberculosis and HIV services began to grow, community health workers also took part in identifying community members likely to have tuberculosis, advising them to seek medical help.

Even in countries with better human resources for health, community volunteers often supplement hospital care.

6.2 Research

In order to achieve high levels of relevance and validity, research projects testing new approaches in the prevention and treatment of HIV must be carried out in the communities for which the given intervention is intended. Although often overlooked, community participation is a key component of HIV research. Clinical trials often require approval from regulatory bodies like Ethics Committees (EC); Data Safety and Monitoring Boards (DSMB); and Institutional Review Boards, all of which include community representatives. In countries with a more developed research agenda, Community Advisory Boards (CAB) also exist. CABs, which are made up entirely of community members, play a role in determining the relevance and safety of research proposals as they affect the community.

Subjects of clinical research are an enormous community contribution to the advancement of science. Large numbers of people are recruited every day into HIV trials. These participants contribute to the development of rapid tests, vaccines, medication and behavioural interventions. Community involvement in HIV vaccine research is necessary for success, as it promotes better enrolment and retention in trials (ICASO, 2007).

6.3 Activism

HIV activists are community members who may or may not be infected with HIV and who promote equal rights and opportunities for PLHIV. They seek to empower PLHIV and decry situations and people that jeopardize their rights and dignity. They fight for the legal rights of PLHIV; availability and accessibility of testing and treatment services; and discourage risky behaviour among vulnerable groups (Senterfitt, 1998). Activists play an important role in changing legislation and policy that work to the disadvantage of PLHIV and vulnerable populations. Through activism and workshops with the medical community, they are able to negotiate for better and specially tailored services. They also contribute to the mitigation of stigma and discrimination by educating journalists to use more appropriate terminology when reporting on HIV-related issues. In many countries, stigma and discrimination against PLHIV are the key reasons that people give for refusing testing, medication and other HIV services. Activism may take the form of education, mass media campaigns, law suits and public demonstrations.

HIV activists made a significant contribution to the development of effective preventive and treatment strategies for HIV by mounting pressure for accelerated research and contributing to the development of clinical guidelines. Many deaths have been prevented thanks to such activism (Harrington, 2009).

A small proportion of activists resort to dramatic demonstrations and sometimes violence. These few should not be used as examples to undermine the positive achievements obtained by community activism.

6.4 Role models

Role models play an important role in catalysing behaviour change. Reducing individual and community vulnerability to HIV relies heavily on bringing about positive behaviour changes. Depending on the context, celebrities, football players, artists and politicians can use their status to encourage positive practices by setting examples for the community. Many people worldwide were moved when United States President Barack Obama publicly did an HIV test. Some role models take part in advertisements and mass media campaigns encouraging abstinence, condom use and testing. Role models can also act as peer educators.

6.5 Peer educators

Peer educators are usually community members with social characteristics similar to a target group. Their function is to transmit a desired health message to achieve positive behaviour changes by speaking in a language and cultural context that their community is more apt to receive. The most common example is the use of students to conduct education among their peers to raise awareness about safe sex. Peer leaders are generally identified within the community they are to work with. They are then trained to educate and encourage positive behaviours that reduce vulnerability to HIV. At the onset of the HIV epidemic in the 1980s, peer education was used to access difficult populations like men who have sex with men, commercial sex workers and injecting drug users. Over time, it has gained momentum and it is now used to reach adolescents worldwide (Ward et al., 1997).

6.6 Associations of PLHIV

PLHIV can play a major role in encouraging testing and disclosure, reducing stigma, providing credible information and raising funds by openly disclosing their status. Depending on legislation, associations of PLHIV can be comprised entirely or partially of HIV-positive persons. Other groups that might participate can include people affected by HIV, such as those living with or related to someone who is HIV-positive. Associations of PLHIV give a face to the disease, while providing comfort and support to persons already living with the disease. These associations are also the ideal forum for PLHIV to focus on their rights and health and demand an adequate response from their governments.

6.7 Community-Based Organisations (CBOs)

Community based organisations (CBOs) represent a more organised effort to combat HIV. These organisations are created by community members, have their headquarters in the community and collaborate with the local health authorities to achieve prevention, treatment, care and support goals. Their range of activities depends on their individual mission statements, but they may be involved in home-based care, voluntary counselling and testing, patient identification and referral, subsidy of health-related costs, research, data collection and local health area decision-making. They are particularly in tune with community needs and have an active presence within their respective communities. For instance, there are CBOs that focus on prevention and treatment efforts among specific vulnerable groups, such as sex workers to injecting drug users. Often the staff of such organisations include members of vulnerable groups (e.g. current/former sex workers or drug users). Their intimate connection to their respective communities provides an essential and invaluable link between service providers and target populations. These CBOs conduct outreach work distributing condoms and/or needles directly to target groups and providing valuable informational materials, counselling and case management to disenfranchised populations.

6.8 The Municipal Council

Over time, the institution known as the Municipal Council has acquired a variety of meanings. For the purposes of this chapter, this term will refer to a small, democratically elected governmental body operating in small communities, the leader of which is often the mayor. This is a formal body representing the community in all areas including health. In some legislations, the mayor or a representative of the council is also a member of the health district management committee. The municipal council determines the community agenda for health and provides estimates of how much of their budget can be allocated for health. These finances can be used to boost community efforts to fight HIV by providing compensation for social mobilisers and community health workers.

6.9 Community health appraisal

Planning health care services requires appraisal and 'community diagnosis', both of which require the direct involvement of community members. Community representatives may be responsible for providing information as well as collecting and analysing collected and existing data. The involvement of community members in validating data collected, both empowers the community and ensures that the data does in fact reflect the given community (Rifkin, 1992). HIV programs require in-depth appraisal of community problems before interventions can be developed. The community's knowledge, attitudes, practices and behaviours must be adequately assessed. Additionally, there must be a thorough study and understanding of local cultures and traditions, including dates and locations of social events, traditional calendars and local means of communication. It is equally important to investigate community demographics, use of services and literacy rates. It is only then, for example, that program managers can determine not only how many condoms are needed, but how to best disseminate them so that the community will receive them. It will also determine when and where to have health talks; what is the best medium for communication; and what kind of language and messaging needs to be used in order to effectively deliver important health messages. The community, therefore, plays an important role in the decision-making process by providing, collecting and validating information pertinent to the development of HIV programs.

7. Challenges to community participation

Community participation in HIV activities is often hampered by a lack of adequate leadership and poor credibility owing to the fact that community members usually have no formal training either in health or community action. For example, without appropriate training, community workers visiting households of PLHIV may disclose patients' status in the community. Support groups are not only difficult to establish and sustain, but retention rates are low due to fear of stigma and status disclosure (Population Council and Health Systems Trust, 2006). Community advisory bodies are also difficult to initiate and sustain (UNAIDS, 2007).

In some countries, community mobilisation may be perceived as opposition to the government and constructive initiatives may be stopped or delayed. In fact, such initiatives can be dangerous for those involved. Political, religious and cultural factors can impede community efforts that appear to contradict accepted social standards, such as the distribution of essential prevention materials (i.e. condoms, needles) and important educational information. Additionally, the governments of many countries are reluctant to fund such initiatives, resulting in fierce competition among CBOs for international funds from the same pool of donors: this often creates an environment that fosters competition rather than collaboration. Further, community participation often ignites power struggles within the community, as members are far from homogenous and can be in bitter disagreement among themselves. All these factors make community participation a highly dynamic and complex process (Olico-Okui, 2004).

Additional challenges to community participation include ensuring that the community takes ownership of the initiative. Rushed programs using community participation as an objective rather than a process are more likely to hamper the long-term success of the initiative. Also, community participation often requires external support. Consistent provision of supplies that cannot be generated from the community is crucial to ensure continuity. Finally, it is also necessary to ensure adequate leadership and representation from community members by retaining their interest in the project, reserving seats for them at important meetings and making them know that their input is valuable.

The integration of health care services is not making community participation any easier. Community volunteers who initially focused on HIV activities now find themselves providing services for tuberculosis and, at times, general reproductive health. There is a need for the development of better conceptual frameworks to determine the extent and scope of community participation in specific projects. Finally, there may be too few examples of success community initiatives to follow from.

8. Examples of community participation in HIV programs

8.1 CBOs and vaccine development in Brazil

In August 1991, the WHO selected Brazil as a preferred site for vaccine trials. Brazilian authorities were less than welcoming to foreign-initiated research and decried the use of Brazilians as "guinea pigs". HIV activists understood the need to be involved in vaccine research and used the opportunity to discuss the development of trial capacity and infrastructure in Brazil, while insisting on the highest standards for research processes and ethics. They even negotiated access to vaccines in the future (ICASO, 2006).

8.2 The AIDS Support Organisation (TASO) in Uganda

In 1987, groups of PLHIV and their families started forming spontaneously throughout Uganda. They came together to share information, comfort one another and cope with the burdens of stigma and discrimination. The new larger group grew rapidly as news spread of their activities. They then sought out external financial and logistic assistance for training volunteers in prevention and care. It is now one of the biggest HIV care organisations in Africa with 150 staff members and 200 volunteers (UNAIDS, 1997).

8.3 The CIHR Canadian HIV Trials Network (CTN) Community Advisory Committee (CAC)

Before the initiation of the CAC for the CTN, very few volunteers participated in the review of HIV clinical trials in Canada. In the late 1980s, PLHIV demanded a bigger role in the decision-making process. In response, scientists and drug companies began adding PLHIV to existing committees. In 1993, the CTN added another level of review by a newly created CAC to reinforce the work of other community members in other CTN committees. The CAC's advice is essential in determining if trials will be attractive to participants. Based on the CAC's recommendations, specific changes can be made without the study losing its scientific value. Now, pharmaceutical companies regularly ask for community input in the development of protocols and informed consent forms. The CAC's activities include ensuring that the proposed research is relevant and of interest to the HIV community; that the research is ethical and protects trial volunteers from unnecessary risk; and that informed consent is clear and understandable. They also provide a forum for the discussion of trials and improve communication between community representatives and researchers (CTN, 2010).

8.4 The Lawyers' Collective, Bombay, India

The Lawyers' Collective is an Indian NGO that devotes considerable resources to the legal needs of PLHIV. It is mostly self-financed, but has fought many legal cases and worked towards changing laws that discriminate against PLHIV. In 1989, they took on the case of Dominic D'Souza, arrested because he was found to be HIV-positive after donating blood. He was considered a 'public threat' under the Goa Public Health Act and was subsequently incarcerated. D'Souza's case reached the High Court, and, with the help of the Collective, he was released and amendments were made to the Public Health Act (UNAIDS, 1997).

8.5 HIV Vaccine Division (HAVD), South Africa

The HAVD developed an extensive and comprehensive community education program in the Soweto community of South Africa. They began teaching community members about

HIV vaccine trials a full year before the onset of the trials. This 'no rush' policy gave the community ample time to absorb the information and make informed decisions about whether they wanted to take part in the trials or not. Their understanding is assessed before they are included in the trials. They also have a representative community advisory board that advises the researchers on community norms and concerns. The board members are democratically elected by their constituents.

9. Conclusion

Community participation has played a fundamental role in the fight against HIV. It has a positive effect on prevention strategies, uptake and availability of treatment and use of services. It has also initiated and guided the research agenda for HIV prevention and treatment. The scope of community participation is much broader than often reported and should not be overlooked. Communities with high burdens of HIV are encouraged to mobilise and participate in a collaborative response to the epidemic.

10. Acknowledgment

This work is supported in part by the CIHR Canadian HIV Trials Network (CTN) in the form of The International Fellowship Program awarded to the first author. This work would not have been possible without the invaluable insights of Lehana Thabane, Kevin Pendergraft, Shari Margolese, Suzanne MacCarthy and many others who prefer to remain anonymous.

11. References

Botterill, L. & Fisher, M. (2002). The rise of the community participation model. *Proceedings of the Jubilee conference of the Australasian Political Studies Association.* Australian National University, Canberra, Australia, October 2002.

CTN. (2010). *A primer for members of community advisory committees and HIV clinical trials and observational studies,* Available from http://www.hivnet.ubc.ca/ctn_hivnet/wp-content/uploads/2010/12/CAC-Primer.pdf

Harrington, M. (2009). Community involvement in HIV and Tuberculosis Research, *Journal of the Acquired Immune Deficiency Syndrome,* Vol. 52, Suppl. 63-66.

International Council of AIDS Service Organizations (ICASO). (2006). *Community involvement in HIV vaccine research: Making it work,* 27 March 2011, Available from http://www.icaso.org/publications/Comm_Involv_VaccineResearch2006.pdf

Morgan, LM. (1993). *Community participation in health: The politics of primary care in Costa Rica.* Cambridge University Press, ISBN 0-521-41898-4, Cambridge.

Olico-Okui. (2004). Community participation: an abused concept? *Health Policy and Development,* Vol 2, No. 1, pp. 7-10, ISSN 1728-6107.

Population Council and Health Systems Trust. (2006). *Understanding barriers to community participation in HIV and AIDS services, Summary Report.* 24 February 2011, Available from <http://www.popcouncil.org/pdfs/AP_BarriersFinalReport.pdf>

Ramirez-Valles, J. (2002). The protective effects of community involvement for HIV risk behaviour: a conceptual framework. *Health Education Research,* Vol. 17, No. 4, pp. 389-403.

Rifkin, S. B. (1992). Rapid appraisals for health: an overview, In: *RRA notes*, Iss. 16, pp. 7-12, IIED London.

Senterfitt, W. (1998). *The Denver Principles : The original manifesto of the PWA self empowerment movement,* 21 February 2011, Available from http://www.aegis.com/pubs/bala/1998/ba980509.html

UNAIDS. (1997). Community mobilization and AIDS: UNAIDS Technical Update, *In: UNAIDS Best Practice Collection: Technical Update*). 28 March 2011, Available from http://www.data.unaids.org/Publications/IRC-pub03/commmob-tu_en.pdf

UNAIDS. (2007). *Good participatory practice guidelines for biomedical HIV prevention trials,* Available from
http://data.unaids.org/pub/Manual/2010/guidelines_biomedical_hiv_prevention_2010_en.pdf

Ward, J; Hunter, G & Power, R. (1997). Peer education as a means of drug prevention and education among young people, *Health Education Journal,* No. 56:251-263.

Werner, D.; & Sanders, D. (1997) Alma ata and the institutionalisation of Primary Health Care. In: *Questioning the solution: The Politics of Primary Health Care and Child Survival,* Health Wrights, pp 18-20, Retrieved from
<http://www.healthwrights.org/hw-dev/books/208-ques-solu>

13

The Culture Inspired Hybrid Interpretations of the HIV/AIDS Lived-Experiences

Uchenna Beatrice Amadi-Ihunwo
Centre for Education Policy Development (CEPD)
St Augustine College, Victory Park
Johannesburg,
South Africa

1. Introduction

Over the past two decades of HIV/AIDS disease, there has been a range of research perspectives concentrating on the health related concerns of the epidemic. Parker (2001) stated that like many other disciplines, anthropology failed to distinguish itself in its initial responses to the HIV/AIDS epidemic. Furthermore, anthropologists, especially in Africa, contributed only irregularly to such early research and mobilisation was on the basis of their own individual research initiatives and publications rather than as part of a formal or organised research response. This is evidenced in the paucity of ethnographic empirical research focusing on the management of HIV/AIDS in public schools. This does not mean that there were no important and valuable contributions made by anthropologists to the study of HIV/AIDS (Bolognone 1986).

The dominant paradigm for the organisation and conduct of AIDS research in Sub-Saharan Africa has begun to be perceptible in the past decades. The paradigm that characterised the prevailing studies during this time had a mainly biomedical emphasis and a largely individualistic bias in relation to the ways in which the social sciences might contribute meaningfully to the development and implementation of an HIV/AIDS research agenda (Parker, 2001).

Much of the social sciences research activity that emerged in response to HIV/AIDS in Sub-Saharan Africa during the mid 80s to late 90s, and up to the present, focused on surveys of risk-related behaviours and on the knowledge, attitudes and beliefs about sexuality that are HIV risk associated. The aims of these studies were in Parker's terms, to collect quantifiable data on numbers of sexual partners, the frequency of different sexually transmitted diseases, and any number of other similar issues that were understood to contribute to the spread of HIV infection (Carballo, Cleland, Carael, & Albrecht, 1989; Cleland and Ferry, 1995). Thus, such studies could only pave the way for prevention policies and intervention programmes designed by government to reduce HIV-related risk behaviours.

The limitations of behavioural intervention based on information and reasoned persuasion as a stimulus for risk reduction became evident. In Sub-Saharan Africa, the emergence of cultural studies that have some traces of ethnographic characteristics began to emerge among researchers in Uganda and South Africa. By the late 1990s, it became clear that a far more complex and wider set of social, structural and cultural factors are likely to mediate

HIV/AIDS risks in every population and that individual psychology cannot be expected to explain fully, let alone produce changes in sexual conduct, without taking these issues into account (Obbo 1988, Herdt & Boxer, 1991).

The 1990s witnessed a growing focus on the interpretation of cultural meanings as central to fuller appreciation of HIV/AIDS transmission. In South Africa then, ethnographic studies began to identify culture as key to understanding practices that impact on the high prevalence of HIV/AIDS. These studies viewed cultural/traditional practices as a problem contributing to transmission rather than examining possibilities that might exist for responding to cultural practices through the design of more culturally appropriate prevention programmes. A matter of paramount concern at this time was to examine and explicate what sexual practices mean to the persons involved, the significant contexts in which they take place, the social scripting of sexual encounters, and the diverse sexual cultures and subcultures that are present within different societies. The researchers sought to go beyond the identification of statistical correlates aimed at explaining sexual risk behaviours and conceptions (Leclerc-Madlala, 2005; Abdul Karim, 2000; Parker, 2001).

The focus on sexuality in relation to HIV/AIDS shifted to the knowledge and what informed the knowledge on HIV/AIDS within the society i.e. the cultural setting within which behaviours take place and to the cultural symbols, meanings and rules that arranged it (Ashforth, 2001; Stadler, 2003; Naeme, 2004). It became evident that not just cultural, but also structural, racial, political and economic factors moulded beliefs and experiences. Emphasis was placed on the fact that racial and economic factors have played a key role in determining the shape and spread of the epidemic in South Africa. These studies also focused on the ways in which societies and communities structured the possibilities of sexual interactions between social actors with whom one may have sex, in what ways and under what circumstances.

Gender inequalities in sub-Saharan Africa were identified as the seeds of social and cultural rules and regulations placing specific limitations on the female's potential for negotiation in sexual interactions. These rules and regulations conditioned the possibilities for the occurrence of sexual violence and the patterns of contraceptive used and sexual negotiation (Visser, Schoeman, & Perold, 2004; Naeme 2004). Consequently, the dynamics of gender power relations have become a major focus for recent research such as mine. Although most studies concentrated on reproductive health, some social anthropological studies voiced concerns about gender relations especially among the rural women. This body of research has drawn attention to the need for structural changes aimed at highlighting, in a wider perspective, a focus on cultural influences. The findings of these studies channel the attentions of these researchers towards critically envisioning the search for effective mediation of HIV/AIDS and People living with HIV/AIDS (PLHIV) towards cultural and religious practices. Similarly, it moves the focus from the usual biomedical constructs investigation to investigation of the lived experiences of the members in order to get clues for the way forward especially now that the existing strategies seem neither effective nor efficient.

In this chapter, I have drawn attention to overlaps between various beliefs and practices that characterised the HIV/AIDS lived experiences of the members of education workplaces. Though some studies refer to these constructs, they do not explicitly identify the combination, or what I identified as 'hybridisation', of these constructs in the understanding and practices around HIV/AIDS and PLHIV. HIV/AIDS academic analysts have rarely looked at these combined lived experiences that characterise HIV/AIDS. However, in the

South African public schools' cases, I saw that there is no one approach or strategy that individuals use to mediate the epidemic. I also note that while there are various ways of experiencing the disease: people combine two or more approaches.

Firstly, there is evidence confirming that members of these education institutions have relatively good biomedical and legal knowledge of the epidemic, such as is provided in the National Policy document. A closer look at the HIV/AIDS lived experiences at the individual level confirms the inadequacy of the biomedical and legal approaches to the epidemic. Although most of the educators and principals draw their experiences mostly from the biomedical and legal approaches, most of them also integrate aspects of religious, gender and indigenous cultural beliefs and practices. Also, despite the fact that biomedical and legal approaches are officially recommended, members of these education institutions see these strategies as insufficient, inefficient and ineffective in providing solutions or answers to several questions. Because these two approaches (biomedical and legal) have some attributes which instead of solving the problems, encourage several forms of emotional torment from their high costs, and because of the culture of secrecy and privacy, alternative measures were incorporated by these individuals to deal with the multifaceted challenges of HIV/AIDS.

The experiences narrated in this chapter have pragmatic implications for how people experience the disease and PLHIV in education workplaces. The first category of the respondents, presents the narratives of an educator who *was* very knowledgeable in biomedical approaches to HIV/AIDS, but who chose to embrace religious beliefs and practices in her lived experiences. This educator seems to have successfully maintained her claim on the religious approaches whilst acknowledging the biomedical and other cultural practices relating to the epidemic and PLHIV. There does not appear to have been any significant disaffirmation by her of HIV/AIDS lived experiences; rather, it is the aspiration to the search for a cure and protection from stigma that led her to choose to give up the biomedical approaches to the disease. Her lived experience with the disease has reinforced her sense of being someone who is able to deal with the HIV/AIDS related circumstances in her school. What emerges very powerfully from this respondent's narrative is the centrality of belief, particularly religious belief in dealing with HIV/AIDS in the work place. This theme appears throughout my research but in a variety of forms. I abandoned the assumption that biomedical and legal constructs are truly accurate versions of a participant's beliefs, actions and practices towards HIV/AIDS and PLHIV. From the above, the challenges seem to revolve around the treatment of the infection and dealing with the stigma associated with it.

The second category that switched from treatment to protection against the infection. One of the educators in this category demonstrated considerable dissatisfaction at the western-medicine approach to protection against the disease. It was his experience of his ethnic practices, which provided understanding and meaning to what he prefers to use to protect himself and his wife. He was able to develop this new protective strategy by adhering to his indigenous cultural practices. With this new experience, he was able to protect his family from the disease which carries unbearable shame for someone like him. From this respondent, I posit that people construct their own beliefs and practices towards protection against the epidemic, some of which are in contrast to the protective strategies laid out by the biomedical discourses.

Another example of religious beliefs is one of extended eschatological Christian beliefs and practices. This notion by some identified Christians suggested that HIV/AIDS is God's ways of venting His anger on the generation that has turned their backs on Him. This view does not necessarily provide opportunity for people to learn from their mistakes. People living with the disease have been condemned to pay for their 'sin' by death which is their 'wage' for not listening to God's messages and instructions.

The fourth category offered an example of an educator who is struggling to accept the challenges of being infected. She started with bitterness, blames and anger towards the society that seems to appreciate the males more than the females. She took this position because it was difficult for her to forgive a man who traditionally married three wives and yet was promiscuous. She has now resigned to a life of shame for her while alive and for her children when she is dead. These narratives highlighted important culturally-related concepts such as 'curses' 'dirt' and 'pollution'. Some educators also see the disease as dirt and the infected as polluted with dirt. Douglas (1966) asserts that such feelings introduce the concept of sacredness whereby the society isolates the sick person who then keeps his or her distance from other people.

Obviously, the practices of '*sacredness*' in relation to the illness and the infected ushered in the understanding of 'dirt' as associated with HIV/AIDS. At this juncture, I must emphasise that those infected are not treated as taboo or outcasts openly but are indirectly stigmatised. Not all respondents treat them so. According to Stein's (2003) theory of the 'latest changing faces of HIV/AIDS stigma', it can be accepted that symbolic stigma (i.e. stigma based on moral condemnation regarding sexual behaviour) is instrumental or useful here because it serves to distance the individual or group from the fear of infection by facilitating denial of own risk (*It will not happen to me because I am a good person/part of a good group of people*).

The fifth respondent's attitude constructs the epidemic as a taboo, not discussed or easily talked about. She suggests that some members of the education sector use blame and resignation to mediate HIV/AIDS. The failure to speak openly about the epidemic, irrespective of biomedical knowledge of the disease acquired through training and based on the construction of gender was revealed. Her responses help highlight the influence of gender according to which the women are socialised not to freely discuss death and sex.

Finally, a new perspective on the disease emerges from the youths which contradict in every way the fears, shame and condemnation consistently found in the responses of the interviewees. Taking different perspectives and routes to understand and mediate the epidemic, they appear to attempt to distance themselves from the entire mystifying HIV/AIDS-related stigma because of death. They provide models for reclaiming their desired HIV/AIDS lived experiences. Their sexual relationships and the socialisation practices they engage in provide completely new and contradictory views of their friends and acquaintances living with HIV/AIDS and the epidemic.

What do we learn from this rather long expedition into the realities of the HIV/AIDS lived experiences? I argue that in order to effectively deal with the challenges people face as a result of the epidemic, we need to know the diverse ways people understand and experience the disease. I have presented information that not only do people mediate the epidemic in diverse ways; they also combine constructs in their HIV/AIDS lived experiences. I also showed that biomedical and legal discourses are not taken very seriously in the practice of HIV/AIDS treatment and protection against the epidemic by the members of education work places. The culture of secrecy and privacy located within the biomedical and legal discourses strengthens the HIV/AIDS-related stigma which I identified in the narratives as '*residential*' (in the epidemic) and '*translated*' (not only for the PLHIV but also their children when they are dead).

The HIV/AIDS and PLHIV understandings have been the subject of avid interest and curiosity in this section. The section presented a significant sampling of responses from the semi-structured interviews and the focus group discussions with the participants, and explored both their HIV/AIDS narratives and meaning.

Many participants would still subscribe to the biomedical theory in understanding HIV/AIDS and PLHIV; many think that there will always be 'confusion, strife and dispute' in making sense of the disease and PLHIV especially considering that there is still no cure for the epidemic. The fact is that today neither biomedical nor legal discourses (common with researchers and policy designers) are satisfactory in explaining issues around HIV/AIDS and PLHIV. But the question is to know whether there are alternative ways people understand or make meaning of the epidemic and those infected that may explain the existing implementation gaps between HIV/AIDS policies and practices in the South African schools.

Biomedical and legal understandings notwithstanding, no one discourse explains the HIV/AIDS and PLHIV understandings of these participants. The truth is that these individuals engage more than one realm of ideas in making sense of the disease. Indeed, even with the most extreme religious and indigenous theories, it is possible to demonstrate the existence of a rivalry between these two discourses and one or two other discourses. It is clear from the extracts discussed in this chapter that there is more than one alternative way people make sense of the disease in their individual schools. But these understandings are very ambiguous and unconventional.

These interpretations do not unfold on a conventional level of understanding of the disease. Further, no one theory has ever seemed sufficient to define how people make meaning of the disease, to furnish in itself the key to human explanations of the disease, or to express the totality of a situation (especially with PLHIV) that it only helps to define. These realms of ideas are products of their lived experiences and belief systems. Based on these systems of understanding, the concept of 'hybridisation' as identified in the lived experiences summarises ways these individuals make sense of the epidemic and PLHIV.

Hybridisation theory in this context suggests that people combine one or more views to make sense of the disease. With biomedical knowledge as top on the list, there is less evidence of or emphasis on the legal discourses in these narratives. People combine one or more of these alternative discourses with their existing biomedical knowledge of the disease. These alternative discourses are; indigenous (including witchcraft), religious, eschatological and racial discourses. It is vain to apportion praise or blame to any of these theories. The hybrid theory for explaining the disease and attitudes towards PLHIV will go on as long as the biomedical discourse fails to discover the cure for HIV/AIDS. These men and women fail to recognise a single system of understanding as the ultimate in explaining the epidemic.

For a long time there have been efforts to disguise this misfortune (complicated understanding of the epidemic and PLHIV) in South Africa. For example, the indigenous theory of the epidemic has been accused of escalating HIV/AIDS transmission. No one has been able to pinpoint the fact that it is first one way individuals make sense of the epidemic and PLHIV; the religious and eschatological views have not received much recognition and the constructions of the racial discourse was not very different from the legacies of apartheid. However, the innumerable conflicts that set biomedical discourse against others (which I described as 'alternatives') come from the fact that neither is prepared to offer credible, effective and efficient explanations for the consequences of this epidemic.

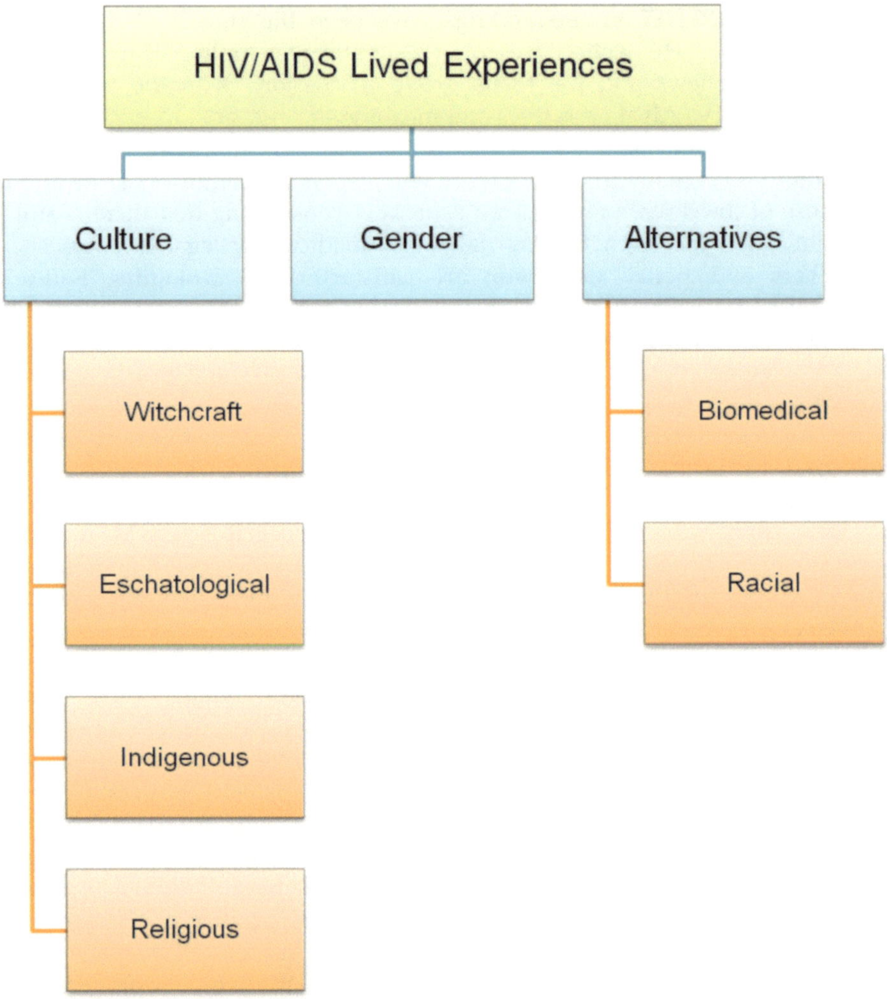

Fig. 1. Diagrammatical representation of the interconnectivity of the impact of culture and gender on HIV/AIDS lived experiences

At the commencement of the research from which this chapter is written, I accepted the premise that there are several factors that directly or indirectly influence the HIV/AIDS lived experiences and how people make sense of the epidemic and PLHIV. Having accepted this, I created relationships and situations which might offer members of South African public schools the possibility of narrating and describing their HIV/AIDS lived experiences in interviews and discussions with me and each other. From the findings, I identified the defining experiences and perceptions as 'conventional' and 'alternatives'. I also identified the systems by which these conventions and alternatives function together, as 'hybridisation' processes. I attempted to create scenarios and situations which would offer the participants opportunities for revealing these. The focus of my attention was on;

- Individual HIV/AIDS lived experiences
- The background events, practices, knowledge and beliefs which might highlight the individual's lived experiences

- The background perceptions and circumstances which might stimulate the likelihood of cultural response to their HIV/AIDS lived experiences
- The respondents' interactions, responses and non-verbal communication

I concluded that culture has immense influence in the HIV/AIDS lived experiences of the majority of the members of South African public schools in the following ways;

- Understanding of the epidemic and PLHIV
- Their treatment approaches
- Their methods of caring
- Their prevention strategies
- Beliefs and practices

I further concluded that;

- Gender constructs are embedded in the cultural discourse so as to impact HIV/AIDS lived experiences of individual members of these institutions
- Biomedical discourse is inadequate in providing detailed explanations for and interpretations of the HIV/AIDS lived experiences of these individuals
- There are alternative realms of ideas and practices that these people engage in making sense of and dealing with the epidemic and PLHIV
- Members of these educational institutions engage in a process of 'hybridisation' of the diverse discourses that are prevalent in HIV/AIDS related study in understanding and experiencing HIV/AIDS and PLHIV
- Most of these 'alternative' approaches are unconventional and may be seen as authentic or contrived. However, they provide these people with other ways of mediating the epidemic than the biomedical discourse
- The National Policy also created conflicts and complications in understanding and dealing with the epidemic through its linguistic constructions

Although I drew these conclusions, my attempts to generalise findings were not successful. Diverse experiences and understandings in a society that is very diversified (such as exists in Gauteng province; South Africa) in terms of culture and beliefs made it impossible. I am therefore forced to accept that the findings in this study may yield different or more consistent results if conducted in a society with the same or similar culture and belief systems.

Theoretical assumptions that inform the research were greatly challenged as I continued to explore these HIV/AIDS lived experiences and how people actually understood the disease and PLHIV. I realised that available ideas and existing metaphors are not adequate in projecting the lived experiences and various interpretations that plagued the research content: HIV/AIDS, culture, gender, and lived-experiences. When I analysed my data, I reacted to more than the few theories that touched on the subjects of my interest. As well, I note during data collection that people react differently from the prescriptions of most of the theories that seemed to offer reasonable interpretations in some aspects. I concluded that there are immense complexities, complications and conflicts in interpreting how HIV/AIDS and PLHIV are experienced and understood. Having adopted this position, I then concluded that no one approach or discourse could offer adequate interpretations to the HIV/AIDS and PLHIV lived experiences and understandings. Individuals make sense and deal with the epidemic and those infected not only through the biomedical paradigm but also following their cultural precedents. I therefore posit that the intricacies associated with HIV/AIDS brought about by lack of a cure would be said to have initiated the combinations of world views in dealing with and understanding the epidemic and PLHIV even among members of the education sector.

I explored the empirical elements of persistent cultural and gender themes in HIV/AIDS transmission and treatment debates vis-à-vis the personal epistemologies of the members of education workplaces that deal with HIV/AIDS and PLHIV. I focused on participants' narratives, to study the identified social and cultural variables that shaped and nurtured the participants' experiences which inform their practices and attitudes towards the disease and PLHIV.

I reviewed the empirical literature for HIV/AIDS culture and gender and the National HIV/AIDS Policy, with particular emphasis on the education workplace. Although there is a paucity of literature in this regard, some high quality evaluation designs informed the methodological strengths of some aspects of the data collection tools and analysis. For example, I borrowed the use of 'rumours and gossip' from an incredible study on HIV/AIDS by Stadler (2003). Most of the HIV/AIDS and culture literature offers exposure to the exacerbated impact of culture in mediating HIV/AIDS especially with respect to gender construction. While I admit that this literature offers extensive insight on the topics, the external validity of these studies for HIV/AIDS lived experiences was difficult to ascertain.

On the HIV/AIDS programmes in the public schools, there is no evidence that cultural issues are considered in the curriculum. However, it is notable that cultural issues influence the transmission of the knowledge especially in the gender, sex and death related topics which chiefly characterise HIV/AIDS. The evidence for cultural effects on learners and other members of the education sector is inconclusive. This is because there is no study that directly examined the concepts of culture, gender, and HIV/AIDS lived experiences in South African public schools. Conclusions were drawn in this area based on the assumptions that members of these education sectors constitute part of the society where most of these studies were carried out. It is very difficult to accept such conclusions as valid considering that most of the studies were conducted in the rural areas and with less educated people. This therefore suggested that if some of those studies were replicated in urban areas where diversity is high and levels of education are of a reasonable standard (such as in Gauteng), the study would yield different results.

Several carefully designed qualitative HIV/AIDS studies demonstrated the considerable effects of cultural influence in the education sector. One of the studies not done in South Africa highlighted that culture impacts not only on the individuals' HIV/AIDS lived experiences but also the ways HIV/AIDS related issues are dealt with in public schools in sub-Saharans Africa (Mirembe and Davis, 2001). My study indicated that because of the intrinsic presence of cultural beliefs and practices in the schools, many HIV/AIDS related programmes and taught curriculum were not effective. Most of these findings locate this deficiency in the gender-related restrictions induced by cultural perceptions of sex and death. Whether the combination of the impact of culture and gender on HIV/AIDS educational programmes in schools is sufficient to justify the schools' inability to openly state how they are dealing with the epidemic and PLHIV (UNESCO/UNAIDS, 2000), there is evidence that the choice to ignore the cultural influence by education sectors does not exclude its presence. It is rather a choice not to deal with the challenges associated with these cultural influences.

The policy decision to allow independent autonomy for implementation guideline design may be based on the cultural diversity that characterises South Africa. Based on the literature on National Policy, there is substantial indirect evidence that there are other factors that may impact the HIV/AIDS implementations in public schools. However, the key question is whether other factors other than biomedical, legal and risk metaphors, would yield any better results in mediating between the HIV/AIDS lived experiences and the practices of the National Policy. On this matter, the literature presented very little evidence. Very few studies have been done on the experimental evaluations of alternative approaches to the National Policy-identified metaphors. Moreover, the study that measured the impact of the National Policy often neglected to collect the additional data needed to obtain information on the influence of cultural beliefs and practices. The literature review on policy implications suggest that more systematic and detailed research is needed to find the most effective way to deal with cultural implications in the implementation of the National Policy in public schools, especially those with high cultural diversity.

My study advanced the existing knowledge in this field of research through the following arguments that proceeded from the findings. First, in this study, I posit that dealing with HIV/AIDS in education workplaces is not only complex and complicated but seems impossible because of the manner in which the members of the public school institutions experience the disease. In other words, the policy documents, the biomedical knowledge, their elitism, exposure and training in relation to the disease seem, perhaps, overshadowed by their cultural backgrounds, other world views and perceptions.

Second, from the findings of this study, I reveal that there are various ways members of the education workplaces in South African mediate HIV/AIDS, the PLHIV and those affected. Most of these strategies are based on individual experiences, personal belief systems, personal attitudes, biomedical exposure and the official policies for understanding and dealing with the disease, PLHIV and those affected. At this juncture, I must reiterate that not all the stakeholders share the same experiences but the extent to which their experiences differ is still based on their various cultural beliefs and practices. Again, no one of them uses one world view to arbitrate the epidemic. They share the strategy of combining more than one world view to deal with the epidemic.

2. Conclusion

I note from the findings that HIV/AIDS lived experiences in public schools are generational. There is significant variation in the ways and manner in which the youths (learners) and educators understand and deal with the epidemic. While there is not much distinction in their understandings, their HIV/AIDS lived experiences are conspicuously different. The conceptions of stigma also differ considerably. While the adults (educators and school governing board members) experience stigma in a more in-depth manner, the youths (possibly because they do not have a really good sense of death) demystified the HIV/AIDS related stigma.

Again, I suggest, based on my findings, that due to the complications, tensions and complexities associated with HIV/AIDS lived experiences, most members of the schools identified boundaries between those who claimed to be HIV/AIDS negative and those they assume to be positive. Identifying these boundaries means creating distinction-maintaining strategies to deal with the PLHIV in these public schools. I conclude therefore that most members of the public schools deal with PLHIV through symbolic boundary maintenance. I judged this boundary maintenance as a complication arising from their inability to deal with the unknown especially when it touches constructs considered culturally as taboo such as death and sex.

3. Acknowledgement

I wish to appreciate Professor Amadi Ogonda Ihunwo for his continual encouragement during the hectic research processes. To Professor Brahm Fleisch, your supervisory roles in this project are not forgotten. Finally, I wish to thank my boys; Glory and Godswill for being so understanding especially while Mummy was literally absent in their lives for four years.

4. References

Abdool, Karim, Q. (2000). Rising to the challenge of the AIDS epidemic. *South African Journal of Sciences, 96*, 262-273.

Ashforth, A. (2001). *AIDS, witchcraft, and the problem of power in post-apartheid South Africa.* (Institute for Advanced Study, School of Social Science Occasional Paper No 10). Retrieved on June 4, 2007 from: http://www.sss.ias.edu/papers/paperten.pdf (May, 2001).

Bolgnone, D. (1986). A Challenge to anthropologists. *Medical Anthropology Quarterly,* 17(2), 36-52.

Carballo, M., Cleland, J., Carael, M., & Albrecht, G. (1989). A cross-national study of patterns of sexual behaviour. *Journal of Sex Research, 26, 287- 99.*

Cleland, J., & Ferry, B. (eds.) (1995). *Sexual behaviour and AIDS in the developing world.* London: Taylor Francis.

Douglas, M. (1966). *Purity and danger: An Analysis of concepts of pollution and taboo.* New York, NY: Routledge, Taylor and Francis.

Herdt, G., & Boxer, A. (1991). Ethnographic issues in the study of AIDS. *Journal of Sex Research, 28*(2), 171 - 87.

Leclerc-Madlala, S. (2005). Rethinking virginity testing. Gender Links Commentaries, Johannesburg, South Africa. Retrieved on 2nd December, 2005, from: www.genderlinks.org.za

Mirembe, R., & Davies, L. (2001). Is schooling a risk? Gender, power relations, and school culture in Uganda. *Gender and Education, 13*, 401 - 416.

Naeme, A. (2004). HIV/AIDS and violence against women. (ACSSA Newsletter No. 3 February 2004). Melborne: Australian Institute of Family Studies.

Obbo, C. (1988). Is AIDS just another disease? In: Kulstad R (eds). (AAAS Symposia Paper). Washington-DC: American association for the advancement of HIV/AIDS research. pp. 191 – 197.

Parker, B. (2001). Roles and responsibilities, institutional landscapes and curriculum mindscape: A partial view of teacher education policy in South Africa: 1999 to 2000. In K. Lewin, M. Samuel, & Y. Sayed (Eds.). Changing patterns of teacher education in South Africa: policy, practice and prospects. *International Journal of Educational Development, 22(3-4),* pp.381-395.

Stadler, J. (2003). Rumours, gossip and blame: Implications for HIV/AIDS Prevention in the South African Lowveld. *AIDS Education and Prevention, 15,* 357 - 368.

Stein, J. O. (2003). HIV/AIDS stigma: The Latest dirty secret. CSSR Working Paper No. 46. University of Cape Town.

Visser, J. M., Schoeman, J. B., & Perold, J. J. (2004). Evaluation of HIV/AIDS prevention in South African schools. *Journal of Health Psychology, 9*, 263 - 280.

14

Seroprevalence of Human Immunodeficiency Virus (HIV) Among Blood Donors in Jos - Nigeria

Egesie Julie and Egesie Gideon
University of Jos
Nigeria

1. Introduction

Human immunodeficiency virus (HIV), the causative agent of Acquired immunodeficiency syndrome (AIDS) is found in pandemic proportions globally (Osmond and Dennis, 1994). HIV is a scourge, progressing and causing devastation to lives and the healthcare system worldwide (Carpenter et al, 2000). HIV accounted for 38.6 million infections worldwide at the end of 2005. As at 2003, there were about 5.0 million people infected with HIV in Nigeria, giving a national prevalence rate of 5.0% (Federal Ministry of Health, 2004). Infection with HIV occurs through the transfer of infected blood, semen, vaginal fluid, pre-ejaculate, or breast milk. The four major routes of transmission are unprotected sexual intercourse, contaminated blood transfusion, breast milk, transmission from an infected mother to her baby at birth (vertical transmission) (http://en.wikipedia.org/wiki/HIV). Millions of lives are saved each year through blood transfusion. Nonetheless people have a risk of becoming infected with HIV through transfusion of infected blood and blood products. Transmission of HIV and other blood-borne infections can occur during transfusion of blood components (ie, whole blood, packed red cells, fresh-frozen plasma, cryoprecipitate, and platelets) derived from the blood of an infected individual (Donegan et al, 1994). Depending on the production process used, blood products derived from pooled plasma can also transmit HIV and other viruses, but recombinant clotting factors cannot (Berkman et al, 2000) This chapter discusses the transmission of HIV through blood products; prevalence; risk of acquisition through blood transfusion, the current estimated safety of blood components and control measures.

2. HIV infection transmitted during blood transfusion

HIV infection resulting from blood transfusion has been documented repeatedly since the first case report in late 1982 (Curran et al, 1984). HIV transmission through unsafe blood accounts for the second largest source of HIV infection in Nigeria (Federal Ministry of Health, 2009). Not all Nigerian hospitals have the technology to effectively screen blood and therefore there is a risk of using contaminated blood. The Nigerian Federal Ministry of Health have responded by backing legislation that requires hospitals to only use blood from the National Blood Transfusion Service, which has far more advanced blood-screening technology (Nigeria Exchange, 2008).

3. Prevalence of HIV infection among blood donors

The prevalence of HIV infection among blood donors varies from one geographical location to another and can provide a reasonable 'proxy' for HIV infection levels in a larger adult population (WHO/UNAIDS, 2000).

As of January 2004 to December 2008, a total of 15,569 blood donors have been screened for HIV antibodies in Jos University Teaching Hospital of which 1070 were positive, giving a seroprevalence rate of 6.9% (Egesie et al, 2011) as shown in table 1. A fluctuating course in the seroprevalence of HIV among blood donors was observed for the period under review. This finding is in agreement with the study by Hassan et al (2008) in Kaduna, North-western Nigeria and the work by Fasola et al (2009) in Ibadan, South-west Nigeria.

Year	Total number screened	Positive	Negative
2004	1473(100%)	95(6.4%)	1378(9.3%)
2005	4547(100%)	294(6.5%)	4253(93.5%)
2006	3299(100%)	184(5.6%)	3115(94.4%)
2007	1443(100%)	61(4.2%)	1382(95.8%)
2008	4807(100%)	436(9.1%)	4371(90.9%)
Grand Total	15,569	1070	14499

Table 1. Blood donors screened for human immunodeficiency virus in Jos

This prevalence rate obtained in Jos is higher than the 0.08% found by Gupta et al (2004) in their study among Indian blood donors. It is also much higher than the 0.004% found by Bhatti et al (2007) in Karachi among Pakistani donors, and the 0.00009% found by Khan et al (2002) in Peshawar among Pakistani donors. These prevalence rates are shown in table 2 below.

Location	Prevalence (%)
Peshawar (Pakistan)	0.00009
Karachi (Pakistan)	0.004
India	0.08
Kenya	5.8
Tanzania	8.7

Table 2. Prevalence of HIV among blood donors in other parts of the world

The HIV infection rate in this study is also higher than 1.0% in the work of Ejele et al (2005) in Port Harcourt, South-south Nigeria; the 3.1% found by Fiekumo et al (2009) in Osogbo, South-west Nigeria; the 3.9% found by Esumeh et al (2003) in another study in Benin city, South-south Nigeria; the 5.8% in the works of Chikwem et al (1997) in Maiduguri, North-eastern Nigeria and that of Abdalla et al (2005) among Kenyan donors. Furthermore, Fasola et al (2009) found an infection rate of 7.7% among their donors in Ibadan, Southwestern Nigeria while Matee et al (1999) in their work among Tanzanian donors, and Kagu et al (2005) in their work in Nguru, North-eastern Nigeria found an HIV infection rate of 8.7%. (Table 3)

Location	Prevalence (%)
Port Harcourt	1.0
Osogbo	3.1
Benin City	3.9
Maiduguri	5.8
Ibadan	7.7
Nguru	8.7

Table 3. Prevalence of HIV among blood donors in other parts of Nigeria

The wide differences in the HIV infection rate among the blood donors in the different regions within Nigeria, and even those outside Nigeria may be due to the differences in geographical locations, age range of donors, sample sizes, the period of time the studies were carried out, and the different socio-cultural practices such as sexual behavior, marriage practices, circumcision, scarification, tattooing etc which take place in these regions. Access to healthcare services and the laboratory test reagent kits used may also be contributory factors.

The high prevalence of HIV infection among blood donors has heightened the problems of blood safety in Nigeria. The implication of HIV in voluntary blood donors is the risk of transmission of these infections to recipients of blood and blood products as safe blood will be more difficult to get. . It also reflects the prevalence of the infection in the general population from which these blood donors are drawn.

An unsafe blood transfusion is very costly both in terms of human and economic costs. Morbidity and mortality resulting from the transfusion of infected blood have far-reaching consequences, not only for the recipients themselves, but also their families, their communities and the wider society (WHO, 2002 and 2007). Since a person can transmit HIV infection during the asymptomatic phase, it can contribute to an ever-widening pool of HIV infection in the wider population. From the study in Jos-Nigeria, it was observed that HIV infection was found among the 20-39 years age range. This finding is in agreement with the study by Ejele et al (2005) in which higher prevalence of transfusion-transmissible viral infections were observed among youths. This observation is worrisome since the most productive and economically viable age group of the populations is worst hit. There is the urgent need for renewed intensification of preventive programmes aimed at reducing the scourge of this infection (Olokoba et al, 2010).

In some resource-rich countries, testing of donated blood for HIV antibodies was not immediately initiated for a variety of reasons. France began HIV antibody testing in June 1985, Canada began testing in November 1985, and Switzerland began testing in May 1986. Germany inconsistently tested plasma products between 1987 and 1993, as did Japan in 1985 and 1986. These delays led to criminal investigations in France, Germany, Switzerland, and Japan, which in some cases led to criminal conviction of those persons found to be responsible (Weinberg et al, 2002). At least 20 countries initiated compensation programs for some individuals infected by transfusion of HIV-contaminated blood and blood products.

4. Risk of acquisition of HIV infection through blood transfusion and estimated safety of components

The risk of HIV transfusion through infected blood products exceeds that of any other risk exposure. Ninety percent of recipients transfused with HIV antibody-positive blood were found to be HIV infected at follow-up (Donegan et al, 1994). The 90% probability of seroconversion is independent of the age or sex of the recipient, the reason for transfusion, and the type of component transfused (excluding washed red blood cells, which transmit HIV at a lower rate) (Donegan et al, 1990).

HIV infectivity of red blood cell components that were not washed before transfusion decreases as storage time increases. HIV-contaminated red blood cells stored for <8 days are 96% infectious, whereas those stored for >3 weeks are 50% infectious (Donegan et al, 1994). The level of a donor's viremia at the time of donation is also an important determinant of HIV transmission risk, but no other donor characteristics have been found to affect transmission (Busch et al, 1996). Of all transfused patients, half die within 6 months after transfusion from the underlying disease that necessitated the transfusion. Currently, cases involving transfusion of HIV-positive blood do not increase the overall 1-year post transfusion mortality rate of recipients in the United States (Donegan et al, 1994). In Zaire, however, patients transfused with HIV-positive blood are 31% more likely to be dead 1 year after transfusion than are patients transfused with HIV-negative blood (Colebunders et al, 1991). This difference is unexplained but emphasizes the importance of screening blood for HIV in developing countries.

HIV disease due to transfusion progresses in the recipient at rates comparable to those in individuals infected for similar duration but by other routes (Donegan et al, 1986). One report found that a transfusion recipient may develop AIDS more rapidly if the infected blood component comes from a blood donor who develops AIDS soon after the time of the blood donation. Other analyses, however, do not confirm this finding.(Busch et al,1990) It is more likely that host factors, particularly the recipient's age and immune status, and perhaps other as-yet-undefined cofactors influence the progression to AIDS (Operskalski et al,1995) The mean time of progression to AIDS is estimated to be 8.2 years for adult transfusion recipients who receive no antiretroviral therapy, with a cumulative prevalence of 20% having AIDS 5 years after infection (Medley et al, 1987). This progression rate may be overestimated, and the mean time to AIDS development underestimated, because these values are based primarily on data from recipients identified because they developed AIDS or because they received blood from donors who subsequently developed AIDS. The data exclude many donors and recipients who have not been identified because they remain asymptomatic.

Transmission of HIV by transfusion has decreased in developing countries since the initiation of voluntary deferral of donors at risk for HIV infection and routine HIV antibody testing of all donations. Continued improvement in donor recruitment practices, donor education, donor screening, and blood testing has resulted in continued decreases in the risk of transfusion transmission of HIV. In 1995, the risk in the United States of HIV-1 transmission per unit transfused was estimated to be between 1 in 450,000 and 1 in 660,000.(Schreiber et al 1996, Lackritz et al,1995). By 2003, this estimated risk had decreased to between 1 in 1.4 million and 1 in 1.8 million units (Busch et al, 2003).

HIV antibody tests fail to identify HIV-infected blood donated by HIV-infected persons who have not yet seroconverted. Exclusion of donors is voluntary. Interviews with HIV antibody-positive donors reveal that most recognize their risk but fail to exclude themselves.(Cleary et al, 1988) As a result, laboratory efforts to eliminate HIV-infected donors have continued and testing has improved. Currently, HIV antibody tests detect both HIV-1 and HIV-2 and detect antibody approximately 22 days (the "window period") after the viremic phase of HIV infection begins. Antigen testing for p24, mandated by the U.S. Food and Drug Administration (FDA) in 1996, shortened the window period to approximately 16 days. The nucleic acid amplification test (NAT), which detects HIV-1 RNA in minipools (16-24 donation samples/pool), was introduced in the United States in 1999 and further reduces the window period of potential HIV transmission to 11 days (Goodnough et al, 2003). As of early 2003, three transfusion recipients are known to have become HIV infected by transfusion of HIV antibody-negative, p24 antigen-negative, and HIV NAT-negative blood from two different blood donors (among 25 million donations) (www.cbsnews.com/stories/2002/07/19/health/main/515694.shtml)

The global perspective is not as bright as that described for resource-rich countries. Worldwide, 75 million units of blood are estimated to be donated annually, compared with 1.5 million donations in Nigeria. Of the 191 WHO member states, only 43% test blood for HIV, hepatitis C, and hepatitis B viruses. Transfusion-transmitted HIV infection is thought to account for 80,000-160,000 infections annually, contributing 2-4% of all cases of HIV transmission (Bharucha, et al, 2002). Only 20% of the world's supply of safe blood is available to countries with 80% of the world's population.

5. Control measures

Significant progress has been made globally by a number of countries in reducing HIV prevalence through sound prevention effort. HIV prevention still remains the most effective strategy towards addressing the global AIDS pandemic. It is for this reason that various groups and organizations have instituted foundations and committee as a necessary step towards that goal. (National Agency for the Control of AIDS, 2010)

In Nigeria, various preventive strategies are being carried out. One of the components of such preventive strategies is the blood safety programme. This is particularly important in view of the fact that the risk of transmission of HIV through infected blood is virtually 100% (Roberts et al, 1994).

Transmission of HIV through infected blood and blood products accounts for approximately 10% in African region (Mvere, 2002) and the second largest source of HIV infection in Nigeria (Federal Ministry of Health, 2009).

Blood safety remains an issue of major concern in transfusion medicine in developing countries like Nigeria where national blood transfusion services, appropriate infrastructure, trained personnel and financial resources are inadequate due to poor budgetary allocation to the health sector. Inadequate funding for HIV testing is only a part of the problem.

Specific issues that urgently need to be addressed include the lack of a sufficient volunteer blood donor pool, inadequate blood donor screening information, counseling, and confidentiality.

Implementation of standardized and monitored test manufacturing practices, inclusion of test validation procedures, ongoing staff training, and continuous internal and external quality assessment programs are all necessary components of an effective program to prevent transmission. Moreover, transfusion practices must be monitored locally so that HIV transmission from unnecessary transfusions does not occur.

Since blood transfusion is an important part of modern medicine, safety of blood and blood products remains a global issue. The continuous monitoring of the magnitude of transfusion transmissible infections in blood donors is important for estimating the risk of transfusion and optimizing infectious diseases transmission (Tessema et al, 2010). Strict selection of blood donors with the emphasis on getting voluntary donors and comprehensive screening of blood donors for HIV and other transfusion transmissible infections using standard methods are highly recommended to ensure the safety of blood for recipient. We therefore recommend the screening of all prospective blood donors for all transfusion transmissible infections. A strict selection criterion for blood donors to exclude those who have multiple sexual partners and those who engage in high risk behaviour and also that blood transfusion should be given only when absolutely indicated.

6. References

Abdalla F, Mwanda OW, Rana F (2005). Comparing walk-in and call-responsive donors in a national and a private hospital in Nairobi. East African Medical Journal. 82(10):532-536.

Bhatti FA, Ullah Z, Salamat N, Ayub M, Ghani E (2007).

Anti-hepatitis B core antigen testing, viral markers, and occult hepatitis B virus infection in Pakistani blood donors: implication for transfusion practice. Transfusion. 47(1):74-79.

Berkman SA, Groopman JE (1988). Transfusion associated AIDS. Transfus Med Rev; 2:18-28.

Bharucha ZS (2002). Risk management strategies for HIV in blood transfusion in developing countries. Vox Sang. Aug;83 Suppl 1:167-71.

Busch MP, Donegan E, Stuart M, et al (1990). Transfusion Safety Study Group: Donor HIV-1 p24 antigenaemia and course of infection in recipients. Lancet;335:1342.

Busch MP, Kleinman SH, Nemo GJ (2003). Current and emerging infectious risks of blood transfusions. JAMA26;289(8):959-62.

Busch MP, Operskalski EA, Mosley JW, Lee TH, Henrard D, Herman S, Sachs DH, Harris M, Huang W, Stram DO (1996). Factors influencing human immunodeficiency virus type 1 transmission by blood transfusion. Transfusion Safety Study Group. J Infect Dis. 174(1):26-33.

Carpenter CC, Cooper DA, Fischi MA et al (2000). Antiretroviral therapy update and recommendation of the international AIDS society- USA panel. JAMA. 28(3):381-390.

CBS News. HIV-tainted blood infects two in Florida. http://www.cbsnews.com/stories/2002/07/19/health/main515694.shtml (accessed March 23, 2003)

Chikwem J.O, Mohammed I, Okara G.C, Ukwandu, N.C, Ola T.O (1997). Prevalence of transmissible blood infections among blood donors at the University of Maiduguri Teaching Hospital, Maiduguri, Nigeria. East African Medical Journal. 74(4):213-216.

Cleary PD, Singer E, Rogers TF, et al (1988). Sociodemographic and behavioral characteristics of HIV antibody-positive blood donors. Am J Public Health; 78:953-957.

Colebunders R, Ryder R, Francis H, et al (1991). Seroconversion rate, mortality, and clinical manifestations associated with the receipt of a human immunodeficiency virus-infected blood transfusion in Kinshasa, Zaire. J Infect Dis; 164:450-456.

Curran JW, Lawrence DN, Jaffe H, et al (1984). Acquired immunodeficiency syndrome (AIDS) associated with transfusions. N Engl J Med; 310:69-75.

Donegan E, Lee H, Operskalski EA, et al (1994). Transfusion transmission of retroviruses: Human T-lymphotropic virus types I and II compared with human immunodeficiency virus type 1. Transfusion; 34:478-483.

Donegan E, Perkins H, Vyas G, et al (1986). Mortality in the recipients of blood in the Transfusion Safety Study. Blood; 68:296A.

Donegan E, Stuart M, Niland JC, et al (1990). Infection with human immunodeficiency virus type 1 (HIV-1) among recipients of antibody-positive blood donations. Ann Intern Med;113:733-739.

Egesie O.J, Joseph D.E, Egesie U.G, Odeh C.I. (2011). Trends in the incidence of hepatitis B, C and human immunodeficiency virus among blood donors in a tertiary hospital in Nigeria. J. Med. Tropics; 13(1) (In press).

Ejele OA, Erhabor O, Nwauche CA (2005). The risk of transfusion-transmissible viral infections in the Niger-Delta area of Nigeria. Sahel Medical Journal. 8(1):16-19.

Fasola FA, Kotila TR, Akinyemi JO (2009). Trend in transfusion transmitted viral infections from 2001 to 2006 in Ibadan, Nigeria. Intervirology; 51:427-431.

Federal Ministry of Health (2004). Summary of findings from 2003 National HIV seroprevalence survey in Nigeria. Information for policy makers.12-38.

Federal Ministry of Health (2009) 'National Blood Transfusion Service - About Us'

Fiekumo I.B., Musa A.M., Jeremiah Z.A (2009). Seroepidemiology of transfusion-transmissible infectious diseases among blood donors in Osogbo, South-west, Nigeria. Blood Transfusion.1:1-10.

Goodnough LT, Shander A, Brecher ME (2003). Transfusion medicine: looking to the future. Lancet. 11;361(9352):161-9.

Gupta N., Kumar V., Kaur A (2004). Seroprevalence of HIV, HBV, HCV, and syphilis in voluntary blood donors. Indian J Med Sci., 58(6): 255-256. (http://en.wikipedia.org/wiki/HIV)

Hassan A, Muktar HM, Mamman AI, Ahmed AJ, Isa AH and Babadoko AA (2008). The incidence of HIV among blood donors in Kaduna, Nigeria. Afr. Health Sc. 8(1); 60.

Kagu MB, Kawuwa MB, Ayilara AO, Ali BZ (2005). Seroprevalence of HIV and hepatitis viruses in directed blood donors: a preliminary report. Highland Medical Research Journal. 3(2):76-80.

Khan Z, Raziq F, Aslam N (2002). Prevalence of HIV in N.W.F.P. Journal of Postgraduate Medical Institute. 16(2):187-189.

Lackritz EM, Satten, GA, Aberle-Grasse J, et al (1995). Estimated risk of transmission of the human immunodeficiency virus by screened blood in the United States. N Engl J Med; 333:1721-1725.

Matee MI, Lyamuya EF, Mbena EC, Magessa PM, Sufi J, Marwa GJ et al (1997). Prevalence of transfusion associated viral infections and syphilis among blood donors in Muhimbili Medical Centre, Dar es Salaam, Tanzania. East Afr Med J. 76(3):167-171.

Medley GF, Anderson RM, Cox DR, et al (1987). Incubation period of AIDS in patients infected via blood transfusion. Nature; 328:719-721.

Mvere DA (2002). A strategy for blood safety in the African region. Afri Health; 24(5): 9-11.

Nigeria Exchange (2008) 'Ministry of health alerts Nigerians to the transfusion of unsafe blood in hospitals'

Olokoba A.B, Tidi S.K, Salawu F.K et al (2010). Human immunodeficiency virus infection in voluntary blood donors in North-Eastern Nigeria. American Journal of scientific and industrial research. 1(3):435-438.

Operskalski EA, Stram DO, Lee H, et al (1995). Human immunodeficiency virus type 1 infection: Relationship of risk group and age to rate of progression to AIDS. J Infect Dis; 172:648-655.

Osmond M, Dennis H (1994). Classification and staging of HIV disease, In The AIDS knowledge base. 2nd Ed. Cohen PT, Sande MA, Volberding PA(eds). New York: Little Brown.

Roberts CR, Longfield JN, Platte RC, Zielmanski KP, Wages J and Fowler A (1994). Transfusion-associated human immunodeficiency virus type1 from screened antibody-negative blood donor. Arch. Pathol. Lab. Med;118(12): 1188-1192.

Schreiber GB, Busch MP, Kleinman SH, et al (1996). The risk of transfusion-transmitted viral infections. N Engl J Med; 334:1686-1690.

Tessema B, Yismaw G, Kassu A, Amsalu A, Mulu A, Emmrich F and Sack U (2010). Seroprevalence of HIV, HBV, HCV and syphilis infections among blood donors at Gondar University Teaching Hospital, Northwest Ethiopia: declining trends over a period of five years. BMC Infectious diseases; 10:111. Also available @http://www.biomedcentral.com/1471-2334/10/111

Weinberg PD, Hounshell J, Sherman LA, Godwin J, Ali S, Tomori C, Bennett CL(2002). Legal, financial, and public health consequences of HIV contamination of blood and blood products in the 1980s and 1990s. Ann Intern Med. 19; 136(4):312-9.

World Health Organization (2002). Blood Safety Strategy for the African Region. Brazzaville, World Health Organization, Regional Office for Africa (WHO AFR/RC51/9 Rev.1).

World Health Organization (2007). Status of blood safety in the WHO African Region: Report of the 2004 Survey WHO Regional Office for Africa, Brazzaville .1-25

WHO/UNAIDS (2000). Guidelines for second generation HIV surveillance. Geneva, Switzerland: World Health Organization and Joint United Nations Programme on HIV/AIDS.

Part 4

Living with HIV/AIDS

15

Living and Working with HIV/AIDS: A Lifelong Process of Adaptation

André Samson and Habib Siam
University of Ottawa,
Faculty of Education
Canada

1. Introduction

Advancements in scientific knowledge and pharmacological therapies have led to the suppression of HIV replication in infected individuals and the concomitant recovery of immune function. This, in turn, has prompted a dramatic decline in the morbidity and mortality rates associated with HIV infection (UNAIDS, 2010; Werth, Borges, McNally, Maguire, & Britton, 2008). As a consequence, the majority of people living with HIV (PWHIV) who have access to anti-retroviral therapy and to the appropriate medical follow-ups experience a higher quality of life and longer life expectancy. A study conducted in Denmark estimated the median survival time for a young person diagnosed with HIV today at 38.9 years (Lohse et al., 2007).

A primary consequence of this evolution is that PWHIV must learn to adapt to their infection over the long term. The etymology of the verb " to adapt" stems from the Latin roots "ad", which means "towards", and "aptus", which signifies "apt," in the sense of something that is suitable. Therefore, "to adapt" literally means to move towards a suitable outcome or resolution. In the case of HIV/AIDS infection, successful adaptation involves restoring a sense of normalcy to one's everyday life, where "normalcy" is defined by PWHIV according to their perceived needs and situation. This process of adaptation involves numerous aspects, including medical/physical, psychological/affective, social, spiritual and vocational. Therefore, it is crucial to gain an in-depth understanding of how this process of adjustment unfolds.

In an effort to develop such an understanding, this chapter presents and describes a comprehensive theoretical model that accounts for the different aspects of this specific adaptive process. This chapter is divided into two main sections: the first is entitled "living with HIV/AIDS" and the second "working with HIV/AIDS". The former of the two sections is dedicated to developing a comprehensive task-based model of adaptation (CTBMA) to HIV/AIDS that incorporates the following five components: source of stress, cognitive appraisal, adaptive tasks, coping skills and outcome. The latter section describes a very specific adaptive task, the vocational one, that stems from the fact that HIV/AIDS is now categorized as a chronic illness that develops over the long term. Since it is now possible to lead an active life while living with HIV/AIDS, it is pertinent to understand how work helps PWHIV adapt to their infection.

2. Living with HIV

A comprehensive understanding of the adaptation process may help guide diagnosed patients, family members and their relatives through the many uncertainties they face and help them find a way to stabilize the sudden disruption they have experienced. Furthermore, health care professionals may be better equipped to understand their patients' efforts to adapt. A comprehensive look at adaptation processes could also provide policy makers with a broader view of the psychosocial ramifications and implications of living with HIV/AIDS in the age of anti-retroviral therapies.

Numerous theoretical models describe the adaptation to major life transitions, in general, and to the onset of chronic illness, in particular (Samson & Siam, 2008; Samson, Siam & Lavigne, 2007). The literature also shows that the slew of approaches can be grouped into two main paradigms, the first of which proposes that individuals adapt by moving through a set of phases. An example of this theoretical paradigm is Kubler-Ross' (1969) stage-based model, which has had a particularly important impact on health care professional working with palliative patients. Staged-based approaches have been subject to numerous critiques, primarily because their rigid linearity is seen as imposing on patients a prescriptive way to adapt to their condition or situation. This normative aspect does not take into consideration the highly subjective manner in which individuals learn to adapt to a HIV diagnosis. Ascribing to stage-based approaches may therefore lead to the exclusion of those patients who do not follow these predetermined stages, as well as to the imposition of unfounded expectations on medical personnel (Corr, 1992).

The second paradigm revolves around the notion that adaptation to change is achieved by accomplishing a non-linear series of adaptation tasks (Samson 2006; Corr et al, 2003; Corr, 1992; Cohen & Lazarus, 1979; Moos & Tsu, 1977). This approach to adaptation appears to present a more effective alternative to the process of psychosocial adaptation to chronic illness and, more specifically, to HIV/AIDS. This theoretical model sets forth the notion that the adaptation process is based on the completion of certain tasks. Corr (1992) defines tasks as "work that may be undertaken by those who are coping"(p.83) and deems such efforts essential to resolving life challenges. In other words, tasks can be understood as efforts undertaken to reconstruct one, or many, specific aspects of life that has been affected by the contraction of HIV/AIDS (Samson, 2006).

3. Task-based model of adaptation to HIV/AIDS

3.1 Core assumptions of the comprehensive task-based model of adaptation (CTBMA)

This comprehensive task-based model of adaptation (CTBMA) to chronic illness, and to HIV/AIDS in particular, is based on five core assumptions, as well as five components that will be described in the coming sections. The first core assumption is based on the fundamental premise that the process of adaptation to chronic illness is highly individual. As Corr (1992) states, health care professionals should avoid normative models like stage-based approaches, because these models exclude patients that do not comply with a prescribed set of phases. In this sense, the task-based model does not delineate an ideal way to adapt – the ideal manner being the one that the patient chooses to follow.

Secondly, the CTBMA is essentially phenomenological and transactional in nature. Indeed, through primary and secondary cognitive appraisal, patients continually evaluate and reevaluate the impact of HIV/AIDS on different aspects of their everyday lives (Cohen & Lazarus, 1979). This is why patients diagnosed with chronic illness do not perceive their condition in a uniform way. The importance given to cognitive appraisal underlies the highly individual nature of this adaptive process. Thirdly, the integrated model is based on the assumption that individuals possess an innate drive to achieve, and subsequently maintain, social and psychological homeostasis with the objective of regaining a sense of normalcy and satisfaction in life (Moos & Tsu, 1977).

The fourth assumption of the CTBMA is that the process of adaptation usually revolves around the reconstruction of aspects of the patients' lives that have been affected by the onset of chronic illness. Through this process of reconstruction, patients attempt to regain a sense of control over their lives. The fifth and final assumption of the CTBMA is that this process moves towards achieving either a positive or a negative outcome. Patients reach a positive outcome when they successfully reconstruct and reintegrate the aspects of their lives that have been affected by the onset of chronic illness. In other words, patients develop a sense of normality that does not deny or ignore the actual or potential physical or psychological consequences of their illness. Negative outcomes occur when patients are unable to cognitively appraise their diagnosis as a challenge that can be overcome. This perception is rooted in patients' belief that they do not possess the personal, social and professional resources to adapt. Negative outcomes can manifest themselves in the form of psychological deterioration, unsatisfactory social relationships, and difficulty to comply with medical treatment.

3.2 Components of the comprehensive task-based model of adaptation (CTBMA)

The framework that underpins the comprehensive task-based model of adaptation hinges on five components. The first component consists of the patient's history and social context; the second of cognitive evaluations of the diagnosis. The third consists of the different adaptation tasks; the fourth of the different coping skills and the fifth of the final outcome (Figure 1).

Component 1: Patient's personal history and social context

The CTBMA accounts for individuals' particular situation, or overall context, when news of the diagnosis is received. The context entails patients' life history, which encompasses ethnic origins, socio-economic status, previous life transitions and the quality of social support networks. It is crucial to account for these different personal aspects, as they have the potential to impact how patients perceive what is occurring to them. In this regard, patients' background and personal history may potentially impact the process of adaptation, both positively and negatively. According to Moos and Tsu (1977), it is the interplay of these factors that may influence the process of adaptation, to some degree at least.

Component 2: Cognitive appraisal of the diagnosis

The initial impact of the diagnosis and the subsequent achievement of adaptation tasks hinges on the individual cognitive appraisal of the stressor – which is the diagnosis itself. As mentioned in the description of the first component, this cognitive appraisal is contingent on patients' personal history and social context. The cognitive evaluation of the diagnosis is a primary determinant of the process of adaptation to chronic illness, in general, and to HIV/AIDS, in particular (Cohen & Lazarus, 1979). Therefore, the diagnosis does not affect individuals in a uniform manner because the experience itself is a function of individual perception or cognitive appraisal.

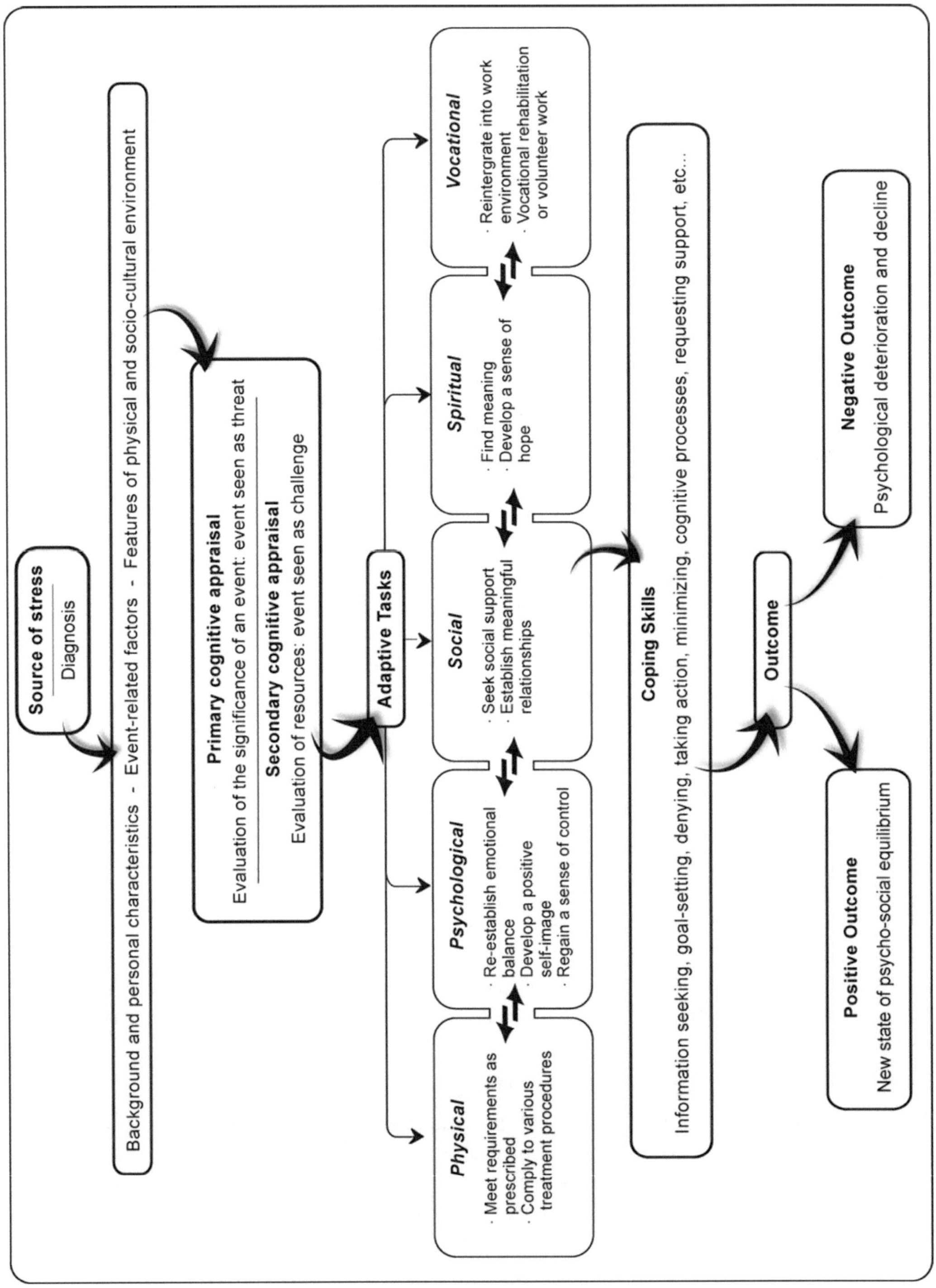

Fig. 1. Comprehensive task-based model of psychosocial adaptation to HIV/AIDS.

Cognitive appraisal can be classified into two categories: (a) primary appraisal and (b) secondary appraisal. Primary appraisal is the initial perception of the impact of the diagnosis, which may be perceived as being threatening, benign-positive, or irrelevant (Cohen & Lazarus, 1979). Primary appraisal is associated with the breaking news of a diagnosis. Perceiving the diagnosis as threatening triggers different psychological responses, such as denial, fear, anxiety, resentment or even anger. These reactions are usually indicators that patients believe that the diagnosis has taxed their resources to the extent that their reality is perceived as being hopeless.

With time, these reactions tend to diminish. The diagnosis gradually becomes a part of patients' lived, daily reality and the perceived threat of diagnosis diminishes. This evolution usually engenders a secondary appraisal, which indicates that patients have begun to perceive their illness as a challenge that requires adaptive efforts. More specifically, secondary appraisal consists of evaluating personal resources and alternatives in order to deal with the challenges, restrictions and demands that the illness imposes. It is the secondary appraisal that mobilizes patient efforts necessary to initiate the adaptation to the new medical condition. This shift in patients' cognitive appraisal of the illness and its impact helps them reconstruct a new sense of normalcy. Furthermore, cognitive appraisal is not a static process; rather, it is fluid and transactional because it evolves depending on patients' personal situation.

Component 3: Adaptive tasks.

Adaptive tasks form the third (and core) component of the CTBMA. These tasks encompass the principal aspects of human functioning that allow the process of adaptation to occur. The adaptive tasks are of a physical, psychological, social, spiritual and vocational nature.

The physical task consists primarily of meeting all medical requirements as prescribed by health care professionals. These may include the intake of medication, compliance to various treatment procedures and a healthier lifestyle that includes regular exercise and a balanced diet. The psychological task involves maintaining satisfactory emotional equilibrium and regaining a sense of control over one's life. The social task aims at gaining effective social support from significant others, friends and family. The spiritual task of adaptation is an effort at giving meaning to the onset of the illness and all the consequences it engenders.

Given the advancements in medical knowledge and interventions, patients living with chronic illness tend to enjoy longer life expectancies and a better overall quality of life. As a result, they are increasingly capable of maintaining an active lifestyle and engaging in meaningful activities. As such, it is important to incorporate a vocational task into the adaptation model. Through this task, which includes work that is both paid and unpaid, patients may resume their professional occupations, give a new orientation to their career or get involved in volunteer work. By accomplishing the vocational task, patients may find meaning in life, forge social status and establish a personal identity (Riverin-Simard, 2002).

The accomplishment of these five adaptive tasks can be achieved simultaneously or in succession, with the accomplishment of a specific task potentially facilitating that of another. This process may vary from one individual to the next, depending on their appraisal of the illness, their personal situation and overall coping skills.

Component 4: Coping skills.

The fourth component of the CTBMA consists of coping skills. If adaptation tasks are seen as the general domains of adjustment, then copings kills may be understood as the specific

means used to accomplish these tasks (Moos & Tsu, 1977). Furthermore, these skills, which embody both a mental and behavioral aspect, are likely to be used in conjunction with one another, rather than individually.
Coping skills include, but are not limited to, denying or minimizing the seriousness of diagnoses, seeking relevant information, requesting reassurance and emotional support, learning specific illness-related procedures, setting concrete limited goals, rehearsing alternative outcomes and finding a general purpose or pattern of meaning in the course of events. According to Cohen and Lazarus (1979) coping is defined as any effort aimed at managing, tolerating, and
minimizing the difficulties, restrictions, and demands typically associated with stressful life events. In summary, a coping skill is a cognitive or behavioral ability used to accomplish a specific task. These skills can be pre-existing at the moment of the diagnosis, or learned during the process of adaptation to the illness.

Component 5: Outcome.

Finally, the concluding component of the CTBMA is that of outcome. According to Moos and Tsu (1977) and Cohen and Lazarus (1979), there are two possible outcomes: (a) positive and (b) negative. While the former is indicative of a new state of psychosocial equilibrium, highlighted by a reestablished sense of normalcy, the latter alludes to a certain degree of psychological deterioration and decline. In other words, a positive outcome is achieved when the illness is seen as less of a disruption and becomes an accepted aspect, among others, of patients' lives. Patients regain a certain sense of control over the course their existence and develop a new perception of life satisfaction (Samson, 2006).
In summary, the CTBMA is predicated on how patients cognitively appraise the impact of illness on their lives. This appraisal is mediated by patients' personal history and context. When patients perceive their illness as a challenge that can be overcome, they begin the process of adaptation. This process is determined by the tasks patients need to accomplish in order to reestablish a sense of normalcy in their lives. These tasks are of a physical, psychological, social, spiritual and vocational nature. The accomplishment of these tasks mobilizes patients' existing coping skills and catalyzes their abilities to learn new ones. At the end of the adaptation process, patients resume a train of life that may be different from the one they led before the diagnosis but is nonetheless a source of satisfaction. Illness is perceived as less of a threatening stranger and more of an unwanted companion: life is different but normal again.
Extensive research has been conducted on the conceptualization and understanding of the first four adaptation tasks. However, little is the vocational aspect of the process of adaptation. This is why the remainder of the chapter focuses on this specific aspect of the CTBMA.

4. Working with HIV/AIDS

4.1 Introduction

This second section describes the content and analyzes the aspects of the vocational task, based on empirical research that has been conducted on the role of paid and unpaid work in the process of adaptation to HIV/AIDS. The rationale behind this section is that the current body of research concerns itself primarily with the physical, psychological, social and spiritual adaptive tasks related to HIV/AIDS. Researchers have paid insufficient attention to the vocational task (Samson, Lavigne & MacPherson, 2009). The dearth in scientific studies is partially explained by the fact that, until the recent past, PWHIV were unable to resume their professional activities or to maintain an active life. With advancements in pharmacological interventions, this is no longer the case. Most PWHIV are now able to lead productive lives, despite their infection, which is why it is important to pay special attention to the vocational task and its contribution to the process of adaptation.

Work is probably one of the most normative activities in individuals' lives. It brings financial autonomy, helps create social networks, allows for self-expression, and provides the possibility to contribute to the common good. In fact, in a globalized economy, work is probably the main aspect of individual identity and a primary contributor to finding meaning in life (Samson, 2006; Riverin-Simard, 2002). This is why one of the principal negative impacts of being diagnosed with a major chronic illness is the deprivation of the ability to work. This, in turn, may lead to social marginalization, a loss of personal identity, and the perception that tangible social contributions are no longer achievable. In this context, the resumption of work activities can therefore be interpreted as an important step in the achievement of a positive outcome in the adaptation process (Samson & Siam, 2008; Samson, 2006).

4.2 The vocational task in the context of adaptation to HIV/AIDS

When it comes to PWHIV, many factors can motivate a return to the job market. A qualitative study identified some of these motivations and showed that working helped the 30 participants feel useful and fulfilled (Brooks & Klosinski, 1999). Work also restores meaning to people's existence, gives them the opportunity to contribute to society, to expand their social network, and to regain a sense of normality. In addition, remunerated work leads to a certain amount of financial independence and can alleviate the social shame and stigma associated with being on social assistance (Conyers, 2004).

In a study conducted by Blalock, McDaniel and Farber (2002), participants living with HIV/AIDS who were also employed reported enjoying a significantly higher quality of life than did their unemployed counterparts. This finding supports the evidence-based notion that work is a contributing factor to recovery and healing (Escovitz & Donegan, 2005). People who successfully return to work after a period of disability have better health indices and shorter durations of disability than people who do not return to work (Martin, Steckart, & Arns, 2006).

Research has shown that there are undeniable benefits to professional reintegration for PWHIV, which positively contributes to the adaptation to HIV/AIDS. The accomplishment of the vocational task can even aid in the completion of other tasks, most notably through the expansion of meaningful social networks, a rise in self-esteem and self-efficacy, and the development of a renewed sense of meaning in life.

Nevertheless, the accomplishment of the vocational task may be complicated by a number of barriers and challenges. Job market re-entry is indeed a complex process and, in certain circumstances, may require professional assistance (Escovitz & Donegan, 2005). According to some researchers, living with HIV/AIDS constitutes a handicap and returning to work may require a form of assistance similar to that which is generally provided to individuals with a physical disability (Arns, Martin, & Chernoof, 2004). The types of obstacles faced by PWHIV can be medical, professional, social, or financial in nature (Goldblum & Kohlenberg, 2005; Martin, Brooks, Ortiz, & Venigas, 2003; Martin et al., 2006; Werth et al., 2008). Over

91% of PWHIV that participated in a 2006 study conducted by Martin et al. (2006) reported experiencing at least one of the above listed barriers during their efforts to return to work.

First, medical barriers are directly related to the consequences of the infection. It remains difficult to predict the rate at which immunodeficiency will develop due to HIV infection and exactly when antiretroviral therapy will be required (Argentier, Fernet, Levy, Bastien, & Fernet, 2003). This uncertainty in prognosis and difficulties in anticipating medical intervention can weigh heavily on PWHIV and their future expectations. Though most PWHIV now enjoy a higher quality of life, many issues, such as resistance to drugs, still cause high levels of uncertainty. This element of the unknown hinders and complicates vocational development and professional reintegration (Brooks & Klosinski, 1999; Hoffman, 1997; Martin et al., 2003).

One of the more significant side effects associated with HIV/AIDS treatment is lipodystrophy or body fat redistribution. Individuals with lipodystrophy lose fat from their face, arms, legs, and buttocks and gain fat in the abdomen and upper back. For some, this fat redistribution can be significant and disfiguring. This may not only affect self-esteem, but can also significantly impact those whose occupation involves interaction with the public (Argentier et al., 2003). In addition, there is fear that stress related to work could be detrimental to overall health or that the workplace could constitute an environment where there is a risk of contracting an infection (Arns et al., 2004).

A realistic return to the job market must take into consideration individuals' health status. The professional activities must be adjusted to the limits and boundaries associated with the illness (Hunt, Jaques, Niles, & Wierzalis, 2003). For the poor or near poor, issues of finding and maintaining a job often take precedence over larger decision-making processes, such as choosing among a variety of job opportunities (Werth et al., 2008).

The second type of barrier is associated with career issues and vocational development. The competitiveness of the job market, fueled by a globalized economy, affects all people, regardless of whether or not they are living with HIV/AIDS. PWHIV, however, face additional challenges that limits their vocational flexibility. For example, PWHIV may require ongoing medical care and monitoring, which are usually provided by specialists and are generally only accessible in large urban centers. Such geographic restrictions on job mobility can affect employability and opportunities for advancement (Timmons & Fesko, 2004).

As supported by existing research, it is obvious that today's economic dynamics can complicate PWHIV's reentry into the job market. Not only do they have to cope with the current economic climate, as do all employees, but they also have to take into account the limitations their medical situation imposes. Furthermore, PWHIV may be forced to find new types of occupations, as their professional activities may have become too physically demanding and their medical status may no longer tolerate the kind of stress generated by their work. Furthermore, this imposed career transition may be difficult to achieve as it may require a certain amount of retraining and the acquisition of new professional skills in a field of activity that is less labor-intensive (Maguire, McNally, Britton, Werth, & Borges; 2008).

The third type of barrier is caused by the social stigma afflicting PWHIV (Herek, Capitanio, & Widaman, 2002). This stigma has the potential to obstruct PWHIV's efforts for job market reentry. In fact, the majority of PWHIV experience some form of rejection or discrimination in the workplace (Brooks et al., 2004). Specifically, they worry that the accidental disclosure of their condition may lead to a form of exclusion, slow the progression of their career, or even lead to job termination (Brooks & Klosinski, 1999; Hoffman, 1997). A recent study confirms that PWHIV not only experience stigma, but also different forms of abuse (Maguire et al., 2008).

Social stigma related to HIV/AIDS manifests itself in a multiplicity of ways. For example, PWHIV may worry about having to explain or justify their medication intake or the recurring physician consultations scheduled during work hours (Hunt et al., 2003). PWHIV may also worry about the possible humiliation they may be subject to because of the bureaucratic procedures necessary to obtain benefits (Conyers, 2004).

The fourth type of barrier is financial in nature. In certain jurisdictions, returning to work may lead to the termination of long-term disability benefits, a drawback that is compounded by PWHIV's inability to regain these benefits in the event that their health begins to deteriorate. Preoccupation with this potential loss of financial security can lead to increased stress and worry, to the point of debilitating PWHIV in their vocational decision-making (Brooks et al., 2004; Ferrier & Lavis, 2003). Brooks et al. (2004) concluded that, of a sample of 536 unemployed PWHIV, 73% of those contemplating a return to work ranked the fear of losing their disability income as the most significant barrier to the resumption of professional activities.

In conclusion, many obstacles confront PWHIV who wish to return to work and further their careers. Even though a number of PWHIV perceives a return to work as a plausible possibility, reentering the job market can be daunting for some and can therefore jeopardize the process of adaptation.

Under these circumstances, volunteer work may constitute a more realistic option. Research has shown that volunteer work in other medical and social contexts can be a form of personal investment and achievement (Conyers, 2004). Samson et al. (2009) conducted a study on PWHIV engaged in volunteer work and the role of these activities in facilitating the adaptation process. Their qualitative analysis showed that volunteer work could be an alternate way to regain an active lifestyle. More specifically, this research found that volunteer work allows participants to enrich their social lives, to regain a sense of psychological wellbeing, and to apply their abilities to the benefit of others.

One of the more interesting conclusions of this qualitative research is that participants justify their choice to volunteer for HIV/AIDS organizations by explaining that they wish to avoid discrimination and social stigma. In other words, when it comes to volunteer work, PWHIV choose to contribute to organizations that deal with their condition. In doing so, they avoid any form of stress associated with social stigma. The participants are driven by a protective instinct that makes them want to be on familiar ground and to be in an environment where HIV/AIDS is not stigmatized.

In comparison to paid work, where secrecy seems to mitigate the social stigma associated with HIV/AIDS, the choice of the right organization appears to be the solution to prevent social alienation when it comes to volunteering engagements. Both of these strategies involve protective measures, the first of which leads to a form of clandestine behavior where PWHIV are forced to hide their condition from their coworkers, while the second limits PWHIV's choices of volunteer organizations. Despite these restrictions, volunteer work provides a certain degree of flexibility and freedom not normally associated with remunerated work.

In summary, the vocational task appears to be an important aspect of the CTBMA, specifically in contexts where there is an increase in the number of PWHIV who are able to maintain an active lifestyle. Empirical data shows that the accomplishment of this specific task enhances the satisfaction and overall quality of life of PWHIV. Nevertheless, there exist a number of barriers that impede professional reintegration and must be overcome for PWHIV to accomplish a successful reentry into the job market. Finally, it seems that volunteer work can be a viable alternative to remunerated employment.

5. Conclusion

Given the advancements in scientific knowledge and the progress in medicine, major chronic illnesses have, and will continue to, become manageable conditions that are no longer considered as debilitating as they once were (Samson & Siam, 2008). Consequently, individuals diagnosed with chronic diseases are increasingly capable of maintaining active lifestyles. This is particularly true for PWHIV. As previously discussed, it is important for people living with chronic illness, in general, and with HIV/AIDS, in particular, to adapt to their condition over the long term. A comprehensive model that theorizes the different aspects of the adaptation process is crucial in enhancing our understanding of how individuals with chronic illness adapt to their new medical reality and strive to reestablish a certain sense of normalcy in their lives.

The CTBMA proposes an exhaustive description of how people adapt to the onset of a chronic illness. The model includes five components and five adaptive tasks, which are medical, social, psychological, spiritual and vocational. The primary strength of this model is that it accounts for the highly individual nature of the adaptation process. Rather than prescribe an ideal way to adapt, the model posits that adaptation should be dictated by the individual context and reality. However, it appears that the vocational task is becoming an increasingly important aspect of the adaptation process. This may be caused by the fact that work is one of the most normative aspects of individuals' lives and that people with chronic illness are more capable of rejoining the workforce than they once were. These trends should invite a renewed focus on the vocational task and the role of work, paid or unpaid, in the adaptation process.

6. References

Argentier, S., Fernet, M., Levy, J. J., Bastien, R., & Fernet, R. (2003). Les médicaments antirétroviraux et al VIH/sida: Entre espoir et scepticisme. *Frontières*, 16(1), 44–56.

Arns, P. G., Martin, D. J., & Chernoff, R. A. (2004). Psychosocial needs of HIV-positive individuals seeking workforce re-entry. *AIDS Care*, 16(3), 377–386.

Blalock, A. C., McDaniel, J. S., & Farber, E. W. (2002). Effect of employment on quality of life and psychological functioning in patients with HIV/AIDS. *Psychosomatics*, 43(5), 400–404.

Brooks, R. S., Martin, D. J., Ortiz, D. J., & Venigas, R. C. (2004). Perceived barriers to employment among persons living with HIV/AIDS. *AIDS Care*, 16, 756–766.

Brooks, R. A., & Klosinski, L. E. (1999). Assisting persons living with HIV/AIDS to return to work: Programmatic steps for AIDS service organizations. *AIDS Education and Prevention*, 11(3), 212–223.

Cohen, F., & Lazarus R. S. (1979). Coping with the stress of illness. In: C. G. Stone, F. Cohen, N., & E. Adler (Eds), *Health psychology: A handbook* (pp. 217–254). San Francisco, CA: Jossey-Bass.

Conyers, L. M. (2004). Expanding understanding of HIV/AIDS and employment: Perspectives of focus groups. *Rehabilitation Counseling Bulletin*, 48(1), 5-18.

Corr, C. A., Nabe, C. M., Corr, D. M. (2003). *Death and dying, life and living*. Belmont, CA: Wadsworth.

Corr, C. (1992). A task-based approach to coping with dying. *Omega*, 24, 81-94.

Escovitz, K., & Donegan, K. (2005). Proving effective employment supports for persons living with HIV: The KEEP project. *Journal of Vocational Rehabilitation*, 22, 105-114.

Ferrier, S.E., & Lavis, J.N. (2003). With health comes work? People living with HIV/AIDS consider returning to work. *AIDS Care*, 15(3), 423-435.

Goldblum, P., & Kohlenberg, B. (2005). Vocational counseling for people with HIV: The client-focused considering work model. *Journal of Vocational Rehabilitation*, 69, 30-36.

Herek, G. M., Capitanio, J. P., & Widaman, K. F. (2002). HIV-related stigma and knowledge in the United States: Prevalence and trends, 1991-1999. *American Journal of Public Health*, 92(2), 371-377.

Hoffman, M. A. (1997). HIV disease and work: Effect on the individual, workplace, and interpersonal contexts. *Journal of Vocational Behavior*, 51, 163-201.

Hunt, B., Jaques, J., Niles, S. G., & Wierzalis, E. (2003). Career concerns for people living with HIV/AIDS. *Journal of Counseling and Development*, 81(1), 55-67.

Kubler-Ross, E. (1969). *On death and dying*. New York, NY: McMillan Publishing Company.

Lohse, N., Hansen, A. B., Pedersen, G., Kronborg, G., Gerstoft, J., Sørensen, H. T., et al. (2007). Survival of persons with and without HIV infection in Denmark. *Annals of Internal Medicine*, 146(2), 87-95.

Maguire, C. P., McNally, C. J., Britton, P. J., Werth, J. L., & Borges, N. J. (2008). Challenges of work: Voices of persons with HIV disease. *The Counselling Psychologist*, 36(1), 42-89.

Martin, D. J., Steckart, M. J., & Arns, P. G. (2006). Returning to work with HIV/AIDS: A qualitative study. *Work*, 27, 209-219.

Martin, D. J., Brooks, R. A., Ortiz, D.J., & Venigas, R. C. (2003). Perceived employment barriers and their relation to workforce entry intent among people with HIV/AIDS. *Journal of Occupational Health Psychology*, 8, 181-194.

Moos, R. H, & Tsu, D.V. (1977). *Coping with physical illness*. NewYork, NY: Plenum Medical Company.

Riverand-Simard, D. (2002). Le sens du travail et la carrièrologie. *Carrièrologie*, 8, 303-320.

Samson, A., Lavigne, R., & MacPherson, P. A. (2009). Self-fulfillment despite barriers: Volunteer work of people living with HIV. *AIDS Care*, 21(11), 1425-1431.

Samson, A., & Siam, H. (2008). Adapting to major chronic illnesses: A proposal for a comprehensive task-model approach. *Patient Education and Counseling*, 70(3), 426-429.

Samson, A., Siam, H. & Lavigne, R. (2007). Psychosocial adaptation to chronic illness: description and illustration of an integrated task-based model. *Interventions*, 127, 16-28.

Samson. A. (2006). L'apport de la carrière au modèle théorique des taches d'adaptation a la maladie chronique: une application au cas des personnes qui vivent avec le VIH. *Canadian Journal of Counselling*, 40, 4-16.

Timmons, J. C., & Fesko, S. L. (2004). The impact, meaning, and challenges of work: Perspectives of individuals with HIV/AIDS. *Health & Social Work*, 29(2), 137–144.

United Nations Programs on HIV/AIDS. (2010). *Global report: UNAIDS report on the global AIDS epidemic 2010*. Geneva, Switzerland: WHO Library.

Werth, J. L., Borges, N. J., McNally, C. J., Maguire, C. P., & Britton, P. J. (2008). The intersections of work, health, diversity, and social justice: Helping people living with HIV disease. *The Counselling Psychologist*, 36(1), 16–41.

16

Factors Associated with Neuropsychological Impairment in HIV Infection

Yogita Rai[1], Tanusree Dutta[2] and Ambak Kumar Rai[3]
[1]*Department of Psychology, Faculty of Social Sciences, Banaras Hindu University (B.H.U.), Varanasi*
[2]*Department of Psychology, Mahila Mahavidyalaya, Banaras Hindu University (B.H.U.), Varanasi*
[3]*Cellular Immunology Division, Department of Transplant Immunology & Immunogenetics, All India Institute of Medical Sciences (A.I.I.M.S.), Ansari Nagar, New Delhi*
India

1. Introduction

In today's world, human immunodeficiency virus (HIV)/acquired immunodeficiency syndrome (AIDS) has poorly affected the vast majority of population and has been declared as one of the worst pandemic. It still remains the major public health burden across the world. The burden of HIV is increasingly progressing and due to lack of adequate knowledge among the population, their management is severely compromised. Advancement in the treatment of these cases are significant. New treatments are capable of reducing plasma viral load and in turn decreasing mortality (Carpenter et al., 1998). The betterment of patients with existing treatment regimen is quite evident, at least clinically and virologically. Here, important question is regarding life threatening impact of virus on various vital functions of the body. That includes central and peripheral nervous system (CNS) function. Such impact of virus becomes more evident, once their number increases to a numeric mark most often at the later stage of infection. However, it is reported that HIV enters the CNS within two weeks of initial infection (Krebs et al., 2000). Neuropsychological compromise are thought to occur secondary to HIV infection (Becker et al., 1997; Bornstein et al., 1993; Grant & A. Martin, 1994; Heaton et al., 1995; Hinkin et al., 1995; Maj et al., 1994a; Maj et al., 1994b; Martin et al., 1992; Stern, 1991; Van Gorp et al., 1989; von Giesen et al., 2001). When cases are presented, HIV-related neurocognitive disfunctioning may remain unnoticed at very early stage of infection. As the disease progress from asymptomatic to symptomatic and then to full blown AIDS, many neuropsychological impairments of clinical relevance appears in daily life of the patient, which may or may not have any functional significance. Especially, individual infected with HIV who is otherwise physically asymptomatic, these deficits may result in significant morbidity, in the sense that infected people may be unable to perform important tasks (e.g. bathing, cleaning, driving, work tasks), that influence their quality of life (QOL) and healthcare management directly. Such impairments may range from less severe unnoticeable defects to frank dementia syndromes that profoundly disrupt an infected individual's functioning and activities of daily living. The neurocognitive deficits typically associated with HIV-1 infection include decrements in motor and information-processing speed, divided attention, memory retrieval processes, and executive functioning. Overall, the gross estimates of people infected HIV who experience neuropsychological impairment is range from 30% to 50% of total infected individuals (Grant & Martin, 1994; Foley et al., 2008).

Neuropsychological impairment can be classified into three subgroups (Grant et at., 1988). First group includes patients with subsyndromic neuropsychological impairment show deficits in at least two neuropsychological domains with no evidence of functional impairment. Second group is mild neurocognitive disorder or minor cognitive/ motor disorder and involve deficits in at least two domains (of ability) of neuropsychological test battery, sufficient affect patient daily functioning. Third group consist of most severe HIV-1 associated dementia which is characterized by moderate to severe cognitive and psychomotor slowing, impaired concentration and attention, memory disturbances and often motor incordination and weakness. Many studies made attempt to found factors associated with neurocognitive impairment in HIV infection. However, factors related to neuropsychological impairment remain poorly understood. Herewith, we have reviewed the possible factors and divided them into three groups depending on their origin. Present chapter is an attempt to review the available literature on the possible factors and to discuss their mechanisms those are associated with neurocognitive impairment (Figure-1).

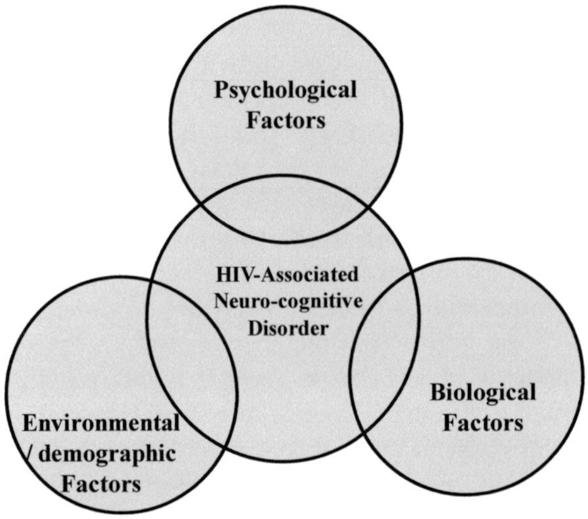

Fig. 1. Factors affecting HIV associated neuro-cognitive impairment

HIV associated neuro-cognitive impairment /disorder are affected by three confounding factors; Biological factors, Psychological factors, Environmental and demographic factors. Initially, HIV does not easily get into the brain. But once it enters through blood-brain barrier and infects the resident microglial cells (a type of macrophage, which harbours the virus). Majority of the influence of biological factors are mediated by direct infection of HIV in brain. Symptoms of HIV associated neuro-cognitive impairments are misjudged with various other psychological problems like depression/ mood disorder, apathy and stress. Environmental and demographic factors like age, gender etc. also influence the HIV mediated neuro-cognitive impairment.

2. Biological factors

2.1 Direct infection of HIV

Earlier, for long time, it was never thought of that HIV can also infect brain cells and that led to poor interpretation of many mental disorders associated with HIV-1 infection. Now, this biological stigma has been resolved. HIV-1 targets the cells of lymphoid and myeloid origin containing major HIV-1 receptors, CD4 and various chemokine receptors considered as HIV-1 co-receptors. These receptors help the attachment of the virus to the cell and the fusion of their membrane resulting in the entry of the virus into the cell (Zaitseva et al., 2003). Infected CD4+ T cells and monocytes, which circulate in the blood, are the potential source of CNS infection (Gonzalez-Scarano & Martin-Garcia, 2005). Many cells, such as T cells and monocytes are infected by HIV-1, these cells circulate in the blood and can cross the blood-brain barrier (BBB) and propagate the infection within the CNS (Figure-2) (Haase, 1986). A major part of HIV-1 associated neurological disfunctioning may be attributed to the entry of HIV-1 into the brain by crossing. The HIV-1 associated neuropathology is characterized by the infiltration of HIV-1 carrying macrophages into the CNS; the formation of microglial nodules; and multinucleated giant cells which result possibly from virus-induced fusion of microglia and/or macrophages in central white and deep gray matter; activation of astrocytes and their damage; neuronal loss particularly in hippocampus, basal ganglia and caudate nucleus. In addition, a variable degree of white matter pathology with evidence of broad range of myelin damage has been reported. HIV-1 has also been detected in the cerebral spinal fluid (CSF) (Gendelman et al., 1994). Imaging of brain using MRI, confirm that HIV infection is associated with progressive cortical atrophy within the gray and white matter, particularly in the later stage of the disease (Hall et al., 1996; Dal Pan et al., 1992; Stout et al., 1998; Aylward et al., 1993). These studies confirm that in the latter stage of infection, the anatomical atrophy in certain parts of brain occurs and many of them proven critical in the daily functioning of the individuals. These studies also report a correlation between the deterioration of cognitive function and the reduction in volume of certain brain structures.

2.2 Immunodeficiency (opportunistic infections, CD4 & plasma viral load)

2.2.1 Level of plasma HIV ribonucleic acid (RNA)

The levels of HIV-1 or its immune-dominant antigens/RNA (viral load) in plasma of infected individuals are the established marker for onset/progress of HIV related pathology. Infection of HIV-1 to brain cells is characterized by their presence in CSF. It is also proven that level of HIV RNA in CSF is elevated in subjects with cognitive impairments (Ellis et al., 1997; McArthur et al., 1997) and it also predicts future neuropsychological impairment (Ellis et al., 2002).The relationship between viral load and the mechanisms of cognitive decline requires further study. Clinically, however, a relationship between plasma HIV RNA levels and cognitive impairment would be more useful for diagnostic point of view. It is postulated that higher plasma HIV RNA levels may be associated with higher levels of circulating HIV-infected monocytes which may enter the blood-brain barrier and affect CNS functioning (Gartner, 2000). However, research on the direct relationship between plasma viral load and cognitive functioning remains equivocal. Various group failed to find a relationship between overall impairment and plasma HIV RNA (Ellis et al. 1997; Reger et al., 2005). However, contradictory reports are also available (Childs et al., 1999; Ellis et al., 2002). In a small neuropsychological battery, Stankoff et al. (1999) found a significant relationship between motor functioning and plasma viral load. It seems that plasma viral load is associated with neuropsychological impairment but a lot is required to confirm its role as a predictive marker for neuropsychological impairment. Contradictory reports suggest that a comprehensive, in-depth and longitudinal approach with a multi-domain tool is needed is required to affirm its role as a marker.

2.2.2 Opportunistic infections

Opportunistic infections (OIs) of HIV patients significantly reduce their immunity to HIV and this majorly compromised their QOL. OIs generally occur in HIV infected patients with CD4 below 200, when their immune system is not sufficient enough to mount required immunity to prevent the OIs. Development of OIs further compromises their immunity, which in turn aggravates the expansion of HIV-1 and it's spillage into CNS. It is also seen that presence of OIs in HIV infected patients are significantly associated with neuropsychological impairment in HIV infection. The determination of causes of neuropsychological impairment in HIV infection becomes more difficult because of various co-infections associated with it. More often heavy and chronic use of neuro-toxic drugs make it more complicated to study about exact cause. While challenging, these are questions that at one time in the HIV pandemic seemed difficult to imagine.

2.2.3 Treatment of disease

The effects of the HAART on neurocognitive functioning have not been assessed, although there have been some scanty studies showing neurocognitive effects of zidovudine (AZT) (Schmitt et al., 1988; Sidtis et al. 1993; Martin et al., 1999). Because drugs (HAART) can cross blood-brain barrier to achieve sufficient concentration to inhibit HIV replication in the CNS (Enting et al, 1998; Tashima, 1998; Limoges et al., 2000). It has also been shown that Zidovudine (AZT) monotherapy at current standard and higher doses can improve neuropsychological performance (Schmitt et al., 1988, Martin et al., 1999) and severity of dementia (Sidtis et al., 1993). However, the benefits of AZT monotherapy may be temporary because of the emergence of viral resistance (Gulevich et al., 1993). It was observed that individuals who are treated with HAART shortly after the first symptoms of dementia appear may show dramatic improvement.

2.2.4 CD4

Several studies reported that CD4 count is negatively related with neuropsychological impairment. Bornstein et al., (1991) found that patients with CD4 levels less than 200 had low scores on measures of motor speed, verbal memory acquisition, visual motor speed and mental tracking in comparison to patients with CD4 counts above 200. Osowiecki, et al. (2000) has reported a significant association of CD4 count with neurocognitive deficits. Perry, et al. (1989) found that among HIV positive patients, those scoring in the impaired range on neuropsychological measures had lower CD4 counts and lower CD4 /CD8 ratios than patients scoring in the normal range. It is also suggested that CD4 level correlates significantly with cognitive functioning. Several other studies have reported no relationship between neuropsychological performance and CD4 cell count (McArthur et al., 1989; Saykin et al., 1988; Martin et al., 1998). According to Honni and Bornstein (2002) there is very little evidence to suggest a significant association between CD4 count and the prediction of impairment.

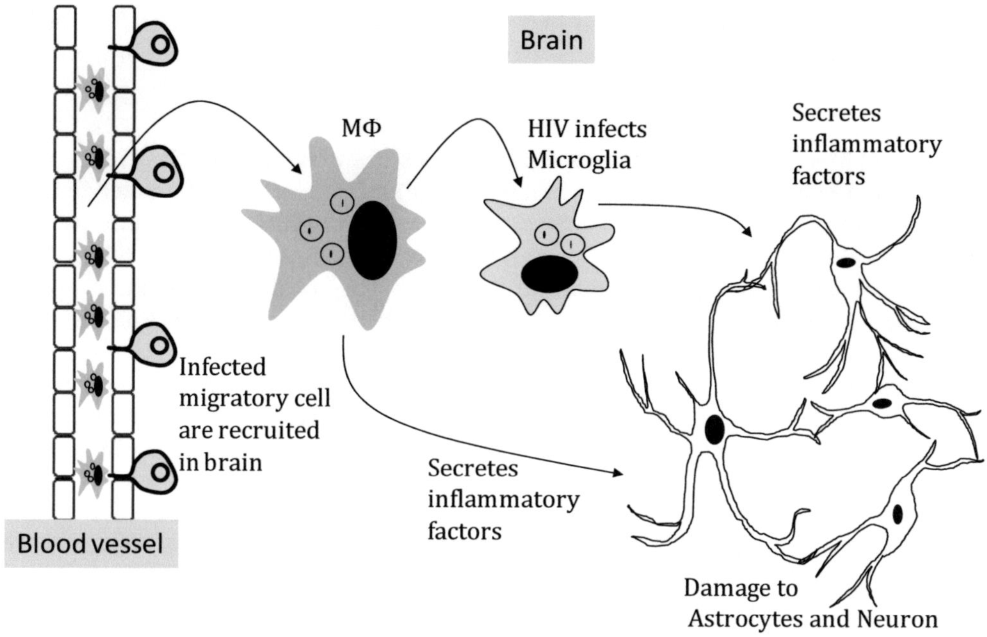

Fig. 2. HIV crosses blood-brain barrier (BBB)

Infected macrophages (carrying HIV) crosses the blood brain barrier and enters into the brain and infects other cells. Infected cells as well as other resident brain cells produce copious amount of mediators (inflammatory factors, various neurotransmitter etc. In the presence of HIV, these factors irreversibly damage the astrocytes and neurons.

3. Psychological factors

3.1 Depression

Neuropsychological impairments are common in HIV infection with major depression although their nature remains partly unclear. Hypothalamic-pituitary-adrenal axis dysfunction is associated with neuropsychological dysfunction in major depressive disorder although evidence of direct causation is not definitive at present. Appearance of symptoms of depression has been significantly reported in patients with HIV-1 infection (Atkinson, et al., 1988; Perry., 1990; Perkins et al., 1994; Rabkin, 2000). However, the causative co-existence of major depression and neuropsychological impairment has not been reported. Additionally, symptoms of depression and neuropsychological impairment may occur together in many HIV-infected persons. Cysique et al., (2007) reported that neurocognitive impairment and major depression should be considered as two independent processes. Moreover, studies have demonstrated that neuropsychological abnormalities observed in HIV infection are distinct and cannot be attributed to depression (Marsh et al., 1994; Mapou et al., 1993; Perkins et al., 1994; Richardson et al., 1999; Bornstein et al., 1993, Claypoole et al., 1998; Goodwin et al., 1996; Goggin et al., 1997; Grant et al 1988; Moore et al., 1997). It has been shown that depressed patients with HIV-1 infection may exhibit deficits in learning and memory (Claypoole et al., 1998; Goggin et al., 1997; Kalechstein et al. 1998), but the contributions/involvement of depression to the impairment and severity of the neuropsychological functioning appear to be minimal. However, more research is needed to confirm and widen these findings, and to expand the knowledge into clinical practice.

3.2 Apathy

Apathy refers to a cluster of symptoms reflecting lack of motivation manifested in motoric, emotional, and cognitive domains. To define here, motoric apathy is characterized by the tendency not to initiate a new motor activity unless externally prompted. Emotional apathy is defined as diminished intensity or persistence of emotion, or placidity, relative to the importance of some goal-directed thought or event. The third one, cognitive apathy is defined as indifference, a generalized loss of interest, decrease in goal-directed thought content diminished motivation associated with executive functions, and sometimes decreased verbal fluency. In context to the subject, Castellon et al., (1998) investigated the relationship between apathy, depression, and cognitive performance in HIV infection. They reported that apathy, but not depression, was found to be associated with working memory deficits among HIV subjects. Higher apathy scores and poorer working memory characterized the subjects with AIDS. Castellon et al., (1998) concluded that apathy is independent of depression and may indicate CNS involvement in HIV infection. In contrast, Rabkin et al., (2000) reported that apathy was consistently related to depression and unrelated to neuropsychological impairment.

3.3 Stress

Life stress has frequently been examined in the context of psychosocial factors in HIV-infected people because of the known adverse effects of stress on immunity of host (Patterson et al., 1995; Evans et al., 1997). In the context of cognitive function among HIV-infected people, the potential importance of stress has gained increased support from available literature. Moreover, these reports have demonstrated its adverse effects on brain structure and function. Several animal studies have reported atrophy in the CA3 region of the hippocampus in response to stress (Kim & Yoon, 1998). The chronic stress induced structural changes in brain is mediated by glucocorticoid hormones and neurotransmitters such as serotonin and the GABA-benzodiazepine system (McEwen, 2000) Furthermore, corticosterone a glucocorticoid appears to regulate levels of internal calcium (Ca2+) and thus may influence synaptic plasticity, aging, and cell death (Kim & Yoon, 1998). In context to patients, It has been demonstrated that atrophy in brain and abnormalities in its function are result of heightened levels of glucocorticoids and severe, traumatic stress (McEwen, 2000). In another study, it is observed that stressful life events were significantly related to cognitive performance only in the HIV-infected subjects (Pukay-Martin et al., 2003).

3.4 Drug addiction

It is well known that the intravenous administration of drugs with shared needles is an important cause for the spread of HIV burden. The persistent use of drugs through other routes (e.g., inhaling crack/cocaine) may also increase the risk for HIV infection. Drug abusers also practice prostitution to support their livelihood, habit and they may also engage in risky sexual behavior while under the influence of drugs or alcohol. But injection drug use with shared needle has also been seen as a main reason for the rapid progression of HIV among drug abusers (Bouwman et al., 1998), and has been found to diminish overall neuropsychological performance and reduce visuomotor processing, executive functioning, motor speed and strength, and sensorimotor perception in persons in the very early stages of HIV infection (Claypoole et al., 1993). It was initially thought that frequent drug usage may impair the cognitive functioning among HIV-seropositive persons for (Wellman, 1992). It was also postulated that drug usage possibly induces CNS impairment independent of that caused by HIV infection. However, this argument does not appear to hold true, asmost studies have found that neuropsychological dysfunction may not be contributed solely or partially by substance abuse, if we do not consider HIV seropositivity (Janssen et al., 1989). It was also suggested that the interaction of HIV infection and drug use might produce additive and synergistic cognitive deficits. Studies suggest that co-presence of HIV infection and drug use does not affect the cognitive functioning (Selnes et al., 1990; Selnes et al., 1992; Goodwin et al., 1996; Bornstein et al., 1993; Bono et al., 1996; Selnes et al., 1995). Cristiani et al., (2004) reported that the effect of marijuana use was greatest in subjects with symptomatic HIV infection. Further inspection suggested that this effect was due primarily to performance on memory tasks. Their finding suggest that although there is minimal impact of marijuana on uninfected individuals or those at early stages of HIV infection, there is a synergistic effect of HIV and marijuana use in patients with advanced HIV disease. Exception to the earlier studies, it was reported that HIV infection and methamphetamine dependence are each associated with neuropsychological deficits, and suggest that these factors in combination are associated with additive deleterious cognitive effects (Rippeth et al., 2004). It is also suggestive of that both HIV infection and methamphetamine dependence can be associated with brain dysfunction.

4. Environmental and demographic factor

4.1 Education

A certain level of education is required for the prevention and cure of HIV infection. It is now established that low education level is an independent risk factor for HIV-1 related cognitive impairment. Stern et al., (1996), Maj et al., (1994), Satz et al., (1993) reported that low educational level (6 years) increases the risk of HIV-1–related cognitive impairment in HIV-1–seropositive persons (asymptomatic and symptomatic). Our own unpublished data is in concordance with their findings. It is important to note that the association between low educational level and HIV-1–related cognitive impairment was independent of all other putative risk factors. In addition to this, another study also suggests that discrepancy in reading and education level is associated with worse neuropsychological performance (Ryan et al., 2005). There are two possible variables related to literacy, those are frequently used to predict the neuropsychological functioning; reading ability and years of education. In a country like India and particularly in its remote rural areas, it is difficult to predict the total year(s) of education. In such situations, it is better to rely on the reading ability of an individual. In other parts of world, previous research has also shown that reading ability is a stronger predictor of cognitive functioning than year(s) of education. Dotson et al., (2009) reported that reading ability predicts cognitive functioning than year(s) of education. They also suggest that influence of literacy and year(s) of education on cognitive functioning may vary among individuals belong to certain racial minority status and low SES group.

4.2 Age

The impact of age on some aspects of neuropsychological performance is well established. In addition, data indicate that age at the time of seroconversion is significantly associated with HIV disease progression and survival time (Babiker et al., 2001). The possibility of an interaction between age and disease level on cognitive function has not been explored thoroughly. Both age and HIV status have been established as independent risk factors for the development of cognitive impairment, it is both reasonable and important to question whether the interaction of these two factors may constitute increased risk of impairment in HIV-infected individuals. While several studies have explored the impact of age on cognitive function in HIV infected subjects (Janssen et al., 1992; McArthur et al., 1993; Kim et al., 2001; Pereda et al., 2000) few have examined the interaction of age and disease status (Van Gorp et al., 1994; Hardy et al., 1999). Kissel et al., (2005) reported that Age and disease status had independent effects on cognitive function, but there were no significant interactions either on a summary measure of performance or on individual test scores.

4.3 Gender

Chiesi et al. and the AIDS in Europe Study Group (1996) reported that rates of cognitive impairment were higher for women. The hypothesis that female seropositive subjects are more vulnerable for neuropsychological impairment than seropositive men, is explained by Satz et al. (1993) that they usually have an extensive pre-morbid history, a history of substance abuse, a lower economic level, a greater psychiatric morbidity and a low educational level (Ickovics & Rodin, 1992; Melnick et al., 1994) variables that could increase the risk of neuropsychological impairment associated with HIV-1 (Stern et al., 1996). Faílde-Garrido et al. (2008) reported different neuropsychological impairment pattern was detected between genders: while HIV+ men had greater impairment in visual memory, attention, psychomotor speed and abstract reasoning, HIV+ women had greater impairment on attention, psychomotor speed and verbal memory for texts. They further reported that there is no difference between the neuropsychological performance of seropositive male and female subjects. Pereda et al. (2000), Rabkin et al. (2000) found same result.

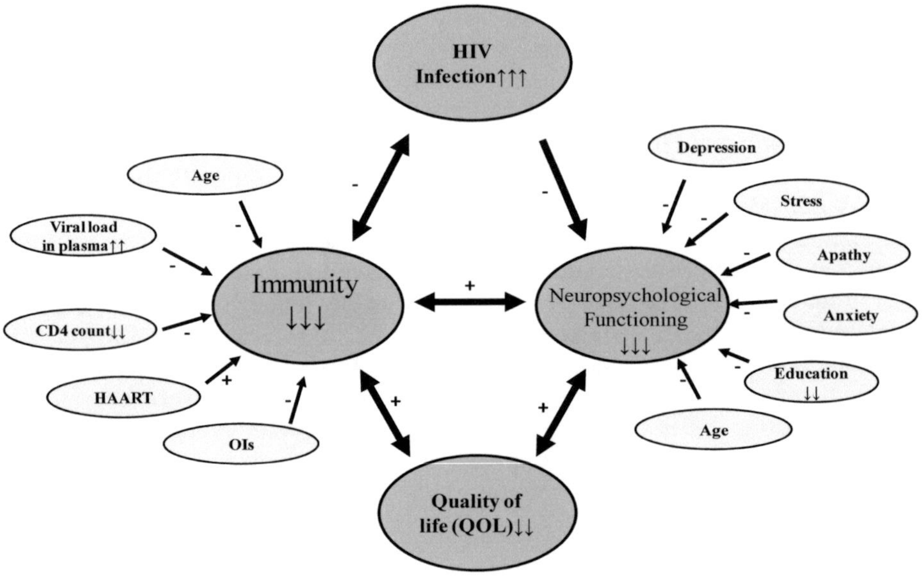

Fig. 3. Figure showing interrelationship among HIV infection, immunity of the host, neuropsychological functioning and quality of life (QOL)

HIV infection, immunity of the host, neuropsychological functioning and QOL are interlinked and affects each other. Various factors may influence neuropsychological functioning and immunity of the host. (-) and (+) sign shows negative association respectively. → and ↔ depicts uni and bidirectional interaction between two.

5. Conclusion

In conclusion, much can learn about factors associated with neuropsychological impairment, a leading cause of morbidity and mortality in persons with HIV infection. It was the intent of this manuscript not only to summarize what we know about factors associated with neuropsychological impairment in HIV infection but also to point out what we don't know and to highlight future directions that this area of research must now address. The adverse effect of HIV on neuropsychological functioning is well established. Manifestations of neurocognitive dysfunction range from subtle and mild cognitive changes to frank dementia syndromes. We have primarily focused on the factors associated with neuropsychological impairment, which is adversely affect QOL and patients' ability demanding daily activities (Figure-3). There are very few studies focusing on factors associated with neuropsychological impairment in HIV infection. This review categorized factors into three broad areas that significantly associated with neuropsychological impairment. There are lacks of consensus among available literature regarding factors associated with neuropsychological impairment in HIV infection, especially psychological and environmental/demographic factors. Contradictory finding have been reported regarding association between neuropsychological impairment and antiretroviral therapy, drug abuse, depression, apathy, stress, age, gender and education. This review help the health care professionals in proper care of HIV seropositive people those are at risk to develop cognitive impairment. Present chapter also mentions the fact that tertiary prevention is urgently needed to improve quality of life of HIV infected people. Comprehensive study is needed to explore the above relationship and is clearly an important area of investigations.

6. Acknowledgement

The authors thank all the patients and control subjects who volunteered participation in their study. We also thank Indian Council of Social Science and Research (ICSSR), Government of India for providing fellowship to Dr. Yogita Rai. The authors also thank Prof. A. K. Gulati, Department of Microbiology, Institute of Medical Sciences, Banaras Hindu University.

7. References

Atkinson, J.H., Jr, Grant, I, Kennedy, C. J., Richman, D. D., Spector, S A, & McCutchan, J A. (1988). Prevalence of psychiatric disorders among men infected with human immunodeficiency virus. A controlled study. *Archives of General Psychiatry*, Vol. 45, No. 9, (Sep 1988), pp. (859-864), ISSN 0003-990X

Aylward, E. H., Henderer, J. D., McArthur, J. C., Brettschneider, P. D., Harris, G. J., Barta, P. E., & Pearlson, G. D. (1993a). Reduced basal ganglia volume in HIV-1-associated dementia: results from quantitative neuroimaging. *Neurology*, Vol. 43, No. 10, (Oct 1993), pp. (2099-2104), ISSN 0028-3878

Babiker, A. G., Peto, T., Porter, K., Walker, A. S., & Darbyshire, J. H. (2001). Age as a determinant of survival in HIV infection. *Journal of Clinical Epidemiology,* Vol. 54, No. 1, (Dec 2001), pp. (S16-21), ISSN 0895-4356

Becker, J. T., Sanchez, J., Dew, M. A., Lopez, O. L., Dorst, S. K., & Banks, G. (1997b). Neuropsychological abnormalities among HIV-infected individuals in a community-based sample. *Neuropsychology,* Vol. 11, No. 4, (Mar 25, 2011), pp. (592-601), ISSN 1573-3254

Bono, G., Mauri, M., Sinforiani, E., Barbarini, G., Minoli, L., & Fea, M. (1996). Longitudinal neuropsychological evaluation of HIV-infected intravenous drug users. *Addiction (Abingdon, England),* Vol. 91, No. 2, (Feb 1996), pp. (263-268), ISSN 0965-2140

Bornstein, R A, Nasrallah, H. A., Para, M. F., Fass, R. J., Whitacre, C. C., & Rice, R. R., Jr. (1991). Rate of CD4 decline and neuropsychological performance in HIV infection. *Archives of Neurology,* Vol. 48, No. 7, (Jul 1991), pp. (704-707), ISSN 0003-9942

Bornstein, R A, Nasrallah, H. A., Para, M. F., Whitacre, C. C., & Fass, R. J. (1993). Change in neuropsychological performance in asymptomatic HIV infection: 1-year follow-up. *AIDS (London, England),* Vol. 7, No. 12, (Dec 1993), pp. (1607-1611), ISSN 0269-9370

Bornstein, R A, Pace, P., Rosenberger, P., Nasrallah, H. A., Para, M. F., Whitacre, C. C., & Fass, R. J. (1993d). Depression and neuropsychological performance in asymptomatic HIV infection. *The American Journal of Psychiatry,* Vol. 150, No. 6, (Jun 1993), pp. (922-927), ISSN 0002-953X

Bouwman, F. H., Skolasky, R. L., Hes, D., Selnes, O. A., Glass, J. D., Nance-Sproson, T. E., Royal, W., et al. (1998c). Variable progression of HIV-associated dementia. *Neurology,*Vol. 50 ,No.6,(Jun 1998), PP.(1814-1820) ISSN 0028-3878

Carpenter, C. C., Fischl, M. A., Hammer, S. M., Hirsch, M. S., Jacobsen, D. M., Katzenstein, D. A., Montaner, J. S., et al. (1998). Antiretroviral therapy for HIV infection in 1998: updated recommendations of the International AIDS Society-USA Panel. *JAMA: The Journal of the American Medical Association,* Vol. *280,* No. 1,(Jul 1, 1998), pp. (78-86) ISSN 0098-7484

Castellon, S. A., Hinkin, C H, Wood, S., & Yarema, K. T. (1998). Apathy, depression, and cognitive performance in HIV-1 infection. *The Journal of Neuropsychiatry and Clinical Neurosciences,* Vol. *10,* No.3, PP. (320-329) ISSN 0895-0172

Chiesi, A., Vella, S., Dally, L. G., Pedersen, C., Danner, S., Johnson, A. M., Schwander, S., et al. (1996). Epidemiology of AIDS dementia complex in Europe. AIDS in Europe Study Group. *Journal of Acquired Immune Deficiency Syndromes and Human Retrovirology: Official Publication of the International Retrovirology Association,* Vol. 11, No. 1, (Jan 1996), pp. (39-44), ISSN 1077-9450

Childs, E. A., Lyles, R. H., Selnes, O. A., Chen, B., Miller, E. N., Cohen, B. A., Becker, J. T., et al. (1999d). Plasma viral load and CD4 lymphocytes predict HIV-associated dementia and sensory neuropathy. *Neurology,* Vol. 52, No. 3, (Feb 1999), pp. (607-613), ISSN 0028-3878

Claypoole, K. H., Elliott, A. J., Uldall, K. K., Russo, J., Dugbartey, A. T., Bergam, K., & Roy-Byrne, P. P. (1998). Cognitive functions and complaints in HIV-1 individuals treated for depression. *Applied Neuropsychology,* Vol. 5, No. 2, (), pp. (74-84), ISSN 0908-4282

Claypoole, K. H., Townes, B. D., Collier, A. C., Marra, C., Longstreth, W. T., Jr, Cohen, W., Martin, D., et al. (1993). Cognitive risk factors and neuropsychological performance in HIV infection. *The International Journal of Neuroscience,* Vol. 70, No. 1-2, (May 1993), pp. (13-27), ISSN 0020-7454

Cristiani, S. A., Pukay-Martin, N. D., & Bornstein, Robert A. (2004). Marijuana use and cognitive function in HIV-infected people. *The Journal of Neuropsychiatry and Clinical Neurosciences*, Vol. 16, No. 3, pp. (330-335), 0895-0172

Cysique, L. A., Deutsch, R., Atkinson, J Hampton, Young, C., Marcotte, Thomas D, Dawson, L., Grant, Igor, et al. (2007). Incident major depression does not affect neuropsychological functioning in HIV-infected men. *Journal of the International Neuropsychological Society: JINS*, Vol. 13, No. 1, (Jan 2007), pp. (1-11), ISSN 1355-6177

Dal Pan, G. J., McArthur, J. H., Aylward, E., Selnes, O. A., Nance-Sproson, T. E., Kumar, A. J., Mellits, E. D., et al. (1992e). Patterns of cerebral atrophy in HIV-1-infected individuals: results of a quantitative MRI analysis. *Neurology*, Vol. 42, No. 11, (Nov 1992), pp. (2125-2130), ISSN 0028-3878

Dotson, V. M., Kitner-Triolo, M. H., Evans, M. K., & Zonderman, A. B. (2009). Effects of race and socioeconomic status on the relative influence of education and literacy on cognitive functioning. *Journal of the International Neuropsychological Society: JINS*, Vol. 15, No. 4, (Jul 2009), pp. (580-589), ISSN 1469-7661

Ellis, R J, Hsia, K, Spector, S A, Nelson, J. A., Heaton, R K, Wallace, M. R., Abramson, I., et al. (1997). Cerebrospinal fluid human immunodeficiency virus type 1 RNA levels are elevated in neurocognitively impaired individuals with acquired immunodeficiency syndrome. HIV Neurobehavioral Research Center Group. *Annals of Neurology*, Vol. 42, No. 5, (Nov 1997), pp. (679-688), ISSN 0364-5134

Ellis, Ronald J, Moore, D. J., Childers, M. E., Letendre, S., McCutchan, J Allen, Wolfson, Tanya, Spector, Stephen A, et al. (2002). Progression to neuropsychological impairment in human immunodeficiency virus infection predicted by elevated cerebrospinal fluid levels of human immunodeficiency virus RNA. *Archives of Neurology*, Vol. 59, No. 6, (Jun 2002), pp. (923-928), ISSN 0003-9942

Enting, R. H., Hoetelmans, R. M., Lange, J. M., Burger, D. M., Beijnen, J. H., & Portegies, P. (1998). Antiretroviral drugs and the central nervous system. *AIDS (London, England)*, Vol. 12, No. 15, (Oct 1998), pp. (1941-1955), ISSN 0269-9370

Evans, D. L., Leserman, J., Perkins, D. O., Stern, R. A., Murphy, C., Zheng, B., Gettes, D., et al. (1997a). Severe life stress as a predictor of early disease progression in HIV infection. *The American Journal of Psychiatry*, Vol. 154, No. 5, (May 1997), pp. (630-634), ISSN 0002-953X

Faílde-Garrido, J. M., Alvarez, M. R., & Simón-López, M. A. (2008). Neuropsychological impairment and gender differences in HIV-1 infection. *Psychiatry and Clinical Neurosciences*, Vol. 62, No. 5, (Oct 2008), pp. (494-502), ISSN 1440-1819

Foley, J., Ettenhofer, M., Wright, M., & Hinkin, Charles H. (2008). Emerging issues in the neuropsychology of HIV infection. *Current HIV/AIDS Reports*, Vol. 5, No. 4, (Nov 2008), pp. (204-211), ISSN 1548-3576

Gartner, S. (2000). HIV infection and dementia. *Science (New York, N.Y.)*, Vol. 287, No. (5453), (Jan 2000), pp. 602-604, ISSN 0036-8075

Gendelman, H. E., Lipton, S. A., Tardieu, M., Bukrinsky, M. I., & Nottet, H. S. (1994). The neuropathogenesis of HIV-1 infection. *Journal of Leukocyte Biology*, Vol. 56, No. 3, (Sep 1994), pp. (389-398), ISSN 0741-5400

von Giesen, H. J., Bäcker, R., Hefter, H., & Arendt, G. (2001). Depression does not influence basal ganglia-mediated psychomotor speed in HIV-1 infection. *The Journal of Neuropsychiatry and Clinical Neurosciences*, Vol. 13, No. 1, pp. (88-94), ISSN 0895-0172

Goggin, K. J., Zisook, S., Heaton, R K, Atkinson, J H, Marshall, S., McCutchan, J A, Chandler, J. L., et al. (1997). Neuropsychological performance of HIV-1 infected men with major depression. HNRC Group. HIV Neurobehavioral Research Center. *Journal of the International Neuropsychological Society: JINS*, Vol. 3, No. 5, (Sep 1997), pp. (457-464), ISSN 1355-6177

González-Scarano, F., & Martín-García, J. (2005). The neuropathogenesis of AIDS. *Nature Reviews. Immunology*, Vol. 5, No. 1, (Jan 2005), pp. (69-81), ISSN 1474-1733

Goodwin, G. M., Pretsell, D. O., Chiswick, A., Egan, V., & Brettle, R. P. (1996a). The Edinburgh cohort of HIV-positive injecting drug users at 10 years after infection: a case-control study of the evolution of dementia. *AIDS (London, England)*, Vol. 10, No. 4, (Apr 1996), pp. (431-440), ISSN 0269-9370

Grant, I, Atkinson, J H, Hesselink, J. R., Kennedy, C. J., Richman, D. D., Spector, S A, & McCutchan, J A. (1988a). Human immunodeficiency virus-associated neurobehavioural disorder. *Journal of the Royal College of Physicians of London*, Vol. 22, No. 3, (Jul 1988), pp. (149-157), ISSN 0035-8819

Grant, I, & Martin, A. (1994). *Neuropsychology of HIV Infection*. New York: Osford Univ Press.

Gulevich, S. J., McCutchan, J A, Thal, L. J., Kirson, D., Durand, D., Wallace, M., Mehta, P., et al. (1993). Effect of antiretroviral therapy on the cerebrospinal fluid of patients seropositive for the human immunodeficiency virus. *Journal of Acquired Immune Deficiency Syndromes*, Vol. 6, No. 9, (Sep 1993), pp. (1002-1007), ISSN 0894-9255

Haase, A. T. (1986). Pathogenesis of lentivirus infections. *Nature*, Vol. 322, No. 6075, (Jul 1986), pp. (130-136), ISSN 0028-0836

Hall, M., Whaley, R., Robertson, K., Hamby, S., Wilkins, J., & Hall, C. (1996). The correlation between neuropsychological and neuroanatomic changes over time in asymptomatic and symptomatic HIV-1-infected individuals. *Neurology*, Vol. 46, No. 6, (Jun 1996), pp. (1697-1702), ISSN 0028-3878

Hardy, D. J., Satz, P., & Jones, F. D. (1999). Age differences and neurocognitive performance in HIV-infected adults. *New Zealand Journal of Psychology, Vol.* 28, pp. (94–101), ISSN 0112-109X

Heaton, R K, Grant, I, Butters, N., White, D. A., Kirson, D., Atkinson, J H, McCutchan, J A, et al. (1995). The HNRC 500--neuropsychology of HIV infection at different disease stages. HIV Neurobehavioral Research Center. *Journal of the International Neuropsychological Society: JINS*, Vol. 1, No. 3, (May 1995), pp. (231-251), ISSN 1355-6177

Hinkin, C H, van Gorp, W. G., Mandelkern, M. A., Gee, M., Satz, P., Holston, S., Marcotte, T D, et al. (1995). Cerebral metabolic change in patients with AIDS: report of a six-month follow-up using positron-emission tomography. *The Journal of Neuropsychiatry and Clinical Neurosciences*, Vol. 7, No. 2, pp. (180-187), ISSN 0895-0172

Honn, V. J., Bornstein (2002). Social support, neuropsychological performance, and depression in HIV infection. *Journal of the International Neuropsychological Society: JINS*, Vol. 8, No. 3, (Mar 2002), pp. (436-447), ISSN 1355-6177

Ickovics, J. R., & Rodin, J. (1992). Women and AIDS in the United States: epidemiology, natural history, and mediating mechanisms. *Health Psychology: Official Journal of the Division of Health Psychology, American Psychological Association*, Vol. 11, No. 1, pp. (1-16), ISSN 0278-6133

Janssen, R. S., Nwanyanwu, O. C., Selik, R. M., & Stehr-Green, J. K. (1992). Epidemiology of human immunodeficiency virus encephalopathy in the United States. *Neurology*, Vol. 42, No. 8, (Aug 1992), pp. (1472-1476) ISSN 0028-3878.

Janssen, R. S., Saykin, A. J., Cannon, L., Campbell, J., Pinsky, P. F., Hessol, N. A., O'Malley, P. M., et al. (1989). Neurological and neuropsychological manifestations of HIV-1 infection: association with AIDS-related complex but not asymptomatic HIV-1 infection. *Annals of Neurology*, Vol. 26, No. 5, (Jan 1989), pp. (592-600), ISSN 0028-3878

Kalechstein, A. D., Hinkin, C H, van Gorp, W. G., Castellon, S. A., & Satz, P. (1998f). Depression predicts procedural but not episodic memory in HIV-1 infection. *Journal of Clinical and Experimental Neuropsychology*, Vol. 20, No. 4, (Aug 1998), pp. (529-535), ISSN 1380-3395.

Kim, D. H., Jewison, D. L., Milner, G. R., Rourke, S. B., Gill, M. J., & Power, C. (2001). Neurocognitive symptoms and impairment in an HIV community clinic. *The Canadian Journal of Neurological Sciences. Le Journal Canadien Des Sciences Neurologiques*, Vol. 28, No. 3, (Aug 2001), pp. (228-231), ISSN 0317-1671.

Kim, J. J., & Yoon, K. S. (1998). Stress: metaplastic effects in the hippocampus. *Trends in Neurosciences*, Vol. 21, No. 12, (Dec 1998), pp. (505-509), ISSN 0166-2236.

Kissel, E. C., Pukay-Martin, N. D., & Bornstein, Robert A. (2005). The relationship between age and cognitive function in HIV-infected men. *The Journal of Neuropsychiatry and Clinical Neurosciences*, Vol. 17 No.2, pp. (180-184) ISSN 0895-0172

Krebs, F. C., Ross, H., McAllister, J., & Wigdahl, B. (2000). HIV-1-associated central nervous system dysfunction. *Advances in Pharmacology (San Diego, Calif.)*, Vol. 49, pp. (315-385), ISSN 1054-3589

Limoges, J., Persidsky, Y., Poluektova, L., Rasmussen, J., Ratanasuwan, W., Zelivyanskaya, M., McClernon, D. R., et al. (2000). Evaluation of antiretroviral drug efficacy for HIV-1 encephalitis in SCID mice. *Neurology*, Vol. 54, *No.* 2, (Jan 25, 2000) ,pp. (379-389), ISSN 0028-3878

Maj, M., Janssen, R., Starace, F., Zaudig, M., Satz, P., Sughondhabirom, B., Luabeya, M. A., et al. (1994). WHO Neuropsychiatric AIDS study, cross-sectional phase I. Study design and psychiatric findings. *Archives of General Psychiatry*, Vol. 51, No. 1, (Jan 1994), pp. (39-49), ISSN 0003-990X

Maj, M., Satz, P., Janssen, R., Zaudig, M., Starace, F., D'Elia, L., Sughondhabirom, B., et al. (1994). WHO Neuropsychiatric AIDS study, cross-sectional phase II. Neuropsychological and neurological findings. *Archives of General Psychiatry*, Vol. 51, No. 1, (Jan 1994), pp. (51-61), ISSN 0003-990X

Mapou, R. L., Law, W. A., Martin, A., Kampen, D., Salazar, A. M., & Rundell, J. R. (1993). Neuropsychological performance, mood, and complaints of cognitive and motor difficulties in individuals infected with the human immunodeficiency virus. *The Journal of Neuropsychiatry and Clinical Neurosciences*, Vol. 5, No.1, pp. (86-93) ISSN 0895-0172

Marsh, N. V., & McCall, D. W. (1994). Early neuropsychological change in HIV infection. *Neuropsychology*, Vol. 8, No. 1, (Jan 1994), pp. (44-48)

Martin, A., Heyes, M. P., Salazar, A. M., Kampen, D. L., Williams, J., Law, W. A., Coats, M. E., et al. (1992). Progressive slowing of reaction time and increasing cerebrospinal fluid concentrations of quinolinic acid in HIV-infected individuals. *The Journal of Neuropsychiatry and Clinical Neurosciences*, Vol. 4, No. 3, pp. (270-279), ISSN 0895-0172

Martin, E. M., Pitrak, D. L., Novak, R. M., Pursell, K. J., & Mullane, K. M. (1999). Reaction times are faster in HIV-seropositive patients on antiretroviral therapy: A preliminary report. *Journal of Clinical and Experimental Neuropsychology*, Vol. 21, No. 5, (Oct 1999) pp. (730-735) ISSN 1380-3395

Martin, E. M., Robertson, L. C., Edelstein, H. E., Jagust, W. J., Sorensen, D. J., San Giovanni, D., & Chirurgi, V. A. (1992). Performance of patients with early HIV-1 infection on the Stroop Task. *Journal of Clinical and Experimental Neuropsychology*, Vol. 14, No. 5, (Sep 1992), pp. (857-868) ISSN 1380-3395

McArthur, J. C., Becker, P. S., Parisi, J. E., Trapp, B., Selnes, O. A., Cornblath, D. R., Balakrishnan, J., et al. (1989g). Neuropathological changes in early HIV-1 dementia. *Annals of Neurology*, Vol. 26, No. 5, (Nov 1989), pp. (681-684), ISSN 0364-5134

McArthur, J. C., Hoover, D. R., Bacellar, H., Miller, E. N., Cohen, B. A., Becker, J. T., Graham, N. M., et al. (1993). Dementia in AIDS patients: incidence and risk factors. Multicenter AIDS Cohort Study. *Neurology*, Vol. 43, *No.* 11, (Nov 1993), pp.(2245-2252), ISSN 0028-3878

McArthur, J. C., McClernon, D. R., Cronin, M. F., Nance-Sproson, T. E., Saah, A. J., St Clair, M., & Lanier, E. R. (1997h). Relationship between human immunodeficiency virus-associated dementia and viral load in cerebrospinal fluid and brain. *Annals of Neurology*, Vol. 42, No. 5, (Nov 1997), pp. (689-698), ISSN 0364-5134

McEwen, B. S. (2000). The neurobiology of stress: from serendipity to clinical relevance. *Brain Research*, Vol. 886, No. 1-2, (Dec 15, 2000), pp.(172-189), ISSN 0006-8993

Melnick, S. L., Sherer, R., Louis, T. A., Hillman, D., Rodriguez, E. M., Lackman, C., Capps, L., et al. (1994). Survival and disease progression according to gender of patients with HIV infection. The Terry Beirn Community Programs for Clinical Research on AIDS. *JAMA: The Journal of the American Medical Association*, Vol. 272, No. 24, (Dec 28, 1994), pp. (1915-1921), ISSN 0098-7484

Moore, L. H., van Gorp, W. G., Hinkin, C H, Stern, M. J., Swales, T., & Satz, P. (1997i). Subjective complaints versus actual cognitive deficits in predominantly symptomatic HIV-1 seropositive individuals. *The Journal of Neuropsychiatry and Clinical Neurosciences*, Vol. 9, No. 1, pp. (37-44), ISSN 0895-0172

Osowiecki, D. M., Cohen, R. A., Morrow, K. M., Paul, R. H., Carpenter, C. C., Flanigan, T., & Boland, R. J. (2000). Neurocognitive and psychological contributions to quality of life in HIV-1-infected women. *AIDS (London, England)*, Vol. 14, No. 10, (Jul 2000), pp. (1327-1332), ISSN 0269-9370

Patterson, T. L., Semple, S. J., Temoshok, L. R., Atkinson, J H, McCutchan, J A, Straits-Tröster, K., Chandler, J. L., et al. (1995). Stress and depressive symptoms prospectively predict immune change among HIV-seropositive men. HIV Neurobehavioral Research Center Group. *Psychiatry, Vol. 58,* No. 4, (Nov 1995), pp. (299-312), ISSN 0033-2747

Pereda, M., Ayuso-Mateos, J. L., Gómez Del Barrio, A., Echevarria, S., Farinas, M. C., García Palomo, D., González Macias, J., et al. (2000). Factors associated with neuropsychological performance in HIV-seropositive subjects without AIDS. *Psychological Medicine*, Vol. 30, No. 1, (Jan 2000), pp. (205-217), ISSN 0033-2917

Perkins, D. O., Stern, R. A., Golden, R. N., Murphy, C., Naftolowitz, D., & Evans, D. L. (1994b). Mood disorders in HIV infection: prevalence and risk factors in a nonepicenter of the AIDS epidemic. *The American Journal of Psychiatry*, Vol. 151, No. 2, (Jun 1990), pp. (233-236), ISSN 0002-953X

Perry, S. W. (1990). Organic mental disorders caused by HIV: update on early diagnosis and treatment. *The American Journal of Psychiatry*, Vol. 147, No. 6, pp. (696-710), ISSN 0002-953X

Perry, S., Belsky-Barr, D., Barr, W. B., & Jacobsberg, L. (1989). Neuropsychological function in physically asymptomatic, HIV-seropositive men. *The Journal of Neuropsychiatry and Clinical Neurosciences*, Vol. 1, No. 3, pp. (296-302), ISSN 0895-0172

Pukay-Martin, N. D., Cristiani, S. A., Saveanu, R., & Bornstein, Robert A. (2003). The relationship between stressful life events and cognitive function in HIV-infected men. *The Journal of Neuropsychiatry and Clinical Neurosciences*, Vol. 15, No. 4, pp. (436-441), ISSN 0895-0172

Rabkin, J. G., Ferrando, S. J., van Gorp, W., Rieppi, R., McElhiney, M., & Sewell, M. (2000). Relationships among apathy, depression, and cognitive impairment in HIV/AIDS. *The Journal of Neuropsychiatry and Clinical Neurosciences*, Vol. 12, No. 4, pp. (451-457), ISSN 0895-0172

Reger, M. A., Martin, D. J., Cole, S. L., & Strauss, G. (2005). The relationship between plasma viral load and neuropsychological functioning in HIV-1 infection. *Archives of Clinical Neuropsychology: The Official Journal of the National Academy of Neuropsychologists*, Vol. 20, No. 2, (Mar 2005), pp. (137-143), ISSN 0887-6177

Richardson, M. A., Satz, P. F., Myers, H. F., Miller, E. N., Bing, E. G., Fawzy, F. I., & Maj, M. (1999j). Effects of depressed mood versus clinical depression on neuropsychological test performance among African American men impacted by HIV/AIDS. *Journal of Clinical and Experimental Neuropsychology*, Vol. 21, No. 6, (Dec 1999), pp. (769-783), ISSN 1380-3395

Rippeth, J. D., Heaton, Robert K, Carey, C. L., Marcotte, Thomas D, Moore, D. J., Gonzalez, R., Wolfson, Tanya, et al. (2004). Methamphetamine dependence increases risk of neuropsychological impairment in HIV infected persons. *Journal of the International Neuropsychological Society: JINS*, Vol. 10, No. 1, (Jan 2004), pp. (1-14), ISSN 1355-6177

Ryan, E. L., Baird, R., Mindt, M. R., Byrd, D., Monzones, J., & Bank, S. M. (2005). Neuropsychological impairment in racial/ethnic minorities with HIV infection and low literacy levels: effects of education and reading level in participant characterization. *Journal of the International Neuropsychological Society: JINS*, Vol. 11, No. 7, (Nov 2005), pp. (889-898), ISSN 1355-6177

Satz, P., Morgenstern, H., Miller, E. N., Selnes, O. A., McArthur, J. C., Cohen, B. A., Wesch, J., et al. (1993). Low education as a possible risk factor for cognitive abnormalities in HIV-1: findings from the multicenter AIDS Cohort Study (MACS). *Journal of Acquired Immune Deficiency Syndromes*, Vol. 6, No. 5, (May 1993), pp. (503-511), ISSN 0894-9255

Schmitt, F. A., Bigley, J. W., McKinnis, R., Logue, P. E., Evans, R. W., & Drucker, J. L. (1988). Neuropsychological outcome of zidovudine (AZT) treatment of patients with AIDS and AIDS-related complex. *The New England Journal of Medicine*, Vol. 319, No. 24, (Dec 1988), pp. (1573-1578), ISSN 0028-4793

Selnes, O. A., Galai, N., Bacellar, H., Miller, E. N., Becker, J. T., Wesch, J., Van Gorp, W., et al. (1995). Cognitive performance after progression to AIDS: a longitudinal study from the Multicenter AIDS Cohort Study. *Neurology*, Vol. 45, No. 2, (Feb 1995), pp. (267-275), ISSN 0028-3878

Selnes, O. A., McArthur, J. C., Royal, W., 3rd, Updike, M. L., Nance-Sproson, T., Concha, M., Gordon, B., et al. (1992l). HIV-1 infection and intravenous drug use: longitudinal neuropsychological evaluation of asymptomatic subjects. *Neurology*, Vol. 42, No. 10, (Oct 1992), pp. (1924-1930), ISSN 0028-3878

Selnes, O. A., Miller, E., McArthur, J., Gordon, B., Muñoz, A., Sheridan, K., Fox, R., et al. (1990). HIV-1 infection: no evidence of cognitive decline during the asymptomatic stages. The Multicenter AIDS Cohort Study. *Neurology*, Vol. 40, No. 2, (Feb 1990), pp. (204-208), ISSN 0028-3878.

Sidtis, J. J., Gatsonis, C., Price, R. W., Singer, E. J., Collier, A. C., Richman, D. D., Hirsch, M. S., et al. (1993). Zidovudine treatment of the AIDS dementia complex: results of a placebo-controlled trial. AIDS Clinical Trials Group. *Annals of Neurology*, Vol. 33, No. 4, (Apr 1993), pp. (343-349), ISSN 0364-5134

Stankoff, B., Calvez, V., Suarez, S., Bossi, P., Rosenblum, O., Conquy, L., Turell, E., et al. (1999). Plasma and cerebrospinal fluid human immunodeficiency virus type-1 (HIV-1) RNA levels in HIV-related cognitive impairment. *European Journal of Neurology: The Official Journal of the European Federation of Neurological Societies*, Vol. 6, No. 6, (Nov 1999), pp. (669-675), ISSN 1351-5101

Stern, R. A., Silva, S. G., Chaisson, N., & Evans, D. L. (1996). Influence of cognitive reserve on neuropsychological functioning in asymptomatic human immunodeficiency virus-1 infection. *Archives of Neurology*, Vol. 53, No. 2, (Feb 1996), pp. (148-153), ISSN 0003-9942

Stern, Y. (1991). The impact of human immunodeficiency virus on cognitive function. *Annals of the New York Academy of Sciences*, Vol. 640, pp. (219-223), ISSN 0077-8923

Stout, J. C., Ellis, R J, Jernigan, T. L., Archibald, S. L., Abramson, I., Wolfson, T, McCutchan, J A, et al. (1998). Progressive cerebral volume loss in human immunodeficiency virus infection: a longitudinal volumetric magnetic resonance imaging study. HIV Neurobehavioral Research Center Group. *Archives of Neurology*, Vol. 55, No. 2, (Feb 1998), pp. (161-168), ISSN 0003-9942

Tashima, K. T. (1998). Cerebrospinal fluid levels of antiretroviral medications: abstract and commentary. *JAMA: The Journal of the American Medical Association*, Vol. 280, No. 10, (Sep 1998), pp. (879-880), ISSN 0098-7484.

van Gorp, W. G., Miller, E. N., Satz, P., & Visscher, B. (1989). Neuropsychological performance in HIV-1 immunocompromised patients: a preliminary report. *Journal of Clinical and Experimental Neuropsychology*, Vol. 11, No. 5, (Oct 1989), pp. (763-773), ISSN 1380-3395

Wellman, M. C. (1992). Neuropsychological impairment among intravenous drug users in pre-AIDS stages of HIV infection. *The International Journal of Neuroscience*, Vol. 64, No. 1-4, (May-Jun 1992), pp. (183-194), ISSN 0020-7454

Zaitseva, M., Peden, K., & Golding, H. (2003). HIV coreceptors: role of structure, posttranslational modifications, and internalization in viral-cell fusion and as targets for entry inhibitors. *Biochimica Et Biophysica Acta*, Vol. 1614, No. 1, (Jul 2003), pp. (51-61), ISSN 0006-3002

17

HIV Infection: Implications on Surgical Practice

Peter M. Nthumba and Paul I. Juma
Kijabe, Plastic, Reconstructive and Hand Surgery,
AIC Kijabe Hospital, Kijabe
Kenya

1. Introduction

The human immune deficiency virus (HIV) may have had its origins in Africa; a large percentage of those infected live in sub-Saharan African. HIV is thought to have started and spread unnoticed through the 1960s and 1970s, developing into epidemic proportions in the 1980s. The HIV/AIDS pandemic is currently a global phenomenon that has especially impacted on sub-Saharan Africans because of the large numbers of those affected, as well as poverty and illiteracy so rampant in the continent.

The initial hopelessness of the 1980s and early 1990s because of the social stigma and lack of affordable anti-retroviral therapy was replaced with fresh hope, as a result of on-going initiatives that have over the last decade availed anti-retroviral drugs to a population that had would have had no other possibility of accessing this treatment; health education, civic activism, advocacy, government and international recognition and support. The recognition of the threat that HIV/AIDS poses to the survival of mankind, and the measures taken to counter this threat have significantly eroded the social stigma and other complications associated with HIV/AIDS.

Fear of whole populations being wiped out, as suggested by the large number of HIV orphans in the 1980s and 1990s was transformed into hope by the availability of ARVs, translating into a large population of patients surviving way beyond what was previously possible. Opportunistic infections, which in the pre-ARV era caused so many deaths, have seen a significant reduction since the introduction of HAART. This improved survival has introduced a number of aspects that have, and are impacting on the practice of surgery globally.

The challenge of availing ARVs to the eligible patient population still exists; of an estimated 2.24 million people living with HIV/AIDS in Latin America and the Caribbean in 2008, only 54% were on ARVs (Fink et al. 2011).

2. Aims and objectives

A large population of HIV/AIDS patients present to the surgeon with a variety different of surgical pathologies: these may be familiar or unfamiliar to the surgeon, creating either a dilemma in management or a delay in diagnosis and treatment. Unusual surgical pathologies may present in the background of HIV/AIDS, and surgeons ought to be vigilant

(Nthumba, 2008, Nthumba et al., 2011b). A large body of research on the different aspects of the management of these patients exists, from the experience of surgeons in different surgical disciplines. However, these are scattered, and have not been previously analyzed and collected together; further, misgivings and misunderstandings from the pre-HAART era still exist, as to what should be done for these patients. This chapter examines the impact of HIV/AIDS on the practice of surgery on the global scene, with a review of important surgical milestones, as well as broad overviews of common surgical pathologies in the different disciplines, and provides a summary of current surgical care of the HIV/AIDS patient.

3. Materials and methods

The authors performed internet/PubMed/Medline/Cochrane database searches on HIV/AIDS and surgical pathology and surgical practice; data so collected was used in providing current information under the following sub-topics: 'Surgery and HIV/AIDS', 'HIV/AIDS-related surgical diseases' and 'the last frontier in surgery of the HIV patient: transplantation surgery'.

4. Surgery and HIV/AIDS

4.1 Surgery in HIV infected patients
4.1.1 Risk to the surgeon

4.1.1.1 Universal precautions in the operating room

The risk of HIV transmission from patient to the surgeon depends on the prevalence HIV/AIDS in the population served by the surgeon, the frequency of accidental injuries with exposure to infected blood or body fluids, availability of HIV tests and post-exposure prophylaxis in the institution in which the surgeon works, and importantly, compliance of the surgeon to post-exposure prophylaxis (PEP).
Philips et al identified the scarcity of adequate safe surgical supply as a major obstacle to African surgeons' safety (Phillips et al., 2007). Perception of 'time-wasting' with needle stick injury protocols and the subsequent disruption of operating schedules, and an *ad hoc* assessment of the injury as insignificant were noted as the biggest challenges to the prevention of occupational transmission (McCann., 2009). The three universal precautions are: double-gloving, use of face shields, and hands-free technique.
The frequency of cutaneous injury with sharp instruments in surgical procedures is between 1.5% and 15%, with an average risk of five injuries per 100 procedures. While the estimated risk of exposure from a single bore needle stick injury is 0.3%, that from a suture needle is significantly smaller; no seroconversions have been reported in surgeons after a suture injury needle stick. Needle stick injuries of healthcare workers with exposure to blood of patients on HAART, while on the one hand low-risk because of the low or absent viral loads, may on the other hand pose a significant risk for the transmission of drug resistant HIV, with the danger of seroconversion in the HCW, even after PEP compliance (Beltrami et al., 2002; Phillips, 2007).
A review of reported occupational exposures to HIV infected blood in Brazil between 1984 and 2004 revealed a total of four seroconversions; two of these despite using post-exposure prophylaxis (Rapparini, 2006). The actual number of exposures is much higher than those

reported/recorded, as many HCW find that the post-exposure protocols interfere with their schedules, or residents and other junior doctors manage their own post-exposure care, rather than reporting it. Non-compliance with needle stick injury protocols is commonest amongst senior surgeons (Adams et al., 2010; Kerr et al., 2009).

Of an estimated three million HCW percutaneous exposures to blood-borne pathogens, 170,000 are to HIV, with approximately 500 seroconversions annually; 90% of these occur in the developing world (WHO. 2003).

As of December 2005, globally, there were 106 documented cases of specific occupational exposures that resulted in HIV transmission and seroconversion of the HCW. A further 238 seroconversions in HCW may have resulted from occupational exposures, a total of 344 seroconversions; 5% of these were surgeons. As of March 2005, there were 26 PEP failures (Health Protection Agency. 2005a; Health Protection Agency. 2005b) Eight of 57 HCW who seroconverted after an occupational exposure to HIV despite having used PEP; only two of these incidences occurred in the setting of an operating room (Do et al., 2003). Further, six surgeons thought to have seroconverted after occupational exposure did not either have identified index cases, or their pre-exposure status was unknown (CDC., 2000). Seroconversion following occupational exposure even after post-exposure prophylaxis, though rare, is an unfortunate reality (Looke & Grove, 1990). There are fortunately no reported seroconversions after a suture needle injury to date. Since the 57 HCW seroconversions were reported in 2001 by the CDC, only one seroconversion has been reported in the USA.

Double gloving substantially reduces the risk of percutaneous contact with blood from a perforation. In a study of 66 consecutive surgical procedures, of 32 glove perforations in the double-gloving group, 22 were in the outer glove, 10 in the inner glove, and 4 in both gloves. Most glove perforations (83.3%) had gone unnoticed (Thomas et al., 2001).

Bennett et al estimated that double-gloving reduced the size of the blood innoculum in a normal phlebotomy needle to less than 5%, effectively reducing the risk of transmission from 0.3% to 0.009% (Bennet & Howard, 1994; Kerr., 2009). The benefits of double-gloving far outweigh the perceived loss of tactile sensation and dexterity. Additionally, the 'hands-free' technique of handling sharps has been reported to reduce sharps injuries and percutaneous contamination by up to 60% (Kerr et al., 2009). Lefebvre et al found that while a single glove removed more than 97% of contaminant off a tapered needle, two gloves were needed to remove about 91% of contaminant from a cutting suture needle. Three gloves offered the same protection as did two (Lefebvre et al., 2007).

The discussion on perioperative HIV testing in surgery has gone full circle - from an initial push because of the need to protect healthcare workers and exclude high risk patients with potentially poor outcomes, through a period when this was viewed as an unnecessary process that may have been used to unjustly segregate and exclude HIV positive patients from optimal care, to a time when official healthcare organs such as the CDC recognize perioperative HIV testing as an important and necessary part of blood work up, that is potentially protective for the patient. The consequences of undiagnosed HIV infection are deadly and pose setbacks to public health care (Mullins & Harrison, 1993; Rothman et al. 2003; Cunningham, 2010).

4.1.2 Risk to the patient

While a theoretical risk of surgeon-to-patient transmission exists, the only such reported case is that of a dentist who infected five of his patients. There was also a documented possible transmission from an HIV infected orthopedic surgeon (Lot et al. 1999). The calculated risk of transmission is less than 1 in 41,667 or 1 in 416,670 (Wittmann et al., 1996). Thus the actual risk for the patient is minimal. Nevertheless, the debate on whether or not an HIV positive surgeon should reveal their serostatus to all potential patients continues to rage, and is unlikely to be resolved any time soon.

4.1.3 Outcomes

Studies have shown that CD4+ counts can be reliably used to predict the outcomes of patients with HIV/AIDS after surgical procedures (Deneve et al., 2010).

HIV infection destroys the immune system: only 12% of patients have a CD4 cell count greater than 500 cells/µL, while 50% have a CD4 cell count below 200 cells/µL (Honda, 2006).

Some surgical disciplines have had conflicting conclusions on the use of the CD4+ counts as a surrogate marker for clinical outcomes. With regard to the gastro-intestinal tract some studies have suggested that CD4+ counts are predictive of outcomes, while some found no relationship (Cacala et al., 2006). Viral load has also been used as a marker, but is not as well established. The lower the CD4+ count, the higher the rates of post-operative infective complications, increased length of hospital stay, and mortality. While urgent surgical operations have been associated with increased morbidity and mortality, the overall post-operative mortality in HIV/AIDS is between 18% and 48% (Deneve et al., 2010).

Patients undergoing oral or transoral surgery have a significantly increased incidence of wound sepsis when compared with those undergoing trans-dermal surgery (Reilly et al., 2009).

Cacala et al in a prospective review of 350 patients in a high HIV prevalence environment concluded that HIV infection did not influence the outcome of general surgical admissions. CD4 counts did not influence in-hospital outcomes in their cohort of patients, findings that concurred with those of a study in a similar environment (Cacala et al., 2006; Kalima et al., 1990).

HIV-infected or exposed pediatric patients may have a higher rate of complications, with poor wound healing and breakdown of reconstructive procedures, although other variables such as the need for emergent surgery, malnutrition and comorbidities including respiratory infections in these children contribute significantly to their poor outcome, besides the HIV infection. Karpelowsky et al found a higher morbidity and mortality amongst HIV positive or exposed children undergoing surgery when compared to HIV negative children. Nevertheless, they noted that life-saving urgent or elective surgery should not be denied children on the basis of their HIV status (Karpelowsky et al., 2009).

4.2 HIV/AIDS-related surgical diseases

4.2.1 Prevention

Male circumcision has been shown to protect men against HIV infection during vaginal sex with women, providing evidence that circumcision has the potential to significantly reduce transmission (Books et al., 2010).

4.2.2 Cardiovascular system

The introduction of HAART has seen an increase in the incidence of deep venous thrombosis, and thrombo-embolic phenomena, with Saber et al (2001) finding a 10-fold increase above that in the general population. Increased incidence of deep venous thrombosis and thrombo-embolism translates to an increased morbidity and mortality (Saber et al., 2001; Monsuez et al., 2009).

There is also evidence that in the HAART era, HIV patients are at an increased risk of coronary heart disease. Also notable is the fact that hypertension may occur in up to 41% of HIV positive patients who survive for longer than 40 years (Kaplan et al., 2007). Lin et al reported an increased morbidity and mortality amongst HIV positive patients undergoing abdominal aortic aneurysm reconstruction. Low CD4 counts and hypoalbuminemia correlated with poor outcomes (Lin et al., 2004).

4.3 Cutaneous and nodal pathology

Persistent generalized lymphadenopathy is a common feature in HIV patients. While a fine-needle aspiration (FNA) of a lymph node may provide the diagnosis in most instances (non-specific inflammatory lymphadenitis, mycobacterial infection, Kaposi's sarcoma, etc), open lymph node biopsies may be needed to define a lymphoma or to evaluate nodes that continue to enlarge over time. Head and neck diffuse lymphoproliferation causing psychological distress to the patient may be treated by open surgical excision, repeated therapeutic aspirations of cystic lesions or even low grade radiation (Reilly et al. 2009).

4.3.1 Trauma

Patel et al evaluated the influence of chronic illness on the outcome of trauma in over 300,000 trauma patients; they concluded that while pre-existing cirrhosis, dialysis, and warfarin therapy were risk factors for both complications and mortality, HIV/AIDS was only a risk factor for complications. Most of these complications were minor, related to urinary tract and wound infections (Patel et al., 2011).

Harrison et al found that wound contamination had a more significant impact on infectious complications than did CD4+ counts. In the management of compound tibial fractures in HIV patients therefore, the authors recommended the use of external fixation in preference to internal fixation, because of higher infection complications in the latter. Internal fixation of closed fractures in HIV positive patients followed up for a year did not show any increase in infectious complications or non-unions (Harrison et al., 2004).

Edge et al in a study on burn injuries found that 5% of their burn patients were HIV positive patients; besides having a higher infection complication rate, length of stay and mortality did not differ from that of HIV negative burn patients. Their conclusion was that HIV-infected patients (without AIDS) who suffer moderate to severe burn injuries, have the same outcomes as HIV negative patients (Edge et al., 2001).

4.3.2 Abdominal surgery

CD4+ counts in patients with HIV/AIDS undergoing surgery are predictive of outcomes, with increased morbidity and mortality for those with low counts (100 to 250 cells/µL), as well as those presenting for emergent surgery. HIV/AIDS patients undergoing emergent surgery may also have lower CD4+ counts than those undergoing elective surgery (Deneve et al., 2010). The commonest complications after major abdominal surgery include wound infection, pneumonia, intra-abdominal abscesses, peritonitis, and sepsis (Rose et al., 1998).

Whereas mortality rates of HIV positive patients undergoing abdominal surgery have been historically high (0% to 80%), with some authors recommending avoidance of laparotomy in this patient population, HAART has significantly improved outcomes, but even then mortality remains unacceptably high; urgent laparotomies are associated with even higher mortality in HIV/AIDS patients (Tran, 2000; Deneve et al., 2010; Davidson et al., 1991).

4.4 HIV-associated immune thrombocytopenic purpura

Splenectomy in non-HIV-infected patients has been shown to have significant morbidity related primarily to overwhelming sepsis from encapsulated bacteria. In HIV-infected patients, early studies indicated potentially beneficial results of splenectomy, including a slowing of the progression/deterioration to AIDS, when performed in patients with asymptomatic HIV infection (Tsoukas et al., 1998; Tsoukas et al., 1993).

HIV-associated ITP, first described by Abrams et al in 1986, is a fairly common finding in HIV patients, occurring in both asymptomatic and symptomatic HIV-infected patients (Abrams et al., 1986; Tyler et al., 1990). Unlike in immunocompetent (HIV-negative patients), ITP in HIV-infected patients does not respond well to steroid therapy, and although it may respond to ARV therapy, surgery may be required for refractory ITP. Platelet and CD4 counts rise significantly after splenectomy. Aboolian et al reported an 83% response to splenectomy in AIDS patients as compared to 100% response in HIV-positive (non-AIDS) patients. Splenectomy has not been shown to lead an acceleration of the progression to AIDS, or to the clinical deterioration of those with AIDS (Aboolian et al., 1999). Importantly, there has been no evidence of an increase in overwhelming post-splenectomy infections (Lord et al., 1998; Brown et al., 1994).

Splenectomy has also shown good results in HIV-positive hemophiliacs with ITP. Splenectomy has likewise been shown to effectively restore hematological parameters and reduce the need for multiple transfusions in HIV-infected patients with visceral leishmanisis and significant splenomegaly. Splenectomy does not, however prevent relapsing visceral leishmaniasis (Troya et al., 2007). Power et al reported remission of multifocal leukoencephalopathy in an HIV-patient after splenectomy and ARV therapy (Power et al., 1997).

4.4.1 Laparotomy

Abdominal discomfort in the HIV-infected patient may present acutely in the emergency room, or with a more chronic history. In those presenting with a chronic history, the abdominal discomfort may be secondary to a variety of causes including organomegaly, lymphadenopathy or space-occupying lesions such as abscesses. Organomegaly and/or lymphadenopathy may be secondary to infections or neoplasia. CT scan or ultrasound-guided or laparascopic biopsies have largely replaced open diagnostic laparotomies, as where available, these are able provide sufficient tissue to for the diagnosis of such lesions as KS and lymphomas, as well as drain pus collections. Open laparotomy should largely be performed only for therapeautic purposes such as resection of neoplasia, relief of obstruction or the drainage of complex abscesses.

4.4.2 Biliary tract

Hepatic dysfunction in the HIV/AIDS patient is common, and has a large number of possible causes, including medication, opportunistic infection, tumors (such as Kaposi's sarcoma and lymphomas) and sepsis, amongst other possible causes.

Hepato-biliary pathology in the HIV/AIDS patient may present with jaundice, hepatomegaly, and/or pain. Abdominal ultrasonography and/or CTScan examination may reveal dilated biliary tracts. ERCP may be useful in defining and/or managing hepatobiliary problems (Rerknimitr & Kullavanijaya, 2001). Narushima et al in 2004 successfully performed hepatic resection for hepatocellular carcinoma in two hemophiliac patients with HCV and HIV co-infection with CD4+ counts lower than 200 cells/µL (Narushima et al., 2004).

4.4.3 Gastro-intestinal tract

Due to the abundance of lymphoid tissue along the GI tract, which may act as a viral reservoir, almost all patients with HIV infection will at some time present with GI symptoms. Common pathologies include candidiasis (oral/esophageal), esophageal cytomegalovirus and idiopathic esophageal ulcer (Rerknimitr & Kullavanijaya, 2001). Upper GI endoscopy is an excellent tool for diagnosis or taking biopsies. Kaposi's sarcoma of the upper GI tract may also be diagnosed.
Abdominal tuberculosis has a similar presentation in HIV/AIDS patients as in the HIV negative patient population, with most patients presenting with fever, weight loss, abdominal tenderness, abdominal lymphadenopathy, ascites and/or hepatomegaly (Sinkala et al., 2009).

4.4.4 Acute appendicitis

Bova and Meagher noted that patients with HIV and a clinical diagnosis of acute appendicitis often had a normal white cell count, a finding that may contribute to delayed diagnosis and therefore increased morbidity and potential mortality (Boya, 1998).

4.4.5 Cardiothoracic surgery

The use of video-assisted thoracic surgery in the management of empyema and pneumothorax in HIV-infected patients has significantly reduced morbidity in the care of these patients.
In the absence of uncontrolled HIV infection, open cardiac surgery, including cardiac valve replacement, has the same outcomes as in HIV-negative patients; however, the lifespan of the replaced valves is compromised in intravenous drug users. Coronary artery bypass surgery in HIV/AIDS patients has also become an established practice. Other surgical indications for surgical intervention include pericardial effusion and tamponade. Heart transplantation has also been reported (Frater et al., 1989; Agaskar et al., 2003; Mestres et al., 2003; Chong et al., 2003; Kumar et al., 2008; Calabrese et al., 2003; Bisleri et al., 2003;).

4.4.6 Obstetrics

Caesarian section is the method of choice for the delivery of babies in mothers known to be HIV positive, as it is known to be protective against mother-to-child transmission (Read & Newell, 2005). It has however been shown, as in other surgical specialties, to be associated with a higher morbidity than in HIV-negative women, with a higher rate of the need for blood transfusion, a higher incidence of post-operative fever and wound infection, even with the use of peri-operative antibiotics (Zvandsara et al., 2007). Fiore et al found higher infection rates amongst HIV positive mothers when compared to HIV negative mothers, irrespective of the mode of delivery, and proposed a modification of antibiotic regimen in HIV positive mothers to counter the increased risk of infective complications (Fiore et al., 2004).

4.4.7 Neurosurgery

It is estimated that 10% of patients with HIV/AIDS develop intra-cerebral mass lesions; majority of these are primary CNS lymphomas and toxoplasmosis. Gliomas also form a significant percentage of primary CNS tumors in the HIV-positive population, as in the HIV-negative patients (Chamberlain, 1994; Hall & Short, 2009).

4.4.8 Otologic surgery

Otologic disease is common in HIV/AIDS patients, with some patients requiring surgical intervention. Otitis media may be the commonest otologic diagnosis in HIV patients. As in other organ systems, CD4 counts appear to be of prognostic value in terms of patient outcomes; while the outcome of patients with HIV infection without AIDS may be equivalent to that of HIV negative patients, patients AIDS have poorer outcomes, with a higher mortality (Kohan & Giacchi, 1999).

4.4.9 Ophthalmic surgery

Retinal disease is the commonest ocular complication in HIV positive patients, affecting between 30% and 70% of patients, while ocular surface squamous neoplasia is the commonest ocular tumor in the HIV patient.

4.4.10 Plastic/cosmetic surgery

HIV-associated lipodystrophy seen most commonly in is HIV patients on HAART, afflicting up 53% of HIV patients. It results in abnormal fat redistribution, with lipoatrophy in the face, limbs and buttocks, and lipohypertrophy of the neck, trunk, and breasts. Accumulation of fat in the cervicodorsal region and anterior neck may also interfere with function, resulting in pain, altered posture, limited range of motion, and sleep apnea (Engelhard, 2006). Surgery is the most effective mode of management.

Cancrum oris is a disease that afflicts children, associated with poverty, malnutrition, poor oral hygiene and infectious disease; in adults, it has been associated with debilitating diseases such as HIV/AIDS, diabetes mellitus and hematological disorders. (Nthumba & Carter, 2009). With the advent of HIV/AIDS, noma appears to be on the increase: successful surgical reconstruction with minimal complications has been reported (Chidzonga & Mahomya, 2008). For lipoatrophy, soft tissue replacement can be achieved by structural fat grafting via autotransplantation, dermal-fat grafts, subperiosteal malar implants, semipermanent soft tissue fillers, off-label silicone injection, and even intramuscular gluteal implants (Nelson & Stewart, 2007; Davison et al., 2008).

4.5 Orthopedics

4.5.1 Musculoskeletal infections

Musculoskeletal infections in HIV-infected or AIDS patients may have a wide spectrum of presentation, including osteomyelitis, septic arthritis, septic bursitis and soft tissue infections such as cellulitis abscesses abscess and pyomyositis, amongst others. Tuberculous infections may likewise involve soft tissue or bones/joints (Tehranzadeh et al., 2004).

While it may be expected that HIV infection would lead to an increase in musculoskeletal infections, some studies have indicated that this may not be so (Bahebeck et al., 2004). Further, these authors reported similar outcomes in both HIV negative and HIV positive patients (with CD4+ counts above 200/µL) when a similar protocol of management was instituted. WHO stages III and IV benefited from ARV therapy, along with appropriate surgical debridement and antibiotic administration.

While cellulitis is easily diagnosed clinically, the full extent of tissue involvement may not be apparent to the clinician, as this may be anywhere from a subcutaneous infection to osteomyelitis. Ultrasonography or a CTScan may be used to assist with this work-up, but in many low income countries, surgical debridement permits the substantive diagnosis, and treatment. Tissue or pus culture and sensitivity, where available is important in directing antibiotic therapy, which may need to be prolonged, depending on the type and depth of infection, as well as the degree of immunosuppression (Tehranzadeh et al., 2004; Bahebeck et al., 2004).

Pyomyositis is characterized by suppuration of skeletal muscle, and may be diagnosed by CTScan, MRI, ultrasound or aspiration of pus from the involved muscle. Prior to the HIV/AIDS pandemic, this was a preserve of tropical regions, hence the term 'tropical myositis' or 'myositis tropicans'.

Most patients with tropical pyomyositis have some history of trauma; *Staphylococcus areus* is the commonest isolate from abscesses or biopsies of patients with pyomyositis, irrespective of geographical region of origin. Most patients with non-tropical pyomyositis are immunosuppressed, with HIV/AIDS, diabetes mellitus and immunosuppressive therapy, amongst other conditions. In HIV epidemic areas, there is a high HIV seropositivity amongst patients with pyomyositis (Tehranzadeh et al., 2004; Ansaloni et al., 19960). HIV infected patients with pyomyositis may not give a history of trauma, and have been shown in some studies to have CD4+ counts less than 150cells/µL; further, HIV infected patients have been shown to have an increased staphylococcus carrier rate, when compared with IV negative populations (Ganesh et al., 1989).

Pyomyositis may present at any of three stages of evolution: early (invasive) stage (fever, induration), suppurative stage (high fever with muscle induration and pus on aspiration), and a late stage (bacteremia, septicemia, shock and metastatic abscesses). Patients presenting in the late stage may die from shock or multi-organ dysfunction/failure (Chauhan et al., 2004; Gambhir et al., 1992). The mortality rate from pyomyositis ranges between 1% and 20% (Biviji et al., 2002).

Broad spectrum intravenous antibiotics should be administered after an adequate incision, drainage and debridement (Chauhan et al., 2004).

4.5.2 Osteomyelitis

Osteomyelitis is associated with a mortality rate of up to 20% in HIV infected patients (Tehranzadeh, et al., 2004). While multiple organisms may be isolated in patients with osteomyelitis, *Staphylococcus aureus,*is the commonest isolate in HIV positive patients, as in the immunocompetent patient. CD4+ counts in patients with osteomyelitis average 250 cells/L. Mycobacterial species and *Bartonella henselae* may cause atypical osteomyelitis in the HIV infected patient (Mycobacterial and bacillary angiomatosis osteomyelitis, respectively); these often occur in the setting of CD4+ counts less than 100 cells/µL.

4.5.3 Tuberculosis

Of the almost two billion tuberculosis infections worldwide, 2% affect the skeletal system; of the skeletal infections, 60% involve the vertebral column (Govender et al., 2001).

4.5.4 Orthopedic implants

Implant surgery can be safely performed in HIV positive patients with closed fractures, regardless of their CD4 counts. The risk of wound sepsis increases significantly with open fractures, and although 7% of patients with external fixators may require removal because of pin-tract infection, recommended over internal fixation because of the higher infection rates when these are used for the stabilization of compound fractures (Harrison et al., 2002; Bahebeck et al., 2009; Norrish et al., 2007).

Brijlall proposed early implant removal after radiological evidence of fracture healing to avoid increased implant sepsis in HIV positive patients (Brijlall, 2008). After a five year follow-up of 14 HIV positive patients with uncemented hip arthroplasties, the same author reported excellent results; there was no infection, prosthetic loosening or dislocation. The author concluded that based on a careful selection of patients: nutritional status, and CD4 counts above 400 cells/µL arthroplasties can have good results in HIV infected patients (Brijlall, 2008). Habermann et al performed 55 total joint replacements in 41 HIV positive patients. These authors found that while functional outcomes of these patients did not that differ from those of HIV negative patients, and total joint replacements appeared safe in hemophiliacs, irrespective of serostatus, intravenous drug users had an increased incidence of infectious complications after total joint replacement. There was no correlation between CD4+ counts and infection (Habermann et al., 2008). The experience with total joint replacements in HIV populations has been generally favorable, (Habermann et al., 2008; Mahoney et al., 2005; Hicks et al., 2001; Mahoney et al., 2005; Hicks et al., 2001), although the experience of some workers has been less than favorable, with most citing high infectious complication rates (Parvizi et al., 2003; Luck Jr, 1994), there is a growing body of evidence that appropriate preoperative screening of patients, availability of HAART, antibiotic cover, and improved technique have seen a gradual improvement in outcomes after joint arthroplasties, with low rates of complications (Yoo et al., 2010). The success in joint replacement must be tempered by the need for correct diagnosis in the face of unusual presentations of disease processes in HIV/AIDS (Agarwal et al., 2005). Failure to recognize osteoarticular tuberculosis as the cause of osteoarthritis, with subsequent placement of a total knee prosthesis in a patient later found to have a multi-drug resistant strain of tuberculosis may have led to the patient's death from disseminated tuberculosis (Marschall et al., 2008).

4.6 Dental and maxilla-facial implants

Dental implants/prosthetics have been used in HIV positive patients. Short term favorable results with dental osteo-intergration implants were equivalent for HIV seropositive and negative patients (Stevenson et al., 2007). Several studies have shown that while mandibular fractures may have higher infection rates in HIV positive patients, midfacial fractures managed with miniplate osteosynthesis have the similar outcomes in HIV positive and HIV negative patients (Martinez-Gimeno et al., 1992; Schmidt et al., 1995; Strietzel et al., 2006).

4.6.1 Malignancy

Patients with HIV/AIDS have a heightened risk for the development of cancer. The duration of HIV infection, age greater than 40 years, and a history of opportunistic infection are the primary risk factors identified for the development of non–AIDS-defining cancers. A complex interplay between variables such as immunosuppression, co-infection with human oncogenic biologic agents, an advanced age and traditional risk factors are thought lead to the evolution of malignancy in HIV/AIDS patients.

Grulich et al found an increased incidence of cancers that are associated with a known infectious cause; human herpes virus 8 (Kaposi's sarcoma), human papilloma virus-associated cancers (cervical, anal, vulvar/vaginal, penis, oral cavity and tongue), Epstein Barr Virus (Hodgkin's lymphoma, Non-Hodgkin's lymphoma, nasopharyngeal cancer), Hepatitis B and C (liver cancer), and *Helicobacter pylori* associated gastric cancer (Gruhlich et al., 2007).

Kaposi's sarcoma (KS), Non-Hodgkin's lymphoma (NHL) and cervical cancer in the setting of HIV infection are regarded as AIDS-defining malignancies. The incidence of other cancers, such as skin, liver, anal, colonic, renal, and lung cancer as well as Hodgkin's lymphoma is higher in HIV positive patients compared to HIV negative patients. Malignant melanoma, leukemia, multiple myeloma and head and neck cancers have also been reported at a higher incidence amongst HIV patients (Silverberg & Abrahams, 2007; Patel et al., 2008; Chiao et al., 2003; Ruiz, 2009; Honda, 2006). The introduction of ARVs has seen a reduction in the incidence of KS and NHL, but not in cervical cancer; the effect of ARVs on non-AIDS defining malignancies has been more inconclusive, with most data suggesting an increase in incidence (Silverberg & Abrams, 2007; Nguyen et al., 2010; Honda, 2006). Notwithstanding the evidence of declining incidences of AIDS-defining malignancies, these remain a significant burden of disease in certain parts of the world; 82% of malignancies in HIV-infected patients in Latin America and the Caribbean in 2008 were AIDS-defining cancers (Fink et al., 2011).

Lung cancer is the commonest non-AIDS defining malignancy in the West, and generally affects patients of a much younger age than in non-HIV infected population. Lung cancer does not appear to have any relationship to levels of CD4 counts. In HIV-infected patients, lung cancer has a poor prognosis because of presentation at an advanced stage, and a poor response to therapy. Surgical resection has a similar outcome as in non-HIV-infected patients. Other forms of treatment include radiotherapy and chemotherapy (Nguyen et al., 2010; Spano et al., 2004). CD4 counts in both AIDS-defining and non-AIDS-defining malignancies are predictive of mortality. Although mortality rates from both AIDS-defining and non-AIDS-defining malignancies in patients on HAART in high income countries have declined, mortality rates remain higher for patients with non-AIDS-defining cancers. Older age, smoking, active Hepatitis B co-infection and a longer cumulative exposure to combination antiretroviral therapy were other variables predictive of mortality in patients with malignancies (Monforte et al., 2008).

4.6.2 Cutaneous malignancies

Skin cancers are the most common non–AIDS-defining cancers in HIV infected patients. Similar to HIV negative patients, sun exposure is the main cause of cutaneous malignancies in HIV infected patients. The risk of skin cancer correlates with the level of immunosuppression and inversely with CD4+ counts (Lobo et al., 1992; Honda, 2006).

Kaposi's sarcoma is the commonest cutaneous malignancy in HIV infected patients. It may develop in up to 20% of patients at any stage of HIV disease, with multifocal KS evident at CD4+ counts of less than 200 cells/μL. While the HIV pandemic has seen an increase in the number of KS cases reported, an expected substantial increase did not occur, even in HIV pandemic areas such as sub-Saharan Africa (Nthumba et al., 2011). In Asians, AIDS-related lymphoma is the commonest cancer in HIV patients. KS is a rare cancer in Asian HIV/AIDS

patients (Phatak et al., 2010; Zhang et al., 2011). Even within the continent of Africa, there is in Eastern Africa evidence that the prevalence of Kaposi's sarcoma is much lower incidence, than in Western Africa (Nthumba et al., 2011). There is no good explanation for this inter- and intra-racial difference.
Malignant melanoma and squamous cell carcinoma have an aggressive behavior in HIV positive patients. Nguyen et al recommended aggressive excision of squamous cell carcinoma in HIV patients, with histological control (Nguyen et al., 2010).
Basal cell carcinoma and squamous cell carcinoma have a higher incidence amongst HIV/AIDS patients than in the general population (Chiao, 2010).

4.6.3 Ocular tumors

Ocular surface squamous neoplasia (conjuctival squamous cell carcinoma) occurs in up to 10% of HIV positive patients in sub-Saharan Africa, making it the most common ocular tumor. A disease of the elderly in HIV-negative populations, an exponential increase has been noted in young HIV positive patients. Surgical resection may be curative, although a 30% recurrence rate has been reported. Other therapies include adjuvant chemotherapy, radiotherapy and cryotherapy (Nkomazana & Tshitswana, 2008). Aspergilloma of the orbit has been reported following orbital excenteration for ocular surface squamous neoplasia (Naik et al., 2006).

4.6.4 Cancer management in HIV/AIDS

The treatment of cancers in HIV/AIDS patients remains difficult. While HAART has been shown to improved outcomes in some AIDS-defining malignancies, with a noted significant decline in incidence, non-AIDS-defining cancers appear to be on the increase, even in the HAART era. Cancers in the setting of HIV/AIDS tend to present at an advanced stage; therapy with chemotherapeautic agents or radiotherapy presents real challenges because of the baseline immunesuppression in these patients. Some novel chemotherapeautic interventions in the treatment of AIDS-related lymphoma have shown promise, with improved outcomes reported, after combination therapies of HAART and different chemotherapeautic agents. The immune reconstitution inflammatory syndrome (IRIS) following HAART in AIDS-related lymphoma after receiving chemotherapy and antiretroviral therapy is evidence of improved immunity and may also signify better outcomes (Phatak et al., 2010; Weiss et al., 2006).

4.6.5 Chemotherapy/radiation therapy and chemoradiotherapy

Judicious use of radiation protocols has shown complete response of cervical cancer, an AIDS-defining cancer, where patients are able to complete the full course of radiotherapy; such patients achieved the same outcomes as HIV-negative patients under the same regimen. The primary concern in AIDS patients on radiotherapy is the possibility of enhanced radiation toxicity due to inherent radiosensitivity and glutathione deficiency in AIDS patients (Mallik et al., 2010).
Combination chemoradiation has registered significant success in the treatment of anal cancer, especially in the HAART era, with better outcomes for patients with CD4 counts above 200 cells/μL than for those with lower counts. Toxicity from the intense chemoradiotherapy is the primary concern (Mallik et al., 2010; Oehler-Janne et al., 2006). To date, there has been no evidence that chemoradiation besides toxicity, causes progression of

the tumor or AIDS, and ought to therefore be considered as a viable therapy for HIV/AIDS patients, especially those with CD4 counts above 200 cells/µL.

HAART is an integral part of the treatment of Kaposi's sarcoma. The administration of chemotherapeautic agents, immunotherapy and anti-angiogenic agents in patients with widespread KS has shown significant benefit, while local control may be achieved with radiation therapy, intralesional chemotherapy, cryotherapy and photodynamic therapy. Electron beam therapy has been used to achieve symptom control (Mallik et al., 2010).

With the use or HAART, standard doses of chemotherapy of radiotherapy may be administered to HIV/AIDS patients, with acceptable toxicity for the treatment of lymphomas; primary CNS lymphomas have been shown to respond to a combination of counts chemoradiation and steroids. These lesions are associated with very low CD4, (50 cells/µL or less) (Schultz et al., 1996).

4.7 The last frontier surgery in HIV patient care: Organ transplantation

Longevity of HIV-infected patients because of improved healthcare, especially the availability of HAART, leading to a large population of HIV survivors, has led to the development of long term organ complications (end-stage solid organ failure) that have created a demand for their effective management, transplantation. Renal and liver transplantation are the most accepted and performed transplant procedures in HIV-infected patients. Successful experience with transplantation of these organs has led to transplantation of other organs, such as pancreas and lungs.

4.7.1 Renal transplantation

In appropriately selected HIV-infected patients, the outcome of renal transplants is similar to that of HIV negative patients. Renal transplantation in HIV positive patients is thus an accepted practice in most centers in the world, with the effect that HIV infection is slowly gaining recognition as a chronic medical condition, rather than a contraindication to surgical interventions, including transplantation (Stock et al., 2004; Landin et al., 2010; Tan-Tam et al., 2009).

Notable continuing challenges are in the realm of the pharmacologic interactions between immunosuppressive therapy and some anti-retroviral agents, as well as a higher rate of acute rejection of the renal transplants when compared to HIV negative recipients.

Muller et al introduced an entirely new and previously unexplored, though controversial concept when they reported on their experience with four HIV positive patients who had received their kidneys from HIV infected donors (Muller et al., 2010).

Simultaneous pancreas-kidney transplantation in HIV positive diabetic patients has been reported (Genzini et al., 2010; Miro et al., 2010).

4.7.2 Liver transplantation

Like renal transplantation in end-stage renal disease, liver transplantation is currently accepted as therapy for end-stage liver failure in HIV positive patients, including hepatocellular carcinoma (Viberst et al., 2011; Di Benedetto et al., 2010). In a meta-analysis, HBV co-infection was found to result in improved transplant outcomes, while HCV co-infection had no effect (Cooper et al., 2011; Narushima et al., 2004). The outcome of liver transplants in HIV patients is similar to that of those of HIV negative patients (Sugawara et al., 2011).

4.7.3 Lung transplantation

Successful lung transplantation in an HIV patient with cystic fibrosis and end-stage respiratory failure has been reported (Bertani et al., 2009).

4.7.4 Heart transplantation

Dilated cardiomyopathy leading to end-stage cardiac failure is a common complication in HIV/AIDS patients; the only viable option is cardiac transplantation. Because HAART has improved survival of HIV/AIDS patients, with a 90% 10-year survival rate, heart transplantation has become attractive in well controlled HIV patients. Heart transplantation is still in its nascent stages in HIV patients; the total number of cases is less than 15 to date. Uriel et al reported excellent short term results of heart transplants in seven patients; they had a mean CD4 count of 554 cells/µL, undetectable viral loads, and no AIDS-defining illnesses (Uriel et al., 2009; Calabrese et al., 2003; Bisleri et al., 2003; Jahangiri & Haddad, 2007).

5. Conclusions

The HIV/AIDS pandemic continues to present significant challenges in the care of the patient in totality. The use of HAART has led to an increase in the survival of HIV/AIDS patients, turning this previously fatal disease into a chronic illness. As a result, malignancy, chronic illnesses, and other emerging surgical diseases presenting in these patients, have continued to challenge the ingenuity of the surgical fraternity. Implant surgery, oncology and organ transplantation are fields in HIV/AIDS in which significant progress has been made, and continues to evolve.

6. References

Aboolian A, Ricci M, Shapiro K, Connors A, LaRaja RD. (1999). Surgical treatment of HIV-related immune thrombocytopenia. Int Surg 84(1):81-5.

Abrams DI, Kiprov DD, Goedert JJ, Sarngadharan MG, Gallo RC & Volberding PA. (1986). Antibodies to human T-lymphotropic virus type III and development of the acquired immunodeficiency syndrome in homosexual men presenting with immune thrombocytopenia. Ann Intern Med 104(1):47-50.

Adams S, Stojkovic SG & Leveson SH. (2010). Needlestick injuries during surgical procedures: a multidisciplinary online study. Occup Med (Lond) 60(2):139-144.

Agaskar M, Ghorpade N, Athan E & Mohajeri M. (2003). AIDS and heart disease: is cardiac surgery justified? Heart Lung Circ 12(3):193-195.

Ansaloni L, Acaye GL & Re MC. (1996). High HIV sero-prevalence among patients with pyomyositis in northern Uganda. *Trop Med Int Health* 1:210–212.

Bahebeck J, Bedimo R, Eyenga V, Kouamfack C, Kingue T, Nierenet M & Sosso M. (2004). The management of musculoskeletal infection in HIV carriers. Acta Orthop Belg 70(4):355-360.

Beltrami EM, Luo CC, de la Torre N & Cardo DM. (2002). Transmission of drug-resistant HIV after an occupational exposure despite postexposure prophylaxis with a combination drug regimen. Infect Control Hosp Epidemiol 23(6):345-348.

Bennett NT & Howard RJ. (1994). Quantity of blood inoculated in a needlestick injury from suture needles. J Am Coll Surg 178:107–110.

Bertani A, Grossi P, Vitulo P, D'Ancona G, Arcadipane A, Nanni Costa A & Gridelli B. (2009). Successful lung transplantation in an HIV- and HBV-positive patient with cystic fibrosis. Am J Transplant 9(9):2190-2196.

Bisleri G, Morgan J, Deng M, Mancini D & Oz M. (2003). Should HIV-positive recipients undergo heart transplantation? *J Thorac Cardiovasc Surg* 126:1639-1640.

Biviji AA, Paiement GD & Steinbach LS. (2002). Musculoskeletal manifestations of human immunodeficiency virus infection. *J Am Acad Orthop Surg* 10:312–320.

Bova R & Meagher A. (1998). Appendicitis in HIV-positive patients. Aust N Z J Surg 68(5):337-339.

Brijlall S. Arthroplasty in HIV infected patients – a 5 year follow up. (2008). *J Bone Joint Surg Br* 90-B (Supp B-III):473.

Brijlall S. Implant sepsis in HIV infected patients (2003). *J Bone Joint Surg Br* 85-B (Supp II):148.

Brooks RA, Etzel M, Klosinski LE, Leibowitz AA, Sawires S, Szekeres G, Weston M & Coates TJ. (2010). Male circumcision and HIV prevention: looking to the future. *AIDS Behav* 14(5):1203-6.

Brown SA, Majumdar G, Harrington C, Bedford M, Winter M, O'Doherty MJ & Savidge GF. (1994). Effect of splenectomy on HIV-related thrombocytopenia and progression of HIV infection in patients with severe haemophilia. Blood Coagul Fibrinolysis 5(3):393-397.

Cacala SR, Mafana E, Thomson SR & Smith A. (2006). Prevalence of HIV status and CD4 counts in a surgical cohort: their relationship to clinical outcome. *Ann R Coll Surg Engl* 88(1):46-51.

Calabrese LH, Albrecht M, Young J, McCarthy P, Haug M, Jarcho J & Zackin R. (2003). Successful cardiac transplantation in an HIV-1-infected patient with advanced disease. *N Engl J Med* 348:2323-2328.

Centers for Disease Control and Prevention. (2000). HIV/AIDS surveillance report. Atlanta, GA: Centers for Disease Control and Prevention. Vol.(12):1.

Chamberlain MC. (1994). Gliomas in patients with acquired immune deficiency syndrome. Cancer 74(7):1912-1914.

Chauhan S, Jain S, Varma S & Chauhan SS. (2004). Tropical pyomyositis (myositis tropicans): current perspective. *Postgrad Med J* 80:267-270.

Chiao EY & Krown SE. (2003). Update on non-acquired immunodeficiency syndrome-defining malignancies. *Curr Opin Oncol* 15:389-397.

Chiao EY. (2010). Epidemiology and Clinical Characteristics of Non-AIDS-Defining Malignancies *in*: Dittmer, DP., Krown SE. (ed.) *Molecular Basis for Therapy of AIDS-Defining Cancers*, Springer-Verlag, New York, pp 1-40.

Chidzonga MM & Mahomva L. (2008). Noma (cancrum oris) in human immunodeficiency virus infection and acquired immunodeficiency syndrome (HIV and AIDS): clinical experience in Zimbabwe. J Oral Maxillofac Surg 66(3):475-485.

Chong T, Alejo DE, Greene PS, Redmond JM, Sussman MS, Baumgartner WA & Cameron DE. (2003). Cardiac valve replacement in human immunodeficiency virus-infected patients. Ann Thorac Surg 76(2):478-480.

Cooper C, Kanters S, Klein M, Chaudhury P, Marotta P, Wong P, Kneteman N & Mills EJ. (2011). Liver transplant outcomes in HIV-infected patients: a systematic review and meta-analysis with synthetic cohort. AIDS 25(6):777-786.

Cunningham CM. (2010). Human immunodeficiency virus/acquired immune deficiency syndrome: the forgotten crisis and implications for the general surgery practice. Am J Surg Sep 25; [Epub ahead of print].

Davison SP, Reisman NR, Pellegrino ED, Larson EE, Dermody M & Hutchison PJ. (2008). Perioperative guidelines for elective surgery in the human immunodeficiency virus-positive patient. Plast Reconstr Surg 121(5):1831-1840.

Deneve JL, Shantha JG, Page AJ, Wyrzykowski AD, Rozycki GS & Feliciano DV. (2010). CD4 count is predictive of outcome in HIV-positive patients undergoing abdominal operations. Am J Surg 200(6):694-699.

Di Benedetto F, Di Sandro S, De Ruvo N, Montalti R, Ballarin R, Guerrini GP, Spaggiari M, Guaraldi G & Gerunda G. (2010). First report on a series of HIV patients undergoing rapamycin monotherapy after liver transplantation. Transplantation 89(6):733-738.

Do AN, Ciesielski CA, Metler RP, Hammett TA, Li J & Fleming PL. (2003). Occupationally acquired human immunodeficiency virus (HIV) infection: national case surveillance data during 20 years of the HIV epidemic in the United States. Infect Control Hosp Epidemiol 24(2):86-96.

Edge JM, Van der Merwe AE, Pieper CH & Bouic P. (2001). Clinical outcome of HIV positive patients with moderate to severe burns. *Burns* 27:111-114.

Engelhard P. (2006). Correction options for lipoatrophy in HIV-infected patients. AIDS Patient Care STDS 20(3):151-160.

Fink VI, Shepherd BE, Cesar C, Krolewiecki A, Wehbe F, Cortés CP, Crabtree-Ramírez B, Padgett D, Shafaee M, Schechter M, Gotuzzo E, Bacon M, McGowan C, Cahn P Masys D; on behalf of The Caribbean Central South America Network for HIV Research (CCASAnet) Collaboration of the International Epidemiologic Databases to Evaluate AIDS (IeDEA) Program. (2011). Cancer in HIV-infected persons from the Caribbean, Central and South America. *J Acquir Immune Defic Syndr* 56:467–473.

Fiore S, Newell ML & Thorne C; European HIV in Obstetrics Group. (2004). Higher rates of post-partum complications in HIV-infected than in uninfected women irrespective of mode of delivery. AIDS 18(6):933-8.

Frater RW, Sisto D & Condit D. (1989). Cardiac surgery in human immunodeficiency virus (HIV) carriers. Eur J Cardiothorac Surg 3(2):146-150.

Gambhir IS, Singh DS, Gupta SS, Gupta PR & Kumar M. (1992) Tropical pyomyositis in India, a clinico-histopathological study. *J Trop Med Hyg* 95:42–46.

Ganesh R, Castle D, Mcgibbon D, Phillips I, Bradbeer C. (1989). Staphylococcus infection and HIV carriage. *Lancet* 334(8662):558.

Genzini T, Noujaim HM, Mota LT, Crescentini F, Antunes I, Di Jura VL, Ferreira FA, Muller BF, Vetorazzo JE & de Miranda MP. (2010). Simultaneous pancreas-kidney transplantation in a human immunodeficiency virus-positive recipient: a case report. Transplant Proc 42(2):591-3.

Govender S, Parbhoo AH, Kumar KP & Annamalai K. (2001). Anterior spinal decompression in HIV-positive patients with tuberculosis. A prospective study. Bone Joint Surg Br 83(6):864-867.

Grulich AE, van Leeuwen MT, Falster MO & Vajdic CM. (2007). Incidence of cancers in people with HIV/AIDS compared with immunosuppressed transplant recipients: a meta-analysis. Lancet 370(9581):59-67.

Habermann B, Eberhardt C & Kurth AA. (2008). Total joint replacement in HIV positive patients. J Infect 57(1):41-46.

Hall JR & Short SC. (2009). Management of glioblastoma multiforme in HIV patients: a case series and review of published studies. *Clin Oncol (R Coll Radiol)* 21(8):591-597.

Harrison WJ, Lewis CP & Lavy CB. (2004). Open fractures of the tibia in HIV positive patients: a prospective controlled single blind study. *Injury* 35:852-856.

Harrison WJ, Lewis CP & Lavy CBD. (2002). Wound healing after implant surgery in HIV positive patients. J Bone Joint Surg Br 84(6):802-806.

Health Protection Agency (2005). Occupational transmission of HIV: summary of published reports. URL: http://www.hpa.org.uk/Publications/InfectiousDiseases/BloodBorneInfections/0503OcctransmissionHIVsummaryofreports/.

Health Protection Agency (2005). URL: http://www.hpa.org.uk/hpa/news/articles/press_releases/2005/050125_needlestick.htm.

Hicks JL, Ribbans WJ, Buzzard B, Kelley SS, Toft L, Torri G, Wiedel JD, York J. (2001). Infected joint replacements in HIV-positive patients with haemophilia. *J Bone Joint Surg Br* 83(7):1050-1054.

Honda KS. (2006). HIV and skin cancer. *Dermatol Clin* 24(4):521-530.

Jahangiri B & Haddad H. (2007). Cardiac transplantation in HIV-positive patients: are we there yet? J Heart Lung Transplan*t* 26(2):103-107.

Kalima P, Luo NP, Bem C &Watters DA. (1990). The prevalence of HIV seropositivity and impact of HIV infection in Zambian surgical patients. *Int Conf AIDS* 6:443.

Kaplan RC, Kingsley LA, Sharrett AR, Li X, Lazar J, Tien PC, Mack WJ, Cohen MH, Jacobson L & Gange SJ. (2007). Ten-year predicted coronary heart disease risk in HIV-infected men and women. Clin Infect Dis 45(8):1074-81.

Karpelowsky JS, Leva E, Kelley B, Numanoglu A, Rode H & Millar AJ. (2009). Outcomes of human immunodeficiency virus-infected and -exposed children undergoing surgery--a prospective study. J Pediatr Surg 44(4):681-687.

Kerr HL, Stewart N, Pace A, Elsayed S. (2009). Sharps injury reporting amongst surgeons. Ann R Coll Surg Engl 91(5):430-432.

Lefebvre DR, Strande LF & Hewitt CW. (2008). An enzyme-mediated assay to quantify inoculation volume delivered by suture needlestick injury: two gloves are better than one. J Am Coll Surg 206(1):113-122.

Kohan D & Giacchi RJ. (1999). Otologic surgery in patients with HIV-1 and AIDS. Otolaryngol Head Neck Surg 121(4):355-360.

Kumar N, Reddy B, Jitendra M, Kumar V. (2008). Cardiac surgery in HIV positive patients : Growing needs and concerns. Single centre experience in an Indian setting. *Ind J Thorac Cardiovasc Surg* 24:5-9

Landin L, Rodriguez-Perez JC, Garcia-Bello MA, Cavadas PC, Thione A, Nthumba P, Blanes M & Ibañez J. (2010). Kidney transplants in HIV-positive recipients under HAART.

A comprehensive review and meta-analysis of 12 series. Nephrol Dial Transplant 25(9):3106-3115.

Lin PH, Bush RL, Yao Q, Lam R, Paladugu R, Zhou W, Chen C & Lumsden AB. (2004). Abdominal aortic surgery in patients with human immunodeficiency virus infection. *Am J Surg* 188(6):690-697.

Lobo DV, Chu P, Grekin RC & Berger TG. (1992). Nonmelanoma skin cancers and infection with the human immunodeficiency virus. *Arch Dermatol* 128(5):623-627.

Looke DF & Grove DI. (1990). Failed prophylactic zidovudine after needlestick injury. Lancet. 335(8700):1280.

Lord RV, Coleman MJ & Milliken ST. (1998). Splenectomy for HIV-related immune thrombocytopenia: comparison with results of splenectomy for non-HIV immune thrombocytopenic purpura. Arch Surg 133(2):205-210.

Lot F, Séguier JC, Fégueux S, Astagneau P, Simon P, Aggoune M, van Amerongen P, Ruch M, Cheron M, Brücker G, Desenclos JC & Drucker J. (1999). Probable transmission of HIV from an orthopedic surgeon to a patient in France. *Ann Intern Med* 130(1):1-6.

Luck Jr JV. (1994). Orthopaedic surgery on the HIV-positive patient: complications and outcome. *Instr Course Lect* 43:543-549.

Mahoney CR, Glesby MJ, DiCarlo EF, Peterson MG & Bostrom MP. (2005). Total hip arthroplasty in patients with human immunodeficiency virus infection: pathologic findings and surgical outcomes. *Acta Orthop* 76:198-203.

Mallik S, Talapatra K & Goswami J. (2010). AIDS: A radiation oncologist's perspective. J Cancer Res Ther 6:432-441.

Marschall J, Evison JM, Droz S, Studer UC & Zimmerli S. (2008). Disseminated tuberculosis following total knee arthroplasty in an HIV patient. Infection 36(3):274-278.

Martinez-Gimeno C, Acero-Sanz J, Martin-Sastre R & Navarro-Vila C. (1992). Maxillofacial trauma: Influence of HIV infection. *J Craniomaxillofac Surg* 20:297-302.

Mestres CA, Chuquiure JE, Claramonte X, Muñoz J, Benito N, Castro MA, Pomar JL & Miró JM. (2003). Long-term results after cardiac surgery in patients infected with the human immunodeficiency virus type-1 (HIV-1) Eur J Cardiothorac Surg 23(6):1007-1016.

Miro JM, Ricart MJ, Trullas JC, Cofan F, Cervera C, Brunet M, Tuset M, Manzardo C, Oppenheimer F & Moreno A. (2010). Simultaneous pancreas-kidney transplantation in HIV-infected patients: a case report and literature review. Transplant Proc 42(9):3887-3891.

Monforte A, Abrams D, Pradier C, Weber R, Reiss P, Bonnet F, Kirk O, Law M, De Wit S, Friis-Møller N, Phillips AN, Sabin CA & Lundgren JD; Data Collection on Adverse Events of Anti-HIV Drugs (D:A:D) Study Group. (2008). HIV-induced immunodeficiency and mortality from AIDS-defining and non-AIDS-defining malignancies. AIDS 22(16):2143-2153.

Monsuez JJ, Charniot JC, Escaut L, Teicher E, Wyplosz B, Couzigou C, Vignat N & Vittecoq D. (2009). HIV-associated vascular diseases: structural and functional changes, clinical implications. Int J Cardiol 133(3):293-306.

Muller E, Kahn D & Mendelson M. (2010). Renal transplantation between HIV-positive donors and recipients. *N Engl J Med* 362(24):2336-2337.

Mullins JR & Harrison PB. (1993). The questionable utility of mandatory screening for the human immunodeficiency virus. Am J Surg 166(6):676-677.

Naik MN, Vemuganti GK & Honavar SG. (2006). Primary orbital aspergilloma of the exenterated orbit in an immunocompromized patient. Indian J Med Microbiol 24(3):233-234.

Narushima Y, Ishiyama S, Kawashima K, Shimamura H, Yamaki T & Yamauchi H. (2004). Operated hepatocellular carcinoma in two HIV- and HCV-positive hemophilic patients. J Hepatobiliary Pancreat Surg 11(3):207-210.

Nelson L & Stewart KJ. (2008). Plastic surgical options for HIV-associated lipodystrophy. J *Plast Reconstr Aesthet Surg* 61(4):359-365.

Nguyen ML, Farrell KJ & Gunthel CJ. (2010). Non-AIDS-Defining Malignancies in Patients with HIV in the HAART Era. Curr Infect Dis Rep 12(1):46-55.

Nkomazana O & Tshitswana D. (2008). Ocular complications of HIV infection in sub-Sahara Africa. Curr HIV/AIDS Rep 5(3):120-125.

Norrish AR, Lewis CP & Harrison WJ. (2007). Pin-track infection in HIV-positive and HIV-negative patients with open fractures treated by external fixation: a prospective, blinded, case-controlled study. J Bone Joint Surg Br 89(6):790-793.

Nthumba P & Carter L. (2009). Visor flap for total upper and lower lip reconstruction: a case report. J Med Case Reports 3:7312.

Nthumba PM, Cavadas P & Landin L. (2011). Primary cutaneous malignancies in sub-Saharan Africa. *Ann Plast Surg* 66(3):313-320.

Nthumba PM, Ngure P, Nyoro P. (2011b) Giant condyloma acuminatum of the scrotum in a patient with AIDS: a case report. J Med Case Reports 5:272.

Nthumba PM. (2008). Giant pyogenic granuloma of the thigh: a case report. *J Med Case Reports* 2:95.

Oehler-Janne C, Seifert B, Lutolf UM & Ciernik IF. (2006). Local tumor control and toxicity in HIV-associated anal carcinoma treated with radiotherapy in the era of antiretroviral therapy. *Radiat Oncol* 1:29.

Parvizi J, Sullivan TA, Pagnano MW, Trousdale RT & Bolander ME. (2003). Total joint arthroplasty in human immunodeficiency virus positive patients: an alarming rate of early failure. *J Arthroplasty* 18(3):259-264.

Patel MS, Malinoski DJ, Nguyen XM & Hoyt DB. (2011). The impact of select chronic diseases on outcomes after trauma: a study from the National Trauma Data Bank. J Am Coll Surg 212(1):96-104.

Patel P, Hanson DL, Sullivan PS, Novak RM, Moorman AC, Tong TC, Holmberg SD & Brooks JT. (2008). Adult and Adolescent Spectrum of Disease Project and HIV Outpatient Study Investigators. Incidence of types of cancer among HIV-infected persons compared with the general population in the United States, 1992-2003. Ann Intern Med 148(10):728-36.

Phatak UA, Joshi R, Badakh DK, Gosavi VS, Phatak JU & Jagdale RV. (2010). AIDS-associated cancers: an emerging challenge. J Assoc Physicians India 58:159-162.

Phillips EK, Owusu-Ofori A, & Jagger J (2007). Bloodborne pathogen exposure risk among surgeons in sub-Saharan Africa. *Infect Control Hosp Epidemiol* 28(12):1334-1336.

Power C, Nath A, Aoki FY & Bigio MD. (1997). Remission of Progressive Multifocal Leukoencephalopathy Following Splenectomy and Antiretroviral Therapy in a Patient with HIV Infection. *N Engl J Med* 336:661-662.

Rapparini C. (2006). Occupational HIV infection among health care workers exposed to blood and body fluids in Brazil. *Am J Infect Control* 34:237-240.

Read JS & Newell MK. (2005). Efficacy and safety of cesarean delivery for prevention of mother-to-child transmission of HIV-1. Cochrane Database Syst Rev (4):CD005479.

Reilly MJ, Burke KM & Davison SP. (2009). Wound Infection Rates in Elective Plastic Surgery for HIV-Positive Patients. *Plast Reconstr Surg* 123: 106-111.

Rerknimitr R & Kullavanijaya P. (2001). Endoscopy in HIV infected patients. J Med Assoc Tha*i* 84(Suppl 1):S26-31.

Rose DN, Collins M & Kleban R. (1998). Complications of surgery in HIV-infected patients. *AIDS* 12(17):2243-2251.

Rothman RE, Ketlogetswe KS, Dolan T, Wyer PC & Kelen GD. (2003). Preventive care in the emergency department: should emergency departments conduct routine HIV screening? a systematic review. Acad Emerg Med 10(3):278-285.

Ruiz M. (2009). Certain non-AIDS-defining cancers higher in HIV population. *HIV Clin* 21(4):13-16.

S, Caplivski D & Bottone EJ. (2005). Disseminated tuberculosis presenting with finger swelling in a patient with tuberculous osteomyelitis: a case report. *Ann Clin Microbiol Antimicrob* 4:18.

Saber AA, Aboolian A, LaRaja RD, Baron H & Hanna K. (2001). HIV/AIDS and the risk of deep venous thrombosis: a study of 45 patients with lower extremity involvement. *Am Surg* 67:645–647.

Schmidt B, Kearns G, Perrott D & Kaban LB. (1995). Infection following treatment of mandibular fractures in human immunodeficiency virus seropositive patients. *J Oral Maxillofac Surg* 53:1134–1139.

Schultz C, Scott C, Sherman W, Donahue B, Fields J, Murray K, Fisher B, Abrams R & Meis-Kindblom J. (1996). Preirradiation chemotherapy with cyclophosphamide, doxorubicin, vincristine, and dexamethasone for primary CNS lymphomas: Initial report of radiation therapy oncology group protocol 88-06. *J Clin Oncol* 14:556-564.

Silverberg MJ & Abrams DI. (2007). AIDS-defining and non-AIDS-defining malignancies: cancer occurrence in the antiretroviral therapy era. Curr Opin Oncol 19(5):446-51.

Sinkala E, Gray S, Zulu I, Mudenda V, Zimba L, Vermund SH, Drobniewski F & Kelly P. (2009). Clinical and ultrasonographic features of abdominal tuberculosis in HIV positive adults in Zambia. *BMC Infect Dis* 9:44.

Spano JP, Massiani MA, Bentata M, Rixe O, Friard S, Bossi P, Rouges F, Katlama C, Breau JL, Morere JF, Khayat D & Couderc LJ. (2004). Lung cancer in patients with HIV Infection and review of the literature. Med Oncol 21(2):109-115.

Stevenson GC, Riano PC, Moretti AJ, Nichols CM, Engelmeier RL & Flaitz CM. (2007). Short-term success of osseointegrated dental implants in HIV-positive individuals: a prospective study. J Contemp Dent Pract 8(1):1-10.

Stock PG, Barin B, Murphy B, Hanto D, Diego JM, Light J, Davis C, Blumberg E, Simon D, Subramanian A, Millis JM, Lyon GM, Brayman K, Slakey D, Shapiro R, Melancon J, Jacobson JM, Stosor V, Olson JL, Stablein DM & Roland ME. (2010). Outcomes of

Kidney Transplantation in HIV-Infected Recipients. *N Engl J Med* 363(21):2004-2014.

Strietzel FP, Rothe S, Reichart PA & Schmidt-Westhausen AM. (2006). Implant-prosthetic treatment in HIV-infected patients receiving highly active antiretroviral therapy: report of cases. Int J Oral Maxillofac Implants 21(6):951-956.

Sugawara Y, Tamura S, Kokudo N. (2011). Liver transplantation in HCV/HIV positive patients. World J Gastrointest Surg 3(2):21-28.

Tan-Tam CC, Frassetto LA & Stock PG. (2009). Liver and kidney transplantation in HIV-infected patients. AIDS Rev 11(4):190-204.

Tehranzadeh J, Ter-Oganesyan RR & Steinbach LS. (2004). Musculoskeletal disorders associated with HIV infection and AIDS. Part I: infectious musculoskeletal conditions. Skeletal Radiol 33(5):249-259.

Thomas S, Agarwal M & Mehta G. (2001). Intraoperative glove perforation - single versus double gloving in protection against skin contamination. Postgrad Med J 77:458–460.

Tran HS. (2000). Predictors of Operative Outcome in Patients with Human Immunodeficiency Virus Infection and Acquired Immunodeficiency Syndrome. *Am J Surg* 180:228-233

Troya J, Casquero A, Muñiz G, Fernández-Guerrero ML & Górgolas M. (2007). The role of splenectomy in HIV-infected patients with relapsing visceral leishmaniasis. Parasitology 134(Pt 5):621-624.

Tsoukas CM, Bernard NF, Abrahamowicz M, Strawczynski H, Growe G, Card RT& Gold P. (1998). Effect of splenectomy on slowing human immunodeficiency virus disease progression. Arch Surg 133(1):25-31.

Tyler DS, Shaunak S, Bartlett JA, & Iglehart JD. (1990). HIV-1-associated thrombocytopenia. The role of splenectomy. *Ann Surg* 211(2):211–217.

Uriel N, Jorde UP, Cotarlan V, Colombo PC, Farr M, Restaino SW, Lietz K, Naka Y, Deng MC & Mancini D. (2009). Heart transplantation in human immunodeficiency virus-positive patients. *J Heart Lung Transplant* 28(7):667-679.

Vibert E, Duclos-Vallée JC, Ghigna MR, Hoti E, Salloum C, Guettier C, Castaing D, Samuel D & Adam R. (2011). Liver transplantation for hepatocellular carcinoma: the impact of human immunodeficiency virus infection. *Hepatology* 53(2):475-82.

Weiss R, Mitrou P, Arasteh K, Schuermann D, Hentrich M, Duehrsen U, Sudeck H, Schmidt-Wolf IG, Anagnostopoulos I & Huhn D. (2006). Acquired immunodeficiency syndrome-related lymphoma: simultaneous treatment with combined cyclophosphamide, doxorubicin, vincristine, and prednisone chemotherapy and highly active antiretroviral therapy is safe and improves survival--results of the German Multicenter Trial. *Cancer* 106:1560-8.

Wittmann MM, Wittmann A & Wittmann DH. (1996). AIDS, emergency operations, and infection control. *Infect Control Hosp Epidemiol* 17(8):532-538.

World Health Organization (WHO) (2003). Aide-Memoire for a strategy to protect health workers from infection with bloodborne viruses. Geneva: Department of Blood Safety and Clinical Technology, WHO; 2003. URL:http://www.who.int/injection_safety/toolbox/en/AM_HCW *Safety_EN.pdf.*

Yoo JJ, Chun SH, Kwon YS, Koo KH, Yoon KS & Kim HJ. (2010). Operations about hip in human immunodeficiency virus-positive patients. *Clin Orthop Surg* 2(1):22-27.

Zhang YX, Gui XE, Zhong YH, Rong YP & Yan YJ. (2011). Cancer in cohort of HIV-infected population: prevalence and clinical characteristics. *J Cancer Res Clin Oncol* 137(4):609-14.

Zvandasara P, Saungweme G, Mlambo JT & Moyo J. (2007). Post Caesarean section infective morbidity in HIV-positive women at a tertiary training hospital in Zimbabwe. Cent Afr J Med 53(9-12):43-7.

Part 5

Ethical Considerations Including Acceptance of HIV Vaccine

18

Ethical and Psychosocial Aspects of HIV/AIDS

N. Cannovo[1], M. Paternoster[1], I. Burlin[1],
M. Colangelo[2] and V. Graziano[1]
[1]*Department of Public Medicine and Social Security - Chair of Legal Medicine -University of Naples Federico II, Naples*
[2]*Psi&Co -La Minerva Association, Potenza*
Italy

1. Introduction

Since its global appearance, the Human Immunodeficiency Virus (HIV) has represented the most evident tear between bioethics/rhetoric and the reality of everyday life.

All AIDS related issues are different in two macro areas, the first pertains to the clinical-psychological aspect, the other a psycho-social dimension.

The first derives from the consideration of current disease and health, and the second one focuses primarily on prevention and spread of the disease, considering that the only way to effectively fight AIDS is by preventing contagion. Over the past years, the approach towards AIDS has changed, from being seen as a social sore to a social-sanitary alarm, this in a certain way has favored the perception of the illness, which now is no longer necessarily associated with death.

However something from the past has managed to survive, medicine and science have both evolved, and there have been numerous studies that highlight the process related to the disease, but the psychosocial perception has not changed, damaging who is affected finding themselves fighting against stigma, prejudice and exclusion.

AIDS is not only an illness, but moreover configured as an attack on civil society, so those affected by it are removed or living in a constant state of discrimination, even if behind media campaigns and legislative measures aimed at supporting their quality of life.

The AIDS epidemic infected more than 50 million and has claimed the lives of more than 20 million people worldwide; its devastating effect is particularly seen in the Third World.

Sub-Saharan Africa is the epicenter of HIV, with 67% of the 33 million infected with HIV in the world and with 75% of deaths due to AIDS (UNAIDS, 2008).

In eastern and southern Africa, infant mortality is one third to two thirds higher than it would have been in the absence of HIV and AIDS, and child mortality continues to rise, leading to a dramatic reduction in life expectancy (De Cock et al., 2000).

Currently the progression of the infection in Western countries is slowing down, both because of the use of more effective therapies and the improvement of information and prevention of infection, and thanks to greater attention paid to early diagnosis.

Furthermore, the rate of neonatal transmission is only about 2% thanks to the introduction of antiretroviral drugs and the use of elective Caesarean section.

However the world is divided into two different approaches concerning HIV infected and AIDS, while in western countries they are slowly abandoning the concept (Ehrenkranz et al., 2009) of exceptionalism, in developing countries this is still the most common approach.
In the meantime, screening tests are performed when requested by the patient only after he or she has signed a formal consent form and after having gone through formal counseling; this means that in Africa where there is a higher prevalence of this infection, one out of five are not aware of their status (World Health Organitation [WHO], 2008).
The opt-out testing is still the subject of heated debate between the philosophical currents of consequentialism, liberalism and free paternalism; however there is no denying that the consequences in terms of social impact, although heavy, collide with the benefits of a precocious intervention which results in being a survival rate for those infected (April, 2010).
Such a chronic, infectious disease offers tremendous opportunities for ethical dilemmas and psychosocial discussions. Our job will be to face different topics about the HIV infection.

2. Clinical research

The clinical trials are increasingly conducted globally and Sponsors tend to shift their activities to developing countries where they can save between 10-50% of their investment compared to the rest of industrialized countries.
Moreover, in countries described as "poor", the laws are less stringent due to a low possibility of checkups and it being easier to enlist patients (Altavilla, 2010) for which, often, researching is the only way to obtain drugs. The European Medicines Agency set up a Work on Third Country Clinical Trials in order to clarify the ethical standards used in clinical trials conducted outside the European Economic Area and which were then introduced to the European market.
The validity of the regulations of good clinical practice is universally recognized, however, there is no denying that they have a different impact between Western countries and so-called developing countries.
Even the simple definition of standard of care and treatment, essential for the comparison of innovative therapies, qualitatively absorbs different connotations when assessed in the Western health care system compared to the rest of the world.
In addition to the traditional principles of Bioethics, HIV/AIDS has added new issues, like: accessibility, affordability, standard of care, stigma and discrimination, post-trial benefits, equity and sustainability of interventions, that have generated intense debates both locally and internationally, which nevertheless, did not reach universal ethical standards in the world.
Indeed, the expansion of studies on HIV throughout the world has helped the issue of the adaptation of ethical standards emerge even more, developed in industrialized countries, and exported to developing countries.
One thing is certain, the potential imbalances in various countries and between communities/groups within countries demand that ethically acceptable clinical trials and strategies are planned in different locations so that communities and countries in need of early interventions can be benefited.
It is no coincidence that the debate on the ethnicity of carrying out clinical trials in developing countries in search of a land "more pliable" is still ardently and culminated in the publication of multiple guidelines from the developed worlds (National Bioethics Advisory Commission [NBAC], 2001), (Nuffield Council on Bioethics, 1999).

In this regard the HIV Preventive Trial Network (HPTN) Ethics guidance document developed by HPTN Ethics Working Group of Family Health International (HIV Prevention Trials Network [HPTN], 2003) has addressed the crucial points of the clinical trial in the so-called "host countries", ranging from the reduction of risk associated with stigmatization, to ensure informed consent for complex research with potentially vulnerable participants, from determining ethical authority and accountability in international collaborative research to design research that meets local needs as challenges.

Incidentally the social contexts and cultural specifications of the host communities and countries should be given due consideration to protect the dignity, safety and welfare of the trial participants (Indian Council of Medical Research, 2000), when it intends to undertake a study of international cooperation, remembering that many countries, such as India (ICRM, 2001), the Philippines (Philippines National Health Council, 2001) and South Africa (South Africa Code of Ethics, 2000), have developed their own guidelines to suit the local requirements.

A typical problem of studies made in poor countries is related to the testing design, because while in industrialized countries generally a comparison between new and old pharmaceuticals is made, in developing countries it is rather difficult to find a pharmaceutical of control, therefore it is preferable placebo confrontation or research with a lower dosage or short-term studies.

Under this aspect, not even Helsinki's 2008 version managed to reach global agreement.

Another peculiar aspect of clinic trials held in developing countries, is represented by the vigorous debate of the necessity to guarantee drug coverage to all of those who take part in the experimentation, after of course having finished the study.

Since 2000, researchers, pharmaceutical companies and international bioethics bodies have engaged in a fierce debate on access to post-treatment trials, culminating in note 30 of the Declaration of Helsinki (World Medical Association, 2004) - which recommends that access to treatments for all participants-and the 2005 European Directive (Commission Directive, 2005), which requires foreseeing the cures that will be adopted after the study right from the initial protocol.

Specifically, US National Institutes of Health Division of AIDS (National Institutes of Health [NIH]) and other international Organizations, such as Council for International Organizations of Medical Sciences (Council for International Organizations of Medical Sciences [CIOMS], 2002) and United Nations Programme on HIV/AIDS (United Nations Programme on HIV/AIDS [UNAIDS], 2001), only state that post-trial access to medications and medical care should be "considered" in the trial planning process.

Indeed, the hesitation of the pharmaceutical dispensing of drugs after the study is due to the need to fill the shortage of adequate health structures well beyond the scheduled period of experimentation. In other words, the Sponsors, attracted by low costs of running an experiment in developing countries, would ultimately leave that decision on the burden of dispensing post-trials (Weijer & LeBlanc, 2006).

According to the UNAIDS report of 2010 (UNAIDS, 2010), the average price of the most common regimens for an adult is about US$ 0.17 per day (the cost of condoms has also declined to as low as US$ 0.04 per unit); while stopping a single case of infection among infants now costs a mere US$ 5.

Besides economical reason many Authors (Macklin, 2001) (Grady, 2005) believe that constituting post-trial services would mean trial sponsors would have to take on many responsibilities, so it would be preferable to perform this task having already appointed a government agency or a non-profit entity with larger budgets.

However many International research ethics guidelines do not specify how post-trial services should be organized and a simple hint is not enough to solve the problem, seeing as every drug has its own specific risk and each one possible beneficence should be taken into consideration.

Whether a post-trial service is present or not should be the topic of the information given to the patient in order to avoid false hopes, which would then undermine the expression of consent.

Currently, trials conducted on antiretroviral drugs do not have the explicit reference to post-trials service as a standard or rule in the Protocol or in the information given to the person who is undergoing clinical trials (Ciaranello et a., 2009).

In this regard, it is wisely stressed "the burden and benefit of any collaborative study should be equally borne by the collaborating countries"; besides "Guidelines, rules, regulations and laws of the participating and sponsoring countries should be equally respected" (Muthuswamy, 2005).

The testing of vaccines is another area of heated controversy, which already has several critical issues in the industrial world, but becomes exacerbated in developing countries.

The above HPTN guidance document (developed by the Ethics Working Group) emphasizes protecting the vulnerable from exploitation, promoting equality through non discriminating access to the benefits of research and minimization of research related harms including medical, psychological, social and economic harms.

However, each of these aspects opens new scenarios that did not find unanimous consent, even more so if we turn our attention to the experiments carried out on pregnant women or infants, which, however, we will discuss in the next section.

The last aspect of the clinical trial, in general, concerns the lack of studies on palliative care and end-of-life in patients with AIDS.

In this area the differences between industrialized countries and developing countries is dramatically incurable; to understand the difference, just think that a comparative study carried out on terminally ill patients in Kenya and the United Kingdom, pointed out that first it was more important to quell the pain while the latter played a primary role of emotional pain.

As Harding et al emphasizes (Harding et al., 2003), there are five critical elements that a clinical trial should consider, namely: availability of pain relieving drugs, pain and symptom control, access to services, extent of coverage programs, education and training (including clinical, administrative and other skills), identification of relevant needs and determination of outcomes for care at the community level, and evaluation of the impact of education of policy makers and program directors about palliative and end-of-life care (sometimes termed advocacy); furthermore relevant outcomes may include policy, strategy, sustainability, availability and utility of education and training, and integration of end-of-life care into health systems.

The context of deaths in developed and developing countries are different, and context matters in end-of-life care.

In industrialized countries, people die of cancer and cardiovascular diseases, in developing countries, HIV / AIDS, TB and malaria cause over 300 million illnesses and more than 5 million deaths each year (WHO, 2000). As a result, projects in support of the terminally ill need to be different. As Singer and Bowman well debate (Singer & Bowman, 2002), the discussion of quality end-of-life care points out that there is a lack of information about the current state of end-of-life care among populations; and this should be seen as a global public health problem, because "it seems difficult to know how to improve quality end-of-life care without any understanding of what the current level of quality is, what determines it, and how improvement could be measured".

This is even more interesting considering that we are entering the third and fourth decade of HIV-infected, which now have a longer life expectancy thanks to current therapies.

2.1 Cultural barriers

HIV prevention trials conducted among disadvantaged vulnerable at-risk populations in developing countries present unique ethical dilemmas.

The inclusion of participants from under-represented or vulnerable populations calls for special consideration because the interests of those populations may conflict with clinical trial objectives (Fouad et al., 2004).

This is especially true when the object of research may cause a degree of stigma for the participating population. Generally, people with HIV are excluded for various reasons, some because they fall into illegal-behavior (for example injection drug users or sex workers); others because they are members of an ethnic minority; many have served time in jail or prison; many are poor.

Protection against discrimination and stigmatization is an important issue with regard to recruiting HIV/AIDS people, so appropriate composition and training of the monitoring recruitment team are particularly relevant to successful recruitment; besides basic comfort at the study site is fundamental.

Next to a perfect organization for what regards the technical aspects of the implementation of a clinical study, it is essential to pay particular attention to the specific characteristics of clinical research conducted on this disease.

Basic ethical principles when recruiting study participants include respect for persons, beneficence and justice (Beauchamp & Childress, 1994), but for this illness, confidentiality and providing safety from abuse are critical.

So the definition of ethical guidelines on the approach to these patients, with particular attention to the confidentiality of data, is essential.

First, a statement about maintaining confidentiality should be included in the informed consent letter, guaranteeing the rights of participants to maintain control over access to information about their health status.

About McNutt et al. (McNutt et al., 2009), "research participants commonly provide limited waivers of confidentiality for many studies. These waivers may be for protected information to be provided to researchers (eg, medical records) or disclosed among research participants (ex: research on couples or family counseling).

In these situations, participants typically provide waivers of confidentiality that are limited to requirements for good scientific research"; so if the requirements for research participation are unacceptable, then individuals can choose not to participate.

Certainly, a study to be ethically valid, must also be scientifically valid and unfortunately introducing a selection bias, only enlisting groups of patients who accept in full the questions of the study, may adulterate the results.

On the other hand, to ensure dignified treatment, it should be guaranteed that study participants are treated with full respect for their dignity and their rights as persons.

Dignity, which may be defined as an achievement or acquisition, not only depends on the individual but also on the other surrounding people who either directly or indirectly interact with the subject (May, 1991).

Unfortunately in the current management of HIV infection is not ethical, the individual loses his dignity, because his rights as a human being are being undermined.

HIV/AIDS affects the most intimate rights (Chummar, 2008) of free expression, such as, life, health, physical expression of love, transforming relationships, requiring a physical and metaphorical wall between man and man.

This social tear then clashes with the territory's culture and economy exacerbating the individual's difficulty to manage the disease and the intervention policies against the spread of infection.

Universal Declaration on Human Rights states that health is a right and that it must be preserved by States (Article 25), but this remains a purely theoretical exercise, where there are places that lack of food and water to ensure minimum subsistence.

Yet, prevention programs and the same international clinical research depart from a European conception of the individual, and therefore end up clashing with local realities, especially when they have totally different approaches to society by the Western schematics.

The implementation of consent to clinical research, preventive vaccine trials and trials preventing vertical disease transmission, had been influenced by several factors like family-centered decision-making; cultural dynamics pertaining to sex; relationship to older persons and the care-giving arrangement.

Furthermore, some principles of individual informed consent may not be in keeping with the cultural norms and practices of non-Western societies.

The requirements of Good Clinical Practice require that the enrollment of a patient in a clinical trial is preceded after giving clear and comprehensive information before taking the consent.

Unfortunately, if you do not have any knowledge of the concept of clinical trials, as in many developing countries, enlistment should be preceded by an intensive information campaign on the basis of research (randomized placebo, responsibilities and rights of the Promoter and the participant etc.) before explaining the protocol study (El Sadr & Capps, 1992).

All this implies the willingness and patience to really want to inform those undergoing clinical trials, as well as clearly being an economic burden for the implementation of information plans, considering the low cultural level which is bound to be encountered.

Moreover, these problems are not easily foreseen by Sponsors who do not include considerations for cultural factors, age, gender and social-economic status in their recruitment strategies .

As a result, many social needs (such as lack of funds for public transport, food etc) prevent their most needy patients to participate in clinical trials; still, in the most depressing areas you will find therapeutic misconception (Slack, 2005), bringing the subject to agree undergoing a clinical trial for a vaccine with the illusion of being able to heal the infection.

Vaccine research is challenging on many fronts and has become the subject of many debates (Guenter, 2000). The case of Kenya AIDS Society vs Arthur Obel (Kenya AIDS, 1997), the Nyumbani incident (Siringi, 2004), the HIV net 012 trials carried out in Uganda (Ahn, 2003) and the debate on the use of placebo during International clinical trials (CIOMS, 2002), are only a few of the examples that testify the complexity of the ethical implications in vaccine trials. The vaccine guidelines provide for Community Advisory Board (CAB), whose role is to facilitate community support for vaccine research and to disseminate information to the community hosting the research.

In order to avoid growing skepticism in the community, Oduwo (Oduwo, 2009) suggests facing the issue regarding vaccine trials focusing attention mainly towards:"a detailed analysis of the dutie in each role should be done to resolve duplicities and conflicts among the roles; the legal frame work for HIV vaccine research trials and the legal basis for each should be clarified; discussions on HIV vaccine trials ought to be encouraged, particularly domestic perspectives as they may provide a nuanced appreciation of the challenges of research environment; the role of state to facilitate and sponsor HIV vaccine research, which is expressed in the HIV vaccine sub-committee and its interaction in the research framework may benefit from further analysis and discussion".

There is therefore the general tendency to exclude women - especially if pregnant-from the clinical trial, forgetting that in fact they are being denied treatment.

Furthermore, the different hormone levels do not permit a full correspondence between the results obtained in men and those obtained in woman.

The Department of Health and Human Services has prohibited the enlistment of pregnant women except in cases where the fetus is exposed to a risk or minimal risk necessary (Federal Register, 1978). The International guidelines (World Medical Association, 2000) for the protection of the subjects in experimentation do not however exclude either fertile women nor pregnant women from the trials, even though recognizing the extra caution that must be taken (45 C.F.R. §46 Subpart B, 2002).

For fear of repercussions on the fetus many drugs are not tested in pregnant women or even on fertile women. In fact, the consequence is that these drugs will enter the health care practices that have no knowledge of how to use them.

The same Declaration of Helsinki (Edinburgh version, 2000) states that "the purpose of biomedical research must be to improve the diagnostic, therapeutic and prophylactic methods and understanding of the etiology and pathogenesis of diseases" (art. 4) .

The lack of reliable data makes it even more complex manage health in everyday life, since it authorizes the use of drugs not tested in extreme situations.

The situation is even more complex for HIV/AIDS; for example, the process of the zivudine drug was troubled long before its arrival and authorized in pregnant women.

Since 1987, when the FDA approved the use of the drug in adults with a concentration of CD4 + cells <200 mmc, it was not until 1994 (Morb Mortal Wkly Rep, 1994) that a study was created to show how the incidence of vertical transmission of HIV had reduced, with adequate safety for the fetus.

In this case, the precautionary principle referred all the fetuses of women who took antiretroviral drugs to risk, however, in the absence of any experimental data on these risks.

Many pregnant women, as in this case, have comorbidities besides the HIV infection and do not have adequate data available making their clinical management more difficult.

Kass et al. (Kass et al., 2000). claim in this regard that clinical decisions should always be taken with caution knowing that what the health of pregnant women needs is usually what is in the best interest of the developing fetus.

The problem of the recruitment of women in clinical trials, besides the scientific and economic justification, is dictated, in poor-countries, especially by cultural barriers.

While the presence of children does not allow them to make appointments on time, those that a search require, on the other, their involvement is strongly influenced by the willingness of men (husbands, fathers or sons) to subsidize their existence.

In fact, women have little freedom to make decisions under the lack of economic independence which is often associated to a cultural level so low, as not to guarantee self-determination. Besides this in many communities there is also the belief that being pregnant imposes fidelity onto the women and the use of contraceptive methods stimulate betrayal (Mills et al., 2006).

2.2 Participants' autonomy

Diminished study participant's autonomy is a common phenomenon in poor-resource countries.

The principle of autonomy is based on the assumption that a capable person, that is capable of self-determination, can responsibly make a free choice, deciding on everything that concerns him, outside of any external interference or overlap. The principle of patient self determination links the person who gives his consent to research in the field of HIV, to the person who first receives the information about the disease in question, and the research itself; all of this because it is dealing with a person who realizes what is happening.

A reduced range of candidates for research is a common phenomenon in developing countries in relation to the problem of obtaining adequate informed consent in these populations. In these countries the application of the research comes up against a widespread low-level socio-cultural phenomena with wide margins and a general attitude of distrust towards the helpers.

This may lead to a reduced perception of the fundamental aspects of research, with a low level of awareness about the candidate's proposed procedures and a general lack of grip of the population participating in the trial.

For these reasons, the research aimed towards people in developing countries must take into account the possible interference of some specific aspects, culturally mediated, that may influence the perception and understanding of issues related to the risk of HIV infection and consequently the autonomy of decision making.

It is true that there is a universal ethics of human research but it is true that the application and interpretation of general ethical principles must take into account, as stated above, the specific factors of stakeholders, such social conventions, the cultural factors and economic conditions.

In developing countries, where access to specialized care is very difficult, HIV infection is usually depicted as a hopeless disease, which inevitably causes suffering and death.

This leads to a dissonance than the messages that speak of a disease potentially preventable and controllable.

In each country, and sometimes in each ethnic group in that country, operators encounter different interpretations of medicine, illness, sexuality, death, shame, reputation; they have to deal with strong differences in male and female roles, and are confronted with diverse cultural beliefs about AIDS.

In some populations, for example, the idea persists that certain blood groups or some people are immune to the virus, or that a god may protect certain individuals more than others.

Information on the trial, then follow a general pattern where, instead, each ethnic group has its own rules and beliefs that dictate the expression of pain, the description of the symptoms and how to communicate, beliefs about the causes of the disease, expectations about the prevention and the practical aspects.

The range of choices of participants in the HIV trial is, in essence, linked to personal variables (personality and socio-cultural characteristics) and environmental (presence of an

adequate social support and in particular the presence of emotionally significant people; characteristics of the facility and ability of professionals dedicated to building a relationship of empathy, understanding and containment).
Mannheim (Mannheim, 1999) points out that there should be no constraints for which the patient or, more generally the free man, should feel constrained in those actions that Goethe had described as the "moving through the various domains of human activity" (Stuart Huges, 1967). According to Wilson (Wilson, 2007), in medical ethics when it comes to autonomy three different concepts are evoked: "the ability to make autonomous choices" free choices and "sphere of privacy decision-making" (meaning "with respect to those decisions made without coercion and interference of third parties "). There are those who think at the time information is received, as when news is given, which puts the subject in a position to express a decision in line with their values. Yet the right of veto in which one substantiates, is not automatically to be respected, because one might be faced with arbitrary decisions.

2.3 Illiteracy, language difficulties or inadequate information

Language barriers, as well, raise significant concerns with regard to candidates' full comprehension of the technical, product and methodological information of the research should be adapted to the context of the developing world or poor people as well, where certainly the notions of 'chance', of 'inactive medical".
The central role of autonomy of the person involved in the research is based on the information that should include the necessary input, appropriate to his level of knowledge, to enable him to actively take part in the various decisions.
The normal asymmetry of information between doctor and patient reaches the apex of developing countries in relation to the lower socio-cultural level and communication difficulties for the difference in language (and sometimes between different tribes of the same country) and cultural barriers. This state of affairs can induce operators to a mere provision of a technical piece of information rather than to create a real relationship of communication. Often the research subjects are not able to understand the purpose, or know the process in which they concretely provide their consent, merely to accept some form of treatment as an alternative to the lack of access to care.
In this case what is being acquired by non-consensus is actually invalid because it is underlying information implemented by a consensus but no qualifying adjectives that can not demonstrate the ability of the participant in the choice of self-determination.
It is therefore necessary to build a common language within the physician-patient relationship through interventions that facilitate conflict resolution and help overcome the cultural barriers that impede communication.
Researchers often work with the community leader to explain the research to the people and obtain informed consent. This expedient however is not sufficient and it is desirable that operators of the trial not only enrich their education in the field of HIV but also of transculture.
They must increase their awareness of cultural, religious, social and political factors that have an impact on patients' lives, fleeing from interpreting according to their own frame of reference, dealing with their own prejudices and stereotypes, confronting them directly.
They must also learn how to translate the discomfort of the patient in their own cultural language and return the message in a language that the patient is able to understand.

3. Status of affected women, young girls and/or pregnant women

The situation of women and cultural context is tragic.
Over the years, 'AIDS is increasingly becoming a disease of gender, in fact, more and more women are infected by the disease, 56% of the population ill are women between 15 and 49 years old.
A disease that is differentiating between the sexes not only in developing countries but also in Europe.
In fact, in 2007, over 30% of people who contract the disease are women and one of the main predisposing factors is the risk behavior of their partner.
According to WHO (WHO, 2000), HIV transmission from man to woman in a sexual relationship has double the chance of contracting it than the transmission from woman to man, with a greater risk for young women.
The impact of disease on women in all aspects of life and women living with HIV are very influenced by the country itself, in all spheres in which they are involved, from the family to take care of their health.
Excluding Western society (where at least formally) there is equality between man and woman, in many traditional cultures there is a subordination of the female gender towards the male gender. This implies a sort of tolerance in women to sexual violence, including both at home and away, exposing them to a higher risk of becoming infected with HIV.
Moreover, the inability to support themselves, restricts the freedom even in sexual matters, so they are forced to give in to having physical relationships with people already knowingly infected. If, however, polygamy exists, albeit in a system free from violence, the risk of infection increases, particularly given the common practice of sexual gratification with sex workers and husbands living away from their wives and whom for economic reasons, can not get home during the weekend.
In addition, the superstition that having sexual intercourse with a virgin provides immunity from the HIV infection, generating real rats of adolescents and children, even at a very early age. Still today, in refugee camps women and girls are victims of violence by their own armed forces that should be defending them, or rather they are "prey" of the barbaric savagery of the soldiers during the civil wars, as it happened in Rwandai (Fynn, 2010), where it is estimated that 250,000 to 500.00 "ETIN rapes" had occurred.
The food is, then, the main reason for surrender in unprotected sex for women, as they may engage in transactional sex to procure food for themselves and their children.
A study from Nigeria reported that 35% of female sex workers are poor and due to the lack of food they had accepted unprotected sex with clients (Oyefara, 2007).
Parallel to this there was a breakdown of family values, with an inclination towards fleeting relationships with people that are almost strangers, increasing the possibility of transmitting the HIV infection, and therefore women are either infected with HIV because of their behavior or due to the "gain" after the debauchery of their peers.
For many Africans HIV/AIDS is an ethical problem, meaning that it is the result of forgetting old values with nature, which enlivened the community before the advent of "intellectual" colonialism of the West.
In Africa, the individual has always been part of a community that has guided the choice of a mate and has alleviated the suffering in times of need. With the individualistic approach introduced by the Western world, the values which underpin the community have

deteriorated and AIDS, a symbol of the corrupt new approach to life, has brought with it a tendency to remove the sick from society.

Discrimination and stigmatization is one of the dramatic consequences HIV/AIDS have to face and a major obstacle to prevention and care.

Women in sub Saharan Africa are more likely to be living with HIV and to access health-care facilities offering testing, but any decision to implement expanded HIV testing in Africa must weight the desired biomedical outcomes of testing against the possibility of discrimination (April, 2010).

Fear of discrimination and stigma causes people to avoid testing and prompts those infected with and affected by HIV/AIDS to remain silent, depriving them from essential treatment and social care. These problems are perhaps magnified by the existing taboos regarding sexuality, affecting more intensively women.

A woman who discovers she is living with HIV risks, in all parts of the world, losing economic support, being abandoned to suffer physical and emotional abuse, of being discriminated against and witness her family relationships be destroyed.

Kilewo et al. (Kilewo et al., 2001) revealed that in Tanzania 77.8% of pregnant women infected with HIV participate in trial clinics to avoid maternal fetal transmission, at a distance of 18 months after diagnosis they had still not communicated the test result to their partners; while during a study carried out in Kenya by Galliard et al.(Galliard et al., 2000), a good 76.1% of the interviewed women did not have any intentions in revealing their status'. The reasons for the reluctance were fear of abandonment, rejection and discrimination, violence, upsetting family members, and accusations of in fidelity (Medley, 2004).

The diversity of findings between and within populations reflected a wide range of different ethnic, cultural and religious groups among the women surveyed, who reported important differences in beliefs and preferences relating to formal and informal maternal health care. These variations were explained by differences in women in autonomy, gender relationships and social networks, which are influenced by embedded social structures, religion and cultural beliefs. A woman with HIV who knows her status can make a better choice with regard to her reproductive life and, if pregnant, may undergo specific interventions, such as prophylaxis with antiretroviral drugs, which significantly reduce the risk of maternal-fetal transmission.

Clearly, this occurs where there are health services that allow you to see a woman with HIV in an appropriate manner in relation to current scientific knowledge.

At a time when a pregnancy is emerging as a threat to the management, to which requires integration of knowledge and technical means, of course we should move to a good environment with qualified staff, able to handle the complex clinical problems that the case imposes and suitably sensitive to its ethical aspects.

Neonatal infection remains a terrible scourge for developing countries to poor women who receive care during pregnancy and childbirth.

This state of things pushed 68 priority countries to consider newborn and child health care that are part of the Countdown to 2015 Initiative.

UNICEF, the United Nations Population Fund (UNFPA) and the World Health Organization (UNICEF, 2008) recommend at least 4 antenatal care visits during pregnancy, during which very little would be sufficient to ensure good health to mother and child, such as treatment of hypertension to prevent eclampsia, tetanus immunization, intermittent preventive treatment for malaria and distribution of insecticide-treated nets, prevention of mother-to-child transmission of HIV, micronutrient supplementation, and birth preparedness, including information about danger signs during pregnancy and childbirth.

Natural childbirth at home is the only opportunity for many women and even where it is possible to perform a Caesarean section, it is unlikely that one may have a proper post-partum check-up.
Prevention of mother-to-child transmission of HIV is most effective when antiretroviral drugs are received by the mother during her pregnancy and continued through delivery and then administered to the infant after birth.
Every year a million women infected with HIV deliver babies without professional help. Marc Bulterys and colleagues suggest here that traditional birth attendants could be involved in preventing perinatal transmission of HIV by offering services such as HIV testing and counseling and short courses of antiretroviral drugs (Marc Bulterys et al., 2002).
Antiretroviral drugs are effective in reducing the risk of mother-to-child transmission of HIV even when prophylaxis is started for the infant soon after birth.
The American Academy of Pediatrics recommends documented, routine HIV testing for all pregnant women in the United States after notifying the patient that testing will be performed, unless the patient declines HIV testing ("optout"consent or "right of refusal") (Committee on Pediatric AIDS, 2008).
Assuming then that we have taken the test and a pregnant woman is affected by HIV, can she refuse to take antiretroviral medicines?
In the absence of specific laws that impose a compulsory treatment, the principle of autonomy recognizes that women have full freedom of choice.
In a recent study (Cannovo et al., 2010) we faced an emblematic case of a woman suffering from HIV who chose to complete her pregnancy notwithstanding a compromised pathological clinical picture (diabetes mellitus complicated by nephropathy, retinopathy and hypertension prior to conception, history of alcohol abuse and prostitution).
In this case the self-determination has prevailed over the woman's prescription.
Another issue that plays a key role in the spread of HIV infection is the FGM / C; For UNICEF estimates that in 27 countries of Africa and the Middle East, 70 million girls and women aged 15–49 have undergone FGM/C.

4. Privacy and confidentiality, stigma and discrimination

The attention to the confidentiality of information towards patients with the human immunodeficiency virus involves complex ethical considerations, especially in individuals in developing countries, that regardless of nationality, race or custom, each case involves, a condition of human confidentiality/secrecy inviolable to be protected if fulfills the conditions for the collection of identification data (concerning the identity in the broad sense) and sensitive (those suitable to detect the state of health and/or sex life) on HIV positive people.
The topic is complex and ethically sensitive under a human aspect, when speaking of subjects located in developing countries and within local communities where the knowledge of an infectious disease can result in exclusion from the patient's environment in which they live.

4.1 Legislative approach

In USA, already in 1997, the Health Insurance Portability and Accountability Act (HIPAA) regulations and the Americans with Disabilities Act (ADA) protect people with HIV and their right to control disclosure of their status (Doyal, 1997), then in 2006, the Centers for Disease Control and Prevention (CDC) issued revised recommendations for HIV testing of adults, adolescents, and pregnant women in health care settings and recommend that opt-out HIV screening, with no separate written consent, be a routine part of care in all health care settings (Hanssens, 2007).

In 2003, India adopted a specific law for HIV/AIDS covering the ethical, legal and social implications of this disease, trying to curb discrimination and stigmatize the disease (The Lawyer's Collective, 2003).

In 2006, the major world experts in human rights and scientific fields created the Joint United Nations Programme on HIV/AIDS and the US President's Emergency Plan for AIDS Relief (PEPFAR) Interim Guidelines on Protecting the Confidentiality and Security of HIV Information (UNAIDS, 2007).

These guide lines focus (Beck et al., 2010) their attention on three aspects, intercurrent privacy, confidentiality and security, all facing the protection of sensitive data.

Privacy has both a legal and ethical concept, since it refers both to data protection provided by regulations and to the regulation of access to one's data referring to human rights. The Confidentiality is identified with the right of individuals to see their data protected during collection, storage, transfer and use in order to prevent unauthorized disclosure of that information to third parties. Security refers to technological means by which data is protected from inappropriate disclosure.

The 2008 European Guideline on HIV testing (Poljak, 2009) (2001 update of European Guideline for Testing for HIV infection (Thorvaldsen, 2001), approved by the European Office of International Union against Sexually Transmitted Infections (IUSTI) and European Office of the World Health Organization with the incorporation of various new developments) recommends giving HIV test after having complete consent by the person who has been informed that the result will remain confidential, but confidentiality is not absolute as health-care providers may be legally bound to disclose HIV status information in exceptional circumstances (Rogstad, 2006).

This means that no health professional and / or hospital can refuse to treat or remove a patient if HIV positive, and also that the data on their health or sex life may not be distributed arbitrarily regardless of the type of experimental study or treatment in place.

Conversely, however, only if there is prevention, investigation and prosecution of these crimes, may it be reported to the competent authorities.

In literature it was proposed to introduce a coding system that will stand the test of time (Sajeev, 2006).

The non-uniqueness of understanding on the issue of confidentiality of data worldwide, is clear thanks to a study conducted in 2007 showing that over 80 countries and UNAIDS offices were divided into groups of those who had already issued guidelines on this matter (G -countries) and others intending to develop them (NG-countries).

This research has shown that few countries scaling up HIV services had developed guidelines on protecting the confidentiality and security of HIV information at the time of completing the survey, but 90% of G-countries had a privacy law against 57% of NG-countries.

It should also be noted that even those who have died are entitled to their privacy, since, for example, in South Africa, the law does not protect the confidentiality of deceased persons (McQuoid-Mason, 2007).

It then follows that control over privacy, or the confidentiality of the best data on HIV-infected patients in the NG-countries, is a huge ethical problem related not only to the socio-cultural-economic, but also to the inadequacy of the health system, unable to operate due to lack of transportation and operators to manage the significant and complex reflections of the disease.

Can one rely on the secrecy, confidentiality, dealing with a phenomenon which is such a widespread social alarm?

It is evident that this extraordinary public importance of HIV obligates behavior, without sacrificing the need for knowledge and discussion, to fully respect the dignity of the patient/citizen (of any nationality, race), and their fundamental rights.

Protecting the patient with HIV means allowing the holder of information to freely and independently decide the extent to which personal data, which reveals his identity and other issues related to his health, can be brought to the attention of others and to control treatments to which such data are submitted.

The HIV epidemic has pushed the affected individuals of the developing world to the margins of their societies. Stigma and discrimination can hamper all AIDS patients.

The secrecy of one's HIV status (crucial point with which people infected with HIV compare themselves due to the fear of stigma and discrimination) in populations in developing countries, the fear of the news being spread into one's community, increasing the possibility of being abandoned, isolated or to alarm and frighten relatives, especially the possibility of causing them shame is pushed to a limit.

This is particularly difficult for some participants because it can lead to the revelation of sexual choices up until then lived in secrecy or hiding (because not tolerated by the community of origin) or extra-marital relations (sometimes subject to severe punishment), with the risk of breaking family ties, loss of economic support or exposed to physical violence.

This condition, in Italy, essentially contains the concept of privacy, according to Rodotà (Rodotà, 1991) it provides a set of actions, behaviors, opinions, preferences, personal information, on which the applicant wishes to maintain exclusive control, not only to ensure confidentiality but to ensure full freedom of choice.

In much of the world, including some US states and European countries, disclosure by a physician of an individual's HIV status without the patient's consent is illegal. In other locations, physicians have a duty to warn partners through mandated notification programs. Further, professional ethics codes may differ from local laws, complicating these issues.

In Italy and other European countries there are multiple and meaningful provisions related to the main aspects for the protection of privacy relating to the implementation of the seropositive and HIV testing.

In Italy the reporting of AIDS cases is also governed by an ad hoc law (DM 15 December 1990 and Circular of the Ministry of Health February 27, 1987, 5 and November 25, 1988, 14 in which restricting the flow of information from the doctor directly to the Regional Operations Center and the Ministry of AIDS is clearly marked) and for any transaction information only the code number assigned will be used for each case.

The doctor, investigator, hospital, pharmaceutical company are obliged to respect the confidentiality of personal data of the patient.

When speaking of scientific publications of clinical data or observations relating to individuals, the physician should ensure their non-identifiability.

The specific consent of the patient applies to any further processing of the data, but only within limits, in form and with the exceptions laid down by any standards.
The assessment must also take into account the historical moment facing the subject (environmental, socio-economic and cultural).
In the event that the subject does not show the capacity of decision to authorize the above, the doctor will have to act ethically, ethically with the utmost respect for the dignity of the human activating only those projections that protect the patient's health condition of which only psycho-physical well-being should result.

4.2 Psychosocial issues

Prejudice, exclusion, stigmatization are the three conditions that are still sadly dominant both from an individual and social point of view, that is where the community, family, friends and the context of membership accepts the condition of the patient with AIDS, it could be the patient to perceive and push himself to the point of isolation.
From a collective point of view, unfortunately, poor information is still a problem that leads people to believe that there is a possibility of infection simply being near a person infected with HIV.
Starting from the stigma, over time there has been a change in communication, in fact we have moved from the definition of risk groups to risk behavior, shifting attention from person to action, with the aim of protecting the individual. Nevertheless, those who contract AIDS are labeled for their behavior, but also because, often, the situations are associated with promiscuity. Hence the effect that the disease is closely related to the condition of homosexuality, therefore, still remains, those who declare their homosexuality live in situations of social exclusion for fear of infection, regardless of whether or not they have been diagnosed with the disease.
The situation worsens when the HIV infection is detected, there is exclusion from the family, not for fear of contagion, but the condition of homosexuality and the subsequent voluntary and conscious exposure to the disease.
Another recurring problem is the exclusion in relation to meeting new people, the person with AIDS avoids meeting new people in order to avoid a situation in which he might have to reveal having the disease . Therefore he/she remains anchored to the people who know his/her condition, closing himself/herself into a secure network, a micro-cosmos from which it is advisable to exit. This is amplified greatly for the couple. For these reasons, it often happens that people with AIDS, who may attend self-help groups, prefer to meet up with each other even outside of group meetings, forming closed groups and that most of the time marginalize themselves from the rest of the community.
The key problem of AIDS is information, in fact, most often incorrect when speaking about infection and transmission, while simultaneously resulting in excessive worry or superficiality. It is worrying to know that there are those who think that simply touching or sharing space with people with HIV can transmit the disease, in other cases, however, actions are taken without considering the risk such as oral sex without using precautions
In recent years, this omission of information led to an increase of the disease in the heterosexual population, as opposed to the homosexual population who have increased awareness and therefore paid more attention to prevention.
In fact, in the case of heterosexuals, not perceiving the risk of infection not belonging to "risk groups", lowers the threshold of concern and risky actions are performed such as

unprotected oral sex. It is not usual to see a heterosexual test for HIV, among gay people, however, the test has become routine every six months, promoting early diagnosis and therefore a more effective treatment, but, above all, preventing the risk of infection for potential partners.

Consequently, even the onset of the disease is different, in fact in many cases it occurs that heterosexual couples discover infection when taking AIDS diagnostic tests related to pregnancy or when clinical problems in either partner occur.

Another equally problematic aspect is thee moment in which the news is given, it may provoke reactions of fear, fear of death and social problems.

The news of the disease can occur in three ways: a) the subject goes to a specialized center for testing; b) the person takes the test in any laboratory and c) the patient performs checks due to medical conditions.

In the first case the news is given to personnel who then takes charge of the patient, providing in-depth information on the disease and on all related issues and support with psychological support.

In the second case, the person often reads the result on a sheet of paper that reads *HIV: positive* and from that moment a long and painful ordeal begins, marked by confusion and disorientation, not knowing, knowing little or not well informed causing more fear,until the person hopingly reaches a structure where people are able to respond and support him.

In this case, unfortunately, the news of the disease may push the patient to respond with suicide.

In the third case the patient receives the news from a point which sends him to specialized facilities that take care of providing assistance and support, but in all cases, the news of the disease results in anxiety due to the severe loss, fear of what is happening and the absence of certainty.

We often associate related disorders such as manic depression, mood disorders and anxiety disorders, however, the psychological effects of the news vary according to previous living conditions, in fact, the more prosperous the person, having had both a safe emotional, social and work condition, the more the disease is the collapse of everything he had built and is plunged into the abyss of self-destruction. This also happens in cases where behavior risks are a reaction of anxiety due to suffering and uncomfortable situations. In any case, following diagnosis is an internal reorganization of forces, not only to address all the threats and fears related to the disease, but to address those old ghosts that re-emerge at this time, all the unresolved issues that suddenly emerge, the fears of abandonment, etc..

After the illness is metabolized and after processing coping strategies, fluctuating moments will follow, alternating from calm periods to periods dominated by the uncertainty that determines hypochondria and panic and every little discomfort is associated with threatening entities.

Studies show that women suffer more prejudice and discrimination than being actually infected with HIV, they are most at risk with regard to the possibility of having more aggressive and dangerous forms of the disease and having a harder time dealing with this situation.

Finally, though in recent years it is increasingly common to see women facing a pregnancy and giving birth to children immune to the virus, it is easy to imagine the effort that a woman must make for such a challenging and important project like having a child, knowing that their health can be a burden, an obstacle during their child's growth, perhaps even during these sensitive stages in which it is essential that a mother is near and present.

It follows that the progress and results discovered about AIDS are important and significant. However, there should be more emphasis on information and communication so as to prevent low levels of attention, while it is important to create a welcoming social network and cooperation that will ensure that those who are infected with HIV are not in situations of isolation, hardship and distress.

5. Role of different stakeholders in improving health care and health information in HIV/AIDS patients

Decision-making about controversial public health projects may thus be primarily a function of emotional reactions to drug addicts of disgust, dehumanization and stigmatization rather than reactions of sympathy, humanity and the right to optimal health for all.
Within a disgust/dehumanization framework, effectiveness and cost-effectiveness are usually not important aspects of a program or policy. Rather, it is the congruency between the symbolic value of the program and the emotions of disgust, dehumanization and stigmatization that is critical.
As well pointed out by Soldini (Soldini, 2001), when speaking about the HIV/AIDS infection, issues of health policy are "the result of the ethical debate" that will have to provide the necessary and essential arguments in order to draft a legislation that provides appropriate solutions to curb the problems that characterize this infection.
We must, therefore, even before acting on a deontological and legal level, with health care professionals, behave ethically responsible towards patients with HIV/AIDS.
They only needs to be respected with dignity as human beings and their rights can not be disregarded in any way, diminished or taken away just because of their infection status.
In the world there is a huge difference between countries on how HIV is handled, specifically when speaking about the laws on testing, the use of informed consent, data confidentiality, notification of decisions, and ultimately support .
The Recommendations (2006) of the Centers for Disease Control and Prevention (CDC) suggest testing for HIV with the tests carried out routinely during the hospitalization of an inmate, serving as a battering ram against the wall of silence that makes being infected by the HIV disease, "exceptional. "
Suffice it is to say that informed consent can be considered valid even if the patient gives a general consent at the moment in which he decides to go under medical activity, starting from the definition provided by the American Medical Association, that informed consent is "a process of communication between a patient and physician that results in the patient's authorization or agreement to undergo a specific medical intervention (American Medical Association, 2008)".
Clearly, this assertion does not consider the difference between informed consent in general and those relative to specific situations, which then contextualizes the patients' expression of will to where they live; there is not an easy application form for these regulatory differences, and it could become a standard care, but we must not forget the elements of the tripod that support its HIV exceptionalism - which, incidentally, we have already spoken of- counseling, informed consent and confidentiality.
Not all states that claim the patient's consent for testing, provide counseling, limiting for example, only positive cases - as in California (Maine Revised Statues, 2008) - wasting the opportunity to help prevention in a slice of the population who still may be at risk, even if the response is negative.

Finally, confidentiality and notification of results to interested parties are issues of fundamental importance that can not be left to the good sense of the person concerned.
In USA (Li et al., 2007) there are ethnic differences with respect to the disclosure process, for example, Hispanics are more likely than African Americans and Caucasians, to communicate a positive diagnosis to their relatives in order to prevent spread of infection in the family clan, while Asian Americans, in relation to their culture, ethnic community and their family role have difficulty coping with the problem. Generally, the reason that drives a person to speak comes from the desire to preserve the family from infection, but there is a difference in how these communities in the U.S and Asian countries of origin behave. It is more difficult than having an unintended revelation in the USA where the reporting guidelines are very strict.
In Asian countries there is more reluctance because discrimination is not only found in the family but also in the community, which also ends up pressuring the family clan.
In China, thanks to the "Four Free One Care" national campaign promoted by the Government, a greater awareness is growing with family involvement in accepting not only infection but also in preventing the spread of infection (UNAIDS, 2004).
On this issue it is worth reporting the example of the State of New York, where the District Health Officer is in charge of tracking the individuals concerned and notifying the results if a patient has received a positive response to the HIV test.
Another case in point is represented in South Africa, where the State guarantees the post-exposure prophylaxis treatment (PEP) only to those who meet the definition of "appropriate victimhood", while complicating access by those regarded as co-responsible for their predicament and accordingly as undeserving of treatment (Pieterse, 2010).
Today, the HIV battle is won with information and training, both of which are attributable to public institutions; providing HIV screening programs will allow a hand to save more lives by ensuring patients right to care and help their partners stay safe, the other to save public funds and assist people with full blown AIDS now no longer negotiable.
Civil rights must be incorporated in the laws as was the case in Iran (Zare & Mortazavifar, 2010) where the constitution (principles 19, 20, 28, paragraph 42 and paragraph 4 of article 6, article 43) have been used in several types of international declarations (es. Universal Declaration of Human Rights, Convention on the Elimination of all types of discrimination against women).
As Brown emphasizes, "as that base of scientific literature and public health practice literature grows, and given emerging scientific evidence supporting increate testing as a cost-effective public health measure, legislators and medical communities must work together to ensure that legislation in all states supports the ability to offer large-scale ED HIV testing" (Brown, 2008).
Therefore only when the government and health professionals can ensure the confidentiality and security of HIV information collected in community or health facilities and information repositories, more people will decide to get themselves tested for HIV and to go to assistance and prevention centers created for people with risk of infection (Hargreaves, 2007). The privacy law serves as a legal blueprint to establish policy practices (Stewart, 1988), but the application of and education about the law may require various strategies, which countries must study and implement. This is perhaps the main task to which the states are called to carry out, and that may eventually be the key to defeating the indiscriminate spread of HIV infection.

6. Conclusions

HIV infection, resulting in AIDS is a special event that involves elements that are very personal to the people who come in contact, which also involves upheavals on the biographical, psychological, social and cultural sphere, not just on the person who contractes the disease (who is also found himself in having to radically change his habits) but also on his family and people who are close, which may not be prepared to face a difficult and delicate problem as far as that treaty.

In fact, the infection can occur through physical contact between two people, mediated or not by a syringe or a bag of blood, or through unprotected sex with people already infected. According to popular imagination, these people belong to that particular category of outsiders, such as drug addicts, prostitutes or persons in serious economic difficulties, which unfortunately in our society tend to be seen as persons "guilty" who deserve to be expelled from the "healthy" community which is regulated by "moral" principles that outsiders would infringe with "disgraceful" conduct.

The Greek word encompasses, through the richness of a language, most of the original concept just said. In fact, this word is translated with the Italian word "brand", therefore something that identifies a person negatively, or even with "tattoo" a particular sign and distinctive easily detectable, or even the "spot", either physical or moral, or, finally, surprisingly, with the word "bite", as if to predict a mode of transmission of this disease.

It is therefore the "stigma" of HIV or AIDS that is pushing away the very people who should be helped and protected by society, the weakest that most easily feel their fundamental rights of equality and health are being mined from those with whom they should be living with, with the consequence of continuously being pushed outside that fundamental network that gives support and relief in such delicate moments. One of these is the shocking moment in which the patient receives the bad news of having contracted an incurable disease. Fearing expulsion from society and from affection, it is logical and natural that people who have a "risky" behavior, are normally not the ones who spontaneously take tests to check something. Something that could make them "outsiders", even at the risk of not knowing whether they have actually contracted the disease and give up immediately to treatment. Treatments that could delay the onset of much of the disease, to avoid infecting people who are close to them and even to give or to unknowingly give their partner an infant that would otherwise be born healthy, since you can prevent the transmission vertical mother-fetus if the virus is recognized beforehand. Another problem then is the "self stigmatization" that can affect those who discover they have contracted the disease and as a result of this discovery decide to isolate themselves because they are considered a danger to their loved ones, or because they feel "ashamed". In addiction, a psychological breakdown is hardly be avoided in the absence of adequate information and assistance for this purpose.

The peculiarities of the consequences of this disease and the difficulties of a curative and preventive approach are exacerbated by the cultural attitude and anthropological-ethical territory in which you are studying, whether it is an industrialized country, or a developing country, because besides the differences already discussed in previous sections, the problem of the "stigma" unites these two heterogeneous realities. If we should promote, from a cultural point of view, a real campaign against the stigma of living with HIV or AIDS, with appropriate counseling offered to those who may be in need, as well as the stigmatization of any other carrier of incurable diseases and, more generally, " different, "the ethical side should be able to resolve a painful impasse, constituted by the problem of how to balance the privacy rights on the highly sensitive data such as those relating to health, or, in other words, the confidentiality of the results of examinations, with the principle of beneficence, which, as evidenced by Ngotho (Ngotho, 2009) , may have both negative and positive aspects. Ngotho writes that the success of the different policies will depend on the mutual entirely respect for confidentiality of the patients' care that flows from the patient to medical practitioner". Assuming that the doctor must always pursue the good of the patient, must he behave as if he knows that the patient is suffering from HIV or AIDS? It is his duty to inform the community and identify those who are ill or who may have been infected to get them to start care and prevent them from spreading the infection, even at the risk of going against the right to self-determination and privacy of his patient? Is it right to leave the doctor alone to face this problem without giving him the measures to make this choice less excruciating?

Or, is it ethically acceptable to transform the HIV test into a routine examination for all admissions or for all pregnant women, perhaps preceded and followed by ad hoc counseling, as discussed by Salari and Azizi (Salari & Azizi, 2009) useful to try to balance the right of women to self-determination with the right to health of the unborn? But if such tests were to become routine, will the request of the informed consent of the patient mark the difference between the bid, rather than the imposition of such a test, or it could it even further stigmatize people with HIV/AIDS, as noted by Bayer and Edingtoni (Bayer & Edington, 2009)?

The Code of Medical Ethics of the American Medical Association (opinion 5.5) and global politics tend to affirm the principle that the health information the doctor comes to learn must remain confidential unless it is ethically and legally justifiable its disclosure, to avoid undermining the doctor-patient relationship which is based primarily on trust. But can the preservation of that relationship based on trust be considered a priority even in the case of HIV or AIDS, where it is not only questioning the patient's health, but also the entire community? It rises so difficult to answer another question that has always interested the discussion on bioethics, one of whose leading exponents is the famous bioethicist Hans Jonas (Jonas, 1997), namely the balance between the interests of the individual with the interests of the entire community, that can be summarized in the question: when must the right to the common good take precedence over the right of the individual?

This problem has already been extensively discussed in bioethics in respect of experimentation with human beings, which so far has always tried to protect the rights of the individual more than the community, except in regard to cases of highly contagious or infectious diseases, where instead it is intended to give precedence to the good of the community over the rights of the individual that necessarily weakens the protection of human health. One may wonder then if this is the case HIV or AIDS.

Still, one may wonder what is respectful of another pivotal principle of bioethics, to allow individuals the freedom to announce or not having the infection, leaving the responsibility to indirectly complicit in a "murder" ? How must doctors react when they do not not agree with the decision of the patient to not inform their partners of the future infection?

As for the principle of autonomy, another key element of bioethics, which has always stressed the importance of self-determination of the patient, can this be protected in cases where the patient's autonomy may be lethal to other human beings?

But these are not the only problems that arise when one is confronted with various and diverse effects of HIV and AIDS.

As noted above, other issues may arise again, but much more complicated because they are linked to economic and historical issues, when considering the differences in approach to the prevention, diagnosis and study of the phenomenon of HIV and AIDS in industrialized and developing countries. In this case, the principle of fairness should never be broken in a society that respects the dignity of human beings, one of its hinges, and it can not take second place in the financial resources of a country. Health is a decisive factor for the development of human beings, families and communities throughout the world and you can not imagine a civil and human progress without respect for the fundamental right to health that is inherent to every human being regardless of his economic possibilities, of the place where he was born or is living or his social status.

No law nor the Universal Declaration can ever resolve the problems and discrimination facing people living with HIV or AIDS until each individual is allowed to heal properly, and while deep divisions continue to exist between ethics and law, between theory and practice, between individual rights and community rights, which can not be resolved by common ethical thinking, but they need the active and conscientious participation of the economically more advanced countries that have more resources to combat this phenomenon.

Only by launching a trans-national dialogue on ethical and social aspects of HIV/AIDS with the aim of building a consensus on policies to be implemented, to address this pandemic and to achieve more shared laws - not only to help the individuals with the disease and the people close to them at risk of infection, but the doctors called for the diagnosis, prevention, treatment and progress of the search for a cure - both the right of individuals to privacy and self-determination and the right to health of the general community can be guaranteed without hateful discrimination based on the economic, historical and social structures of a country.

7. References

Addictional protections for pregnant women, human fetuses and neonates involved in research (2002). *45 C.F.R. §46 Subpart B*

Ahn, M.J. (2003). Ethics and the AIDS pandemic in the developing world, *Journal International Association Physicians AIDS*, Vol. 2, No.2, pp. 81-87, doi: 10.1177/154510970300200205

Altavilla, A. (2010). Ethical Standards for clinical trials conducted in third countries: the new strategy of the European Union, pp. 34, *Proceedings of 18th World Congress on Medical Law*, , Zagreb, Croatia, August 8-12, 2010, ISBN 978-953-270-046-6

American Medical Association (2008). *Informed consent*, Retrieved from http://www.ama-assn.org/ama/pub/category/4608.html

April, MD. (2010). Rethinking HIV exceptionalism: the ethics of opt-out HIV testing in sub-Saharan Africa. *Bull World Health Organ*, Vol. 88, pp. 703-708, doi: 10.2471/BLT.09.073049

Bayer, R. & Edington C. (2009) HIV Testing, Human Rights, and Global AIDS Policy: Exceptionalism and Its Discontents, J Health Polit Policy Law, Vol. 34, No 3, pp. 301–323, DOI:10.1215/03616878-2009-002

Beauchamp, T.L.& Childress, J. (1994). *Principles of biomedical ethics* (4th edn). Oxford University Press, New York,

Beck E.J., Mandalia, S., Harling, G., Santas X.M., Mosure D. & Delay P.R. (2011). Protecting HIV information in countries scaling up HIV services: a baseline study. *Journal of the International AIDS Society*, Vol.14, No.6, doi:10.1186/1758-2652-14-6

Brown, J. (2008). The changing landscape of state legislation and expanded HIV testing, *Public Health Reports*, Vol. 123, No 3, pp 16-19

Bulterys, M., Fowler, M.G., Shaffer, N., Tih P.M., Greenberg, A.E., Karita, E., Coovadia, H. & De Cock, K.M. (2002). Role of traditional birth attendants in preventing perinatal transmission of HIV, *BMJ*, Vol. 324, pp. 222–225, doi: 10.1136/bmj.324.7331.222

Cannovo, N., Aganti, A., Sansone, M., Buccelli, P. & Pasquale Martinelli. (2010). Ethic, medical and legal reflections about the fetal protection by a pregnant woman suffering, in comorbidity, from HIV infection, *The Journal of Maternal-Fetal and Neonatal Medicine*, Vol. 23, No.7, pp. 593–594, doi: 10.3109/14767050903192200

Centers for Disease Control and Prevention (1994). Zivudine for the prevention of HIV transmission from mother to infant, *MMWR Morb Mortal Wkly Rep*, Vol. 43, pp. 285-287

Chummar, P. (2009). HIV/AIDS in Africa: a bioethical hard blow to human dignity and human rights. *Proceedings of the International Conference on Bioethics*, pp11-21, ISBN , Egerton University, Kenya, August 12-14, 2008, Retrieved from http://unesdoc.unesco.org/images/0018/001841/184159e.pdf

Ciaranello, A.L., Walensky, R.P., Sax, P. E., Chang, Y., Fredberg, K.A. & Weissman, J.S. (2009). Access to medications and medical care after participation in HIV clinical trials: a systematic review of trial protocols and informed consent documents, *HIV Clin Trials.*, Vol 10, No.1, pp. 13-24, doi: 10.1310/hct1001-13

Commission Directive 2005/28/EC of 8 April 2005 laying down principles and detailed guidelines for good clinical practice as regards investigational medicinal products for human use, as well as the requirements for authorisation of the manufacturing or importation of such products, *Official Journal of the European Union*, L 91, April 9, 2005

Committee on Pediatric AIDS (2008). HIV Testing and Prophylaxis to Prevent Mother-to-Child Transmission in the United States, *Pediatrics*, Vol. 122, pp.1127–1134, doi:10.1542/peds.2008-2175

Council for International Organisations of Medical Sciences (CIOMS) in collaboration with the World Health Organisation (WHO) (1993). *International Guidelines for Biomedical Research Involving Human Subjects*. CIOMS, Geneva.

Council for International Organizations of Medical Sciences (2002). *International ethical guidelines for biomedical research involving human subjects*. Retrieved from http://www.fhi.org/training/fr/Retc/pdf_files/cioms.pdf

De Cock, K.M., Fowler, M.G., Mercier, E., De Vincenzi, I., Saba, J., Hoff, E. et al. (2000). Prevention of mother-to-child HIV trasmission in re source poor countries: translating research into policy and practice. *Jama*, Vol. 283, pp. 1175-82, doi: 10.1001/jama.283.9.1175

Doyal, L. (1997). Good ethical practice in the dental treatment of patients with HIV/AIDS, *Oral Dis*, Vol.3, pp. S214-S220, PMID: 9456692

Ehrenkranz, P.D. et al. (2009) Written Informed-Consent statutes and HIV testing. *Am J Prev Med* , July, Vol. 37, No 1, pp. 57-63, doi:10.1016/j.amepre.2009.03.011

El Sadr, W. & Capps, L. (1992). Minorities in AIDS Clinical Trials. *Jama*, Vol. 267, No. 7 (February 1992), pp. 954-957

Federal Register, *45 C.F.R. Sect. 46.102(I)*

Fouad, M.N., Corbie-Smith, D., Curb D et al (2004). Special populations recruitment for the women's health initiative: successes and limitations, *Control Clin Trials*, Vol. 25, pp. 335-52, ISSN 0197-2456

Fynn, V. (2010). Where there is failing laws: sexual violence against women and children in conflict communities of Africa. *Proceedings of the 18th World Congress on Medical Law*, pp. 34-40, ISBN , Zagreb, Croatia, August 8-12, 2010, ISBN 978-953-270-046-6

Galliard, P. Melis, R., Mwanyumba, F. et al. (2000). Consequences of announcing HIV seropositivity to women in an African setting: lessons for the implementation of HIV testing and interventions to reduce mother-to-child transmission. *Proceedings of the XIII International AIDS Conference*, p. 334, , Durban, South Africa, July 9-14, 2000

Grady, C. (2005). The challenge of assuring continued post-trial access to beneficial treatment, *Yale J Heslth Policy Law Ethics*, Vol. 5, pp.425-435, PMID: 15742586

Guenter, D., Esparza, J. & Macklin, R. (2000). Ethical considerations in international HIV vaccine trials: summary of consultative process conducted by the joint United Nations Programme for HIV/AIDS, *J Med Ethics*, Vol. 26, pp. 37-43 doi:10.1136/jme.26.1.37

Hanssens, C. (2007). Legal and Ethical Implications of Opt-Out HIV Testing. *CID*, Vol. 45, (Suppl 4), pp. S232-S239, doi: 10.1086/522543

Harding, R., Stewart, K., Marconi, K., O'Neill, J.F. & Higginson, I.J. (2003). Current HIV/AIDS end-of-life care in sub-Saharan Africa: a survey of models, services, challenges and priorities, *BMC Public Health*, Vol. 3, p. 33, doi:10.1186/1471-2458-3-33

Hargreaves, S. (2007). New guidance issued on HIV data collection. *The Lancet Infectious Diseases*, Vol. 7, No. 508, doi:10.1016/S1473-3099(07)70171-8

HIV Prevention Trials Network (HPTN) Ethics Working Group (2003). *Ethical Guidance for HIV Preventive trials, Family Health International*, North Carolina, USA.

Indian Council of Medical Research (ICMR) (2000). *Ethical guidelines for biomedical research involving human subjects*, New Delhi, Retrieved from www.icmr.nic.in/Report_socio.pdf

Indian Council of Medical Research (ICMR) & WHO (2001) *Ethical Guidelines for Biomedical and Behavioural Research on HIV/AIDS*, (Unpublished), New Delhi, Retrieved from www.icmr.nic.in/Report_socio.pdf

Joint United Nations Programme on HIV/AIDS (2000). *HIV and AIDS related stigmatization, discrimination and denial: forms, contexts and determinants: research studies from Uganda and India*, Geneva, Retrieved from: http://data.unaids.org/Publications/IRC-pub01/JC316-Uganda-India_en.pdf

Joint United Nations Programme on HIV/AIDS (UNAIDS) (2001). *Ethical Considerations in HIV Preventive Vaccine Research: UNAIDS Guidance Document*, Geneva, Retrieved from www.unaids.org

Joint United Nations Programme on HIV/AIDS (UNAIDS) (2007). Guidelines on Protecting the Confidentiality and Security of HIV Information, *Proceedings of the Workshop*, Geneva, Switzerland, May 15-17, 2006, Retrieved from www.unaids.org

Joint United Nations Programme on HIV/AIDS (UNAIDS) (2008). *Report on the global AIDS epidemic*, Geneva, ISBN 978 92 4 150039 5

Joint United Nations Programme on HIV/AIDS (UNAIDS) (2010). *Global report: UNAIDS report on the global AIDS epidemic*, WHO Library, ISBN 978-92-9173-871-7

Jonas, H. (1997). *Tecnica, Medicina ed etica. Prassi del principio responsabilità*, Einaudi, Torino

Kass, N., Taylor, H.A. & Anderson, J. (2000). Treatment of human immunodeficiency virus during pregnancy: the shift from an exclusive focus on fetal protection to a more balanced approach. *Am J Obstet Gynecol*, Vol. 182, pp. 856-859

Kenya AIDS Society vs Arthur Obel H.C.C.C. 1079 of 1997 & C. A. 188 of 1997.

Kilewo, C. et al (2001). HIV counselling and testing of pregnant women in sub-Saharan Africa, *Journal of Acquired Immune Deficiency Syndromes*, Vol. 28, pp. 458-462

Li L., Sun S., Wu S., Lin C., Wu Z. & Yan Z. (2007). Disclosure of HIV Status Is a Family Matter: Field Notes From China, *J Fam Psychol.*, Vol. 21, No. 2, pp. 307–314, doi:10.1037/0893-3200.21.2.307

Macklin, R. (2001). After Helsinki: unresolved issues in international research. *Kennedy Inst Ethics J*, Vol. 11, pp. 17-36

Maine Revised Statues (MRS) *5§19203-A 2*, In: Brown, J. (2008). The changing landscape of state legislation and expanded HIV testing, *Public Health Reports*, Vol. 123, No 3, pp 16-19

Mannheim, K. (1999). *Ideologia ed utopia*, Mulino Editor, ISBN 978-88-15-07126-2, Milan

May, W.E. (1991). *An introduction to moral Theology*, Out Sunday visitor, Huntington, ISBN

McNutt, L.A., Gordon, E.J. & Uuskula, A. (2009). Informed recruitment in partner studies of HIV transmission: an ethical issue in couples research, *BMC Medical Ethics*, Vol.10, No.14. Doi:10.1186/1472-6939-10-14

McQuoid-Mason, D. (2007). Disclosing the HIV status of deceased persons - ethical and legal implications, Vol. 97, No. 10, *SAMJ Forum*, Retrieved from www.samj.org.za/index.php/samj/article/view/559/92

Medley, A. et al (2004). Rates, barriers and outcomes of HIV serostatus disclosure among women in developing countries: implications for prevention of mother-to-child transmission programmes, *Bulletin of the World Health Organization*, Vol. 82, pp. 299-307

Mills, E., Nixon, S., Singh, S., Dolma, S., Nayyar, A. & Kapoor, S. (2006). Enrolling Women into HIV Preventive Vaccine Trials: An Ethical Imperative but a Logistical Challenge, *Epub*, Vol. 3, No. 3 (e94), DOI: 10.1371/journal.pmed.0030094, Available from www.plosmedicine.org

Muthuswamy, V. (2005). Ethical issues in HIV/AIDS research Indian, *J Med Res*, Vol. 121, pp. 601-610

National Bioethics Advisory Commission (NBAC) (2001). *Ethical and Policy Issues in International Research: Clinical Trials in Developing Countries*, Washington DC

National Institutes of Health (2005). *Guidance for addressing the provision of retroviral treatment for trial participaticipants following their completion of NIH-funded HIV antiretroviral treatment trials in developing countries*. Retrieved from http://grants.nih.gov/grants/guide/notice-files/NOT-OD-05_038.html

Ngotho, D.K. (2009). HIV/AIDS - A major medical ethics dilemma, *Proceedings of the International Conference on Bioethics*, pp. 14-20, Egerton University, Kenya, August 12-14, 2008

Nuffield Council on Bioethics. (1999). *The Ethics of clinical research in Developing Countries*, London

Oduwo, E.A. (2009). Rethinking state participation in HIV vaccine trials, *Proceedings of the International Conference on Bioethics*, pp. 31-39, Egerton University, Kenya, August 12-14, 2008

Oyefara, JL. (2007). Food insecurity, HIV/AIDS pandemic and sexual behaviour of female commercial sex workers in Lagos metropolis, Nigeria. *SAHARA J: Journal of Social Aspects of HIV/AIDS Research Alliance*, Vol. 4, pp. 626–635

Philippines National Health Council (2001). *Ethical Guideline in AIDS Investigations in Philippines*, Manila

Pieterse, M. (2010). Impeding access? Stigma, individual responsibility and access to post HIV exposure prophylaxis (PEP) treatment in South Africa, *Proceedings of 18th World Congress on Medical Law*, p 173, Zagreb, Croatia, August 8-12, 2010, ISBN 978-953-270-046-6

Poljak, M., Smit, E. & Ross, J. (2009). 2008European Guideline on HIV testing. *International Journal of STD & AIDS*, Vol. 20, pp. 77–83

Rodotà, S. (1991), Privacy e costruzione della sfera privata, In: Rodotà, S. (1995). *Tecnologie e diritti*, il Mulino, Bologna, pp. 101-122

Rogstad, K.E., Palfreeman, A., Rooney, G. et al. (2006). *United Kingdom National Guidelines on HIV Testing 2006*, Retrieved from www.bashh.org/documents/63/63.pdf

Salari, P. & Azizi M. (2009). The necessity of HIV testing in Iranian pregnant women and its ethical considerations, *J Med Ethics Hist Med*, Vol. 2, No 1, Available from http://journals.tums.ac.ir/upload_files/pdf/12484.pdf

Sajeev, M.A. (2007). The HIV code. *Arch Dis Child*. Vol. 92 (1), No. 91, doi: 10.1136/adc.2006.107573.

Singer, P.A. & Bowman, K.W. (2002). Quality end-of-life care: A global perspective. *BMC Palliative Care*, Vol. 1, p.4, Available from http://www.biomedcentral.com/1472-684X/1/4

Siringi, S. (2004). British scientists face lawsuit, *The Lancet Infectious Disease*, Vo.4 , No. 7

Slack, C. et al (2005). Provision of HIV treatment in HIV preventive vaccine trials: a developing country perspective, *Soc Sci Med*, Vol. 60, pp.1197-1208.

Soldini, M. (2001). *Bioetica della vita nascente. In puero homo*. CIC Edizioni internazionali, Roma.

South Africa Code of Ethics in HIV/AIDS (2000), In: Muthuswamy, V. (2005). Ethical issues in HIV/AIDS research Indian, *J Med Res*, Vol. 121, pp. 601-610

State Council AIDS Working Committee Office and United Nations Theme Group on HIV/AIDS (UNAIDS) in China (2004). *A joint assessment of HIV/AIDS prevention, treatment and care in China*. Beijing, China, Retrieved from www.chinaids.org.cn/worknet/download/2004/report2004en.pdf

Stewart, R.S. (2007). Protective Measures for Private Health Information. *Perspectives in Health Information Management*, Vol.4, No.5,

Stuart Huges, H. (1967). *Coscienza e società,. Storia delle idee in Europa dal 1980 al 1930*, Einaudi, Torino

The Lawyer's Collective (2003). *Legislating an Epidemic, HIV/AIDS in India*, Universal Law Publishing Co. Private Ltd, New Delhi, OL3337658M

Thorvaldsen, J. (2001). European guideline for testing for HIV infection. *Int J STD AIDS* Vol. 12 (Suppl. 3), pp.7–13

UNICEF (2008). *Progress for Children. A Report Card on Maternal Mortality*. UNICEF, No.7, Retrieved from http://www.unicef.org/childsurvival/files/Progress_for_Children-No._7_Lo-Res_082008.pdf

Weijer, C. & LeBlanc, G. (2006). The Balm of Gilead: Is the provision of treatment to those who seroconvert in HIV prevention trials a matter of moral obligation or moral negotiation?, *J Law Med Ethics*, Vol. 34, pp. 793-808

Wilson, J. (2007). Is respect for autonomy defensible?, *J. Med Ethics*, Vol. 33, pp. 353-356

World Health Organitation. (2008). Towards universal access: scaling up priority HIV/AIDS interventions in the health sector (progress report 2008), Available from http:www.who.int/hiv/pub/towards_universal_access_report_2008.pdf

World Health Organization (WHO) (2000). *Fact Sheet: Backgrounder No. 1*. Retrieved from http://www.who.int/inf-fs/en/back001.html]July

World Medical Association (2000). *Declaration of Helsinki: ethical principles for medical research involving human subjects*. 52nd WMA General Assembly, Edinburgh, Scotland

World Medical Association. (2004) *Declaration of Helsinki*. Available from http://www.wma.net/e/policy/b3.htm

Zare, M. & Mortazavifar, N. (2010). AIDS: human rights and government responsibility, *Proceedings of 18th World Congress on Medical Law*, p 174, Zagreb, Croatia, August 8-12, 2010, ISBN 978-953-270-046

19

Acceptability of HIV Vaccine - Efficacy Trials in Drug Users and Sexual Partners of HIV Infected Patients in Barcelona, Spain

Arantza Sanvisens et al.*
Department of Internal Medicine - HIVACAT,
Hospital Universitari Germans Trias i Pujol,
Universitat Autònoma de Barcelona
Spain

1. Introduction

The epidemiology of HIV infection in Spain has changed during the past decade. Surveillance of HIV infection occurs in 15 of the country's 17 regions, and 2,264 new HIV infections were diagnosed in 2009 (Ministerio de Sanidad y Política Social, Ministerio de Ciencia e Innovación, 2010).

As previously reported (Hernandez-Aguado, 1999), the HIV epidemic in Spain has been largely driven by injecting drug users (IDUs). Reductions in the rates of new infections among drug users were reported a decade ago for the first time since the beginning of the epidemic (Castilla, 2006). In 2009, 77.0% of new infections were acquired through sexual transmission, and IDUs represented less than 10% of reported cases (Ministerio de Sanidad y Política Social, Ministerio de Ciencia e Innovación, 2010).

The HIV epidemic among IDUs continues to develop heterogeneously across different parts of Europe. In the European Union, the reported rates of newly diagnosed cases of HIV infection in IDUs are mostly stable or in decline (European Monitoring Centre for Drugs and Drug Addiction, 2009). Data on newly reported cases of HIV infection in IDUs for 2007 suggest that rates of infection are still declining in Europe following a peak in 2002, which was caused by outbreaks in Estonia, Latvia and Lithuania. In 2007, the overall rate of newly reported infections of HIV among IDUs in the 24 EU member states for which national data

* Inmaculada Rivas[2], Rosa Guerola[3], Patricia Cobarsi[3], Rayen Rall[1,4], Daniel Fuster[1], Joan Romeu[3], Bonaventura Clotet[5], Jordi Tor[1] and Robert Muga[1]
[1]*Department of Internal Medicine - HIVACAT, Hospital Universitari Germans Trias i Pujol, Universitat Autònoma de Barcelona, Spain*
[2]*Municipal Center for Substance Abuse Treatment (CAS Delta), Badalona, Spain*
[3]*HIV/AIDS Unit - HIVACAT, Hospital Universitari Germans Trias i Pujol, Badalona, Spain*
[4]*Centro de Salud Juana Azurduy, Rosario, Argentina*
[5]*IrsiCaixa - HIVACAT, Hospital Universitari Germans Trias i Pujol, Badalona, Universitat Autònoma de Barcelona, Spain*

were available was 4.7 cases per million population, slightly lower than the 5.0 per million population reported in 2006.

Non-injecting drug users are not parenterally exposed to HIV infection, but they remain at risk of acquiring HIV through sexual transmission. Several studies regarding risky sexual practices suggest an association between the abuse of cocaine, amphetamines, and alcohol and sexual transmission of HIV (Wang, 2010; Baliunas, 2010; Booth, 2000; de Azevedo, 2007; Colfax, 2010; Van Tieu, 2009). For these reasons, it is clear that drug users, independent of the route of administration, are a population at risk of HIV infection. Therefore, they are candidates for participation in studies on the efficacy of a preventive vaccine.

In Spain in 2009, the most prevalent route of acquisition of HIV was through transmission among men who have sex with men (MSM) (42.5%), followed by heterosexual transmission, who represented 34.5% of cases. Among men, over 50% of new HIV diagnoses are associated with MSM transmission. There has been a downward trend in the proportion of cases from heterosexual transmission (44.4% of cases in 2004 and 34.5% of cases in 2009). In contrast, MSM transmission accounts for a growing proportion of cases, increasing from 28.8% in 2004 to 42.5% in 2009 (Ministerio de Sanidad y Política Social, Ministerio de Ciencia e Innovación, 2010). Several risk factors contribute to the sexual transmission of HIV, including socioeconomic status and individual factors such as having multiple sexual partners or unprotected sex (Staras, 2009; Hallfors, 2007; Adimora, 2006).

The development of effective vaccines against HIV is the main focus of HIV research and provides hope for limiting the epidemic. In phase III clinical trials of a vaccine, the involvement of thousands of people and a measure of the background incidence of HIV infection are necessary to establish population efficacy (Celentano, 1995; Vanichseni, 2001; Newman, 2010b). Cohorts with less than 2 × 100 person-years (p-y) of HIV incidence and less than 90% retention are considered inappropriate for these trials partly because they are not likely to provide sufficient statistical power to demonstrate an effect of the intervention. The HIV incidence rate in a vaccine efficacy trial performed among IDUs from Thailand showed an HIV incidence rate of 3.4 per 100 p-y (Suntharasamai, 2009); in IDUs from metropolitan Barcelona, incidence is half that shown in the vaccine efficacy trial performed in Thailand in the same type of population (Muga, 2010). In other studies, the rate has varied by geographic area (Kozlov, 2006; Kellogg, 2001; Bruandet, 2006; Duan, 2009).

Globally, cohorts of HIV-negative individuals at high risk of HIV infection have been extensively studied to monitor the incidence of HIV-1 and assess their involvement in vaccine efficacy studies. Currently, there are three international phase III HIV vaccine studies (Table 1). Spain participates in an increasing number of European and North American initiatives to prepare for preventive HIV vaccine trials, but few studies have evaluated the acceptability of a preventive vaccine against HIV/AIDS among potential recipients and their willingness to participate in clinical trials (Etcheverry, 2011).

Factors positively correlated with a decision to participate in a HIV vaccine trial may include altruism, higher education level, suspected exposure to HIV, protection against HIV infection, and free medical care and economic incentives (Strauss, 2001; Golub, 2005). Barriers to participation include little information about the vaccine trials, vaccine-induced seropositivity to HIV in tests, and associated stigma or discrimination (Strauss, 2001; Golub, 2005). Given the historical underutilization of existing preventive vaccines, such as the hepatitis B vaccine, among MSM (in part due to a lack of information (Jacobson, 2007; Schutten, 2002)), it is important to anticipate and understand the characteristics of potential volunteers for an HIV vaccine trial in detail.

Trial ID	Strategy	Group of risk	Start Date	Volunteers
RV 144	Viral vector-Pox/Protein	HIV-uninfected Thai adults	10/2/2003	16,403
VAX 003	Protein	Intravenous drug users in Bangkok	3/1/1999	2,500
VAX 004	Protein	Adults at risk of sexually transmitted HIV in North America	6/1/1998	5,400

Table 1. Characteristics of current phase III clinical trials. Information was taken from the Database of AIDS Vaccine Candidates in Clinical Trials available at http://www.iavireport.org.

The main objective of this study was to assess HIV risk behavior in drug users and sexual partners of HIV-infected patients and to analyze the degree of acceptance and willingness to participate (WTP) in HIV vaccine efficacy trials in metropolitan Barcelona.

2. Patients and methods

Drug addicts were recruited in two centers for substance abuse treatment located in Badalona, Spain (Hospital Universitari Germans Trias i Pujol and the Municipal Center for Substance Abuse Treatment, known as CAS Delta) between November 2007 and May 2010. During the same period, sexual partners of HIV-infected patients were recruited in an HIV/AIDS unit at the Hospital Universitari Germans Trias i Pujol.
The three patient enrollment sites in the study were located in Badalona, north of Barcelona. The CAS Delta treats patients with substance abuse who live in two cities, Badalona (220,000 inhabitants) and Santa Coloma de Gramenet (110,000 inhabitants). The Hospital Universitari Germans Trias i Pujol is a tertiary teaching hospital with 600 beds in Badalona; the HIV/AIDS Unit at Hospital Universitari Germans Trias i Pujol treated in 2010 more than 1,500 HIV-positive patients.
Drug users were diagnosed with drug dependence disorders according to the Diagnostic and Statistical Manual of Mental Disorders, 4th ed. (DSM-IV) (American Psychiatric Association, 2000) and had been referred for substance abuse treatment. The primary drugs of abuse were stimulants (cocaine) and depressants (opiates and alcohol). To be considered for inclusion in the study, drug users had to 1) be 18 years of age or older, 2) be actively using drugs, 3) have HIV-negative status at the time of inclusion, and 4) give informed consent. Drug users at risk of infection who met the inclusion criteria answered a 56-question survey, which collected data on personal history (age, sex, place of origin, educational level, and employment status), drug use (the quantity, frequency, and treatment history for alcohol, cocaine, heroin, and other substances), sexual behavior (sexual orientation, number of partners, characteristics of the sexual partners regarding drug use

and paid sex, and condom use), history of sexually transmitted diseases, knowledge and opinions about a potential HIV vaccine, WTP, and the subject's availability for an extended follow up. The survey questions were presented by doctors and nurses from both recruiting centers, individually and in a quiet setting with no other people present.

To be considered for inclusion in the study, sexual partners of patients with HIV infection had to 1) be 18 years old or older, 2) have been a stable partner for at least 6 months, 3) be HIV-negative at the time of inclusion, and 4) give informed consent. Participants were given a shortened version of the previously described questionnaire that collected data on personal history, sexual behavior, and WTP. The questionnaire was given in the HIV/AIDS unit and was conducted by trained personnel.

In both groups at risk for HIV infection, the degree of WTP in a potential HIV vaccine-efficacy trial was assessed on a four-point scale questionnaire:

a. I am definitely willing to participate [definitely yes];
b. I want to participate, but need to think about it [probably yes];
c. I do not want to participate but will think about it [probably not];
d. I am not at all willing to participate [definitely not].

The group of drug users was given an additional question related to the possibility of receiving remuneration for participating in a vaccine study: If you were paid, would you agree to volunteer in a potential HIV vaccine efficacy trial?

After the questionnaires were completed, participants were scheduled for a blood draw to detect possible HIV, hepatitis C virus (HCV), and hepatitis B virus (HBV) infections. The blood samples were tested by enzyme immunoassay (EIA) for antibodies to HIV infection (Genetic Systems, Bio-Rad Laboratories, Seattle, WA or Abbot HIVAB, Abbot Laboratories, North Chicago, IL) and confirmed by western blot. Infection with HCV was determined by EIA (Ortho HCV, Ortho Diagnostics, Raritan, NJ). Blood samples were tested for the HBV surface antigen (Auszyme Monoclonal EIA or AxSYM microparticle enzyme immunoassay (MEIA), Abbott Laboratories, North Chicago, IL), anti-HBs (Ausab (EIA) or AxSYM (MEIA), Abbot Laboratories, North Chicago, IL), and anti-HBc (Corzyme (EIA) or AxSYM (MEIA), Abbot Laboratories, North Chicago, IL).

The methods used to conduct this study met the ethical standards for medical research and the principles of good clinical practice.

2.1 Statistical analysis

Data from the two groups at risk of HIV infection were pooled. A total of 21 variables were common to both risk groups.

For drug users, we developed an index that evaluated the level of risk of infection based on 10 questions:

1. Have you ever used drugs intravenously?
2. Have you shared elements to inject?
3. How many sexual partners have you had in the past year?
4. Have you had sex for drugs?
5. Have you ever had sex with people who were under the influence of drugs?
6. Have you ever had sex with prostitutes?
7. Have you ever had sex with someone infected with HIV?
8. Have you had sex under the influence of drugs?

9. When you have a steady partner, do you use condoms?
10. When you do not have a steady partner, do use condoms?

For each of the questions, we created an indicator, 0/1, corresponding to no risk/risk. We then summed the indicators obtained for all ten questions. A value between 0 and 3 points was defined as low risk, between 4 and 6 points as moderate risk, and more than 6 points as high risk.

We performed a descriptive analysis and a bivariate analysis by risk group for HIV infection, WTP, and other variables of interest. The outcome variable of WTP was dichotomized so that there were enough subjects in each category for comparison: the variable was "yes" if WTP was "definitely willing" or "probably willing" and "no" if the answer was "probably not" or "definitely not".

We used the chi-square test, Fisher's F-test, and Student's t-test when appropriate to detect significant differences. In addition, we calculated the odds ratio to quantify the probabilities of WTP. Logistic regression methods were used to determine predictive factors for participation in a phase III clinical trial. Variables that were statistically significant in the bivariate analysis were used as co-variables in the regression. Data were entered into a Microsoft Access 2003 database. All statistical analyses were performed using Stata software (version 8.0; StataCorp, College Station, TX). Values of $p < 0.05$ were considered statistically significant.

3. Results

A total of 232 HIV-seronegative individuals were analyzed. The median age at study entry was 39 years (interquartile range (IQR), 33-45 years), and 64% were men. Almost 17% of participants had attained at least a high school education. Seventy-nine individuals (34%) were drug users, and 153 (66%) were sexual partners of HIV-positive patients. Among drug users, 82.3% were men, the median age was 35.4 years (IQR, 29.4 - 40.0 years), most (57.7%) had finished elementary school, and 96.2% were heterosexual. Among the sexual partners, 54.2% were men, the median age was 41 years (IQR, 35.6 - 46.6), 40% had completed middle school, and 67.5% were heterosexual. These and other results can be seen in Table 2, which summarizes the characteristics of the study population overall and by risk group.

The overall prevalence of HCV was 20.5%. This prevalence was higher among drug users than in the other group (41.6% vs. 8.3%). Among drug users, 22.4% (11/49) had a serologic pattern of HBV-vaccine-induced immunity [i.e., HBsAg (-), HBsAb (+), and HBcAb (-)], and the serology of 7 of 49 (14.3%) users reflected immunity from natural infection.

None of the sexual partners of the HIV-positive patients had the three serological markers of HBV. In the same blood sample, we confirmed that all participants were negative for HIV. Table 3 summarizes the HCV and HBV statuses of participants at the time of inclusion in the study.

With regard to risky behaviors of drug users, it was noted that 46% (36/78) were or had been IDUs, and 50% admitted to having shared injecting equipment at some point. In addition, 45% of IDUs reported that they drank alcohol daily, 35.5% had been to jail, and 14.7% had never used condoms despite not having had a stable sexual partner. In general, the level of risk of HIV infection was low for approximately 55% of drug users (43/78) and elevated in 7.7% (6/78). These and related findings on risky behavior among drug users are summarized in Table 4.

	Drug users N = 79 n (%)	Sexual partners of HIV+ patients N = 153 n (%)	Total N = 232 n (%)
Gender			
Male	65 (82.3)	83 (54.2)	148 (63.8)
Female	14 (17.7)	70 (45.8)	84 (36.2)
Age (median [IQR])	35.4 [29.4-40.0]	41.1 [35.6-46.6]	39.3 [33.0-44.8]
Education (n=128)			
None	8 (10.3)	2 (1.4)	10 (4.4)
Primary school	45 (57.7)	50 (34.0)	95 (42.2)
Middle school	23 (29.5)	59 (40.1)	82 (36.4)
High school	2 (2.5)	36 (24.5)	38 (16.9)
Last consumption of drugs (n=231)			
Never	0 (0)	123 (80.4)	123 (53.2)
< 1 month	54 (69.2)	25 (16.3)	79 (34.2)
1-12 months	19 (24.4)	2 (1.3)	21 (9.1)
> 12 months	5 (6.4)	3 (2.0)	8 (3.5)
Sexual behavior (n=128)			
Homosexual	1 (1.3)	49 (32.5)	50 (21.8)
Heterosexual	75 (96.2)	102 (67.5)	177 (77.3)
Bisexual	2 (2.6)	0 (0.0)	2 (0.9)
Willingness to participate			
No	48 (60.7)	1 (0.7)	49 (21.1)
Yes	31 (39.3)	152 (99.3)	183 (78.9)

Table 2. Characteristics of drug users and HIV-positive sexual partners.

	Drug users n / N (%)	Sexual partner of HIV+ patients n / N (%)	Total n / N (%)
HCV+	32/77 (41.6)	11/133 (8.3)	43/210 (20.5)
HBsAg+	0/72 (0)	1/77 (1.3)	1/149 (0.7)
HBcAb+	13/62 (21.0)	11/42 (26.2)	24/104 (23.1)
HBsAb+	19/52 (36.5)	16/42 (38.1)	35/94 (37.2)

Table 3. Serological status of the study population according to risk of infection.

	N=79 n (%)
Recent (< 1 year) usage of IV drugs (n=78)	14 (17.9)
History (> 1 year) of IV drug use (n=78)	22 (28.2)
Have you shared injecting equipment? (n=36)	
Yes	18 (50.0)
No	18 (50.0)
Do you go to the needle-exchange locations? (n=32)	
Yes	14 (43.7)
No	18 (56.3)
Are you in a methadone program? (n=77)	
Yes	29 (37.7)
No	48 (62.3)
Have you consumed alcohol in the past year? (n=78)	
Yes	47 (60.3)
No	31 (39.7)
Do you consume alcohol daily? (n=47)	
Yes	22 (46.8)
No	25 (53.2)
Have you required medical attention for drug use in the past year? (n=74)	
Yes	26 (35.1)
No	48 (64.9)
Have you been in prison? (n=76)	
Yes	27 (35.5)
No	49 (64.5)
How many sexual partners have you had in the past year? (n=78)	
0	17 (21.8)
1-5	55 (70.5)
6-10	3 (3.8)
11-20	1 (1.3)
>20	2 (2.6)
Have you had sex for drugs? (n=78)	
Yes	4 (5.1)
No	73 (93.6)
Don't know/refused	1 (1.3)

Table 4. Risk behaviors in drug users at risk of HIV infection.

	N=79 n (%)
Have you had sex with people who were under the influence of drugs? (n=78)	
Yes	51 (65.4)
No	26 (33.3)
Don't know/refused	1 (1.3)
Have you had sex with prostitutes? (n=74)	
Yes	40 (54.0)
No	33 (44.6)
Don't know/refused	1 (1.4)
Have you had sex with someone infected with HIV? (n=78)	
Yes	9 (11.5)
No	60 (76.9)
Don't know/refused	9 (11.6)
Have you had sex while under the influence of drugs? (n=78)	
Yes	68 (87.2)
No	10 (12.8)
Don't know/refused	0 (0)
Do you currently have a steady partner? (n=78)	
Yes	34 (43.6)
No	44 (56.4)
When you have a steady partner, do you use condoms? (n=76)	
Always	14 (18.4)
Sometimes	27 (35.5)
Never	35 (46.1)
When you have no steady partner, do you use condoms? (n=75)	
Always	43 (57.3)
Sometimes	21 (28.0)
Never	11 (14.7)

Table 4. (Cont.). Risk behaviors in drug users at risk of HIV infection.

Notably, nearly 30% of the stable partners of HIV-infected people did not consistently use condoms, and 23.2% acknowledged having had sex under the influence of drugs. Table 5 summarizes risk behaviors in this population.

Overall, 47.4% of participants answered that they would definitely be willing to participate in HIV vaccine efficacy trials, 31.5% were probably willing, 9.1% wrote they were probably not willing, and 12.1% indicated they were definitely not willing to join vaccine trials. Among drug addicts, 13.9% were definitely willing to participate, in contrast to 64.7% of sexual partners of HIV-infected patients ($p<0.05$). Figure 1 shows the characteristics of WTP according to both study populations. Among drug users, it should be noted that only one person indicated a shift in WTP from "probably no" to "probably yes" if the study were to involve remuneration.

	N=153 n (%)
Have you used drugs in the past month?	
Yes	30 (19.6)
No	123 (80.4)
Do you have a history of IV drug use?	3 (2.0)
Have you had sex with people under the influence of drugs? (n=56)	
Yes	13 (23.2)
No	42 (75.0)
Don't know/refused	1 (1.8)
Have you had sex with prostitutes? (n=67)	
Yes	14 (20.9)
No	52 (77.6)
Don't know/refused	1 (1.5)
Have you had sex while under the influence of drugs? (n=150)	
Yes	16 (10.7)
No	134 (89.3)
When you have a steady partner, do you use condoms? (n=146)	
Always	104 (71.2)
Sometimes	29 (19.9)
Never	13 (8.9)

Table 5. Sexual risk behaviors of sexual partners of HIV-infected patients.

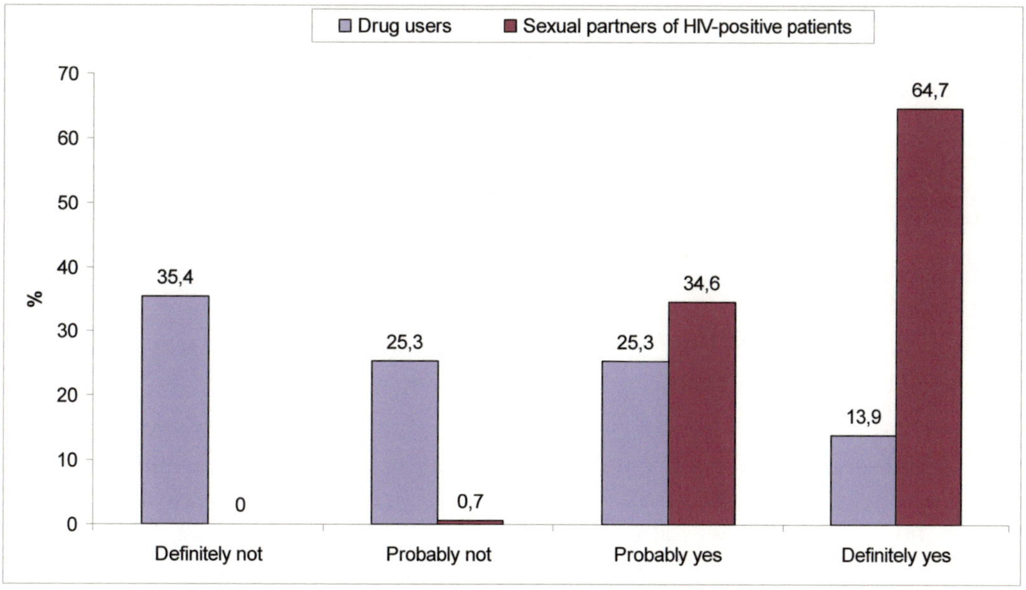

Fig. 1. Willingness to participate in HIV vaccine efficacy trials among drug addicts and sexual partners of HIV-positive patients in Badalona, Spain.

Table 6 summarizes WTP in both risk groups. This table shows that WTP in drug users is more common in women, in those with elementary-school education, in those who have recently used drugs, and in those who show a high number of risk behaviors. In sexual partners of HIV-positive patients, the vast majority (>95%) would be willing to participate in a clinical trial.

	Willingness to participate			
	Drug users N=79		Sexual partners of HIV-positive patients N=153	
	n (%)	p-value	n (%)	p-value
Gender				
Male	22 (33.8)	0.034	83 (100.0)	0.458*
Female	9 (64.3)		69 (98.6)	
Age (mean ± SD)	34.9 ± 9.5	0.944	41.6 ± 8.3	0.872
Education (n=128)				
None	3 (37.5)	0.647	2 (100.0)	1.000*
Elementary school	19 (42.2)		50 (100.0)	
Middle	8 (34.8)		58 (98.3)	
High	0 (0)		36 (100.0)	
Last consumption of drugs (n=231)				
Never	--	0.588	122 (99.2)	1.000*
< 1 month	23 (42.6)		25 (100.0)	
1-12 months	7 (36.8)		2 (100.0)	
> 12 months	1 (20.0)		3 (100.0)	
Sexual behavior (n=128)				
Homosexual	1 (100.0)	0.059*	101 (99.0)	1.000*
Heterosexual	28 (37.3)		49 (100.0)	
Bisexual	2 (100.0)		--	
Risk behavior				
Low	10 (23.8)	0.003		
Moderate	16 (55.3)			
High	5 (83.3)			

* F-test

Table 6. Willingness to participate in HIV vaccine trials among drug users and sexual partners of HIV-positive patients.

There were also significant differences between drug users by gender. The probability that a female drug user agreed to participate in a future vaccine trial for HIV was more than three times higher than in men (OR = 3.52, 95% CI: 1.05-11.77). Having a moderate or high risk of HIV infection (> 3 points) was also associated with WTP (OR = 4.48, 95% CI: 1.70-11.83). Figure 2 shows WTP according to the level of risk of HIV infection in drug users.

In the multivariate analysis, being female (OR = 5.6, 95% CI: 1.4-22.4) and having a moderate-to-high level of infection risk (OR = 6.6, 95% CI: 2.2-19.6) were predictors of participation in a phase III vaccine trial among drug users.

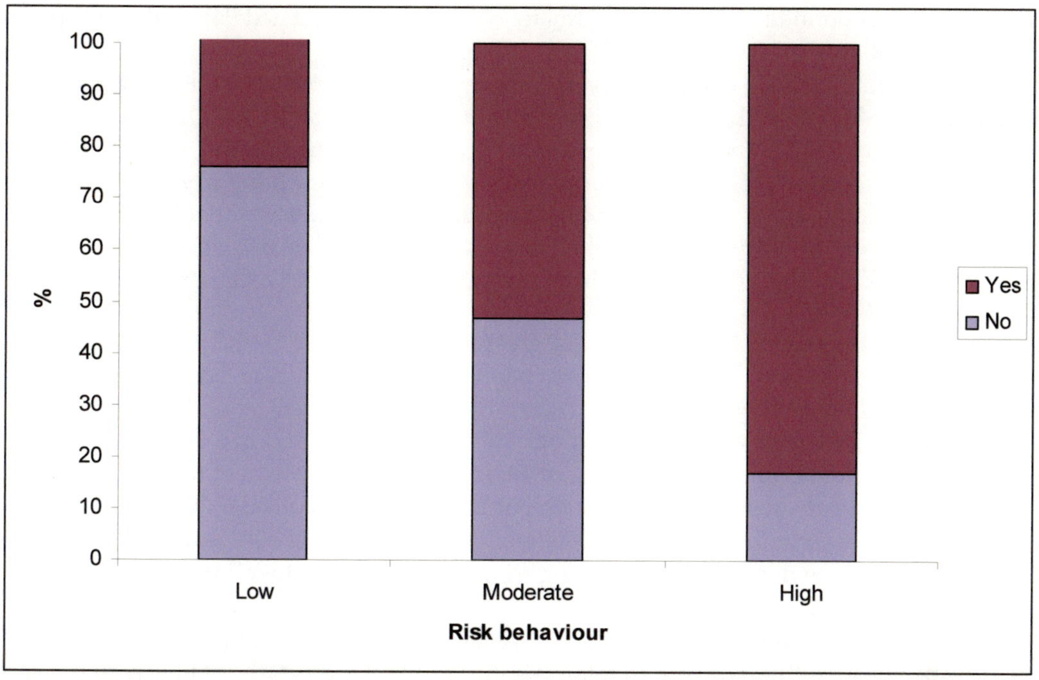

Fig. 2. Willingness to participate according to the level of risk of HIV infection in drug users.

4. Conclusion

Understanding the candidate population of volunteers is crucial for analyzing the efficacy of a potential preventive vaccine trial. In Spain, drug users have exhibited an elevated risk of HIV infection. In anticipation of a safe and effective vaccine candidate, it is appropriate to assess potential sites and populations for future vaccine trials. Accordingly, this study was developed to analyze WTP in a hypothetical HIV vaccine efficacy trial among current drug users in an urban area, many of whom have been affected by HIV/AIDS and parenteral drug addiction for many years. Sexual partners of HIV-infected patients are, by definition, another population at risk and therefore also potential trial participants.

In this study, we observed that WTP is clearly higher in sexual partners of HIV-positive patients and falls far short of 40% in potentially eligible drug users. To the best of our knowledge, this is the first study to report WTP in HIV vaccine trials in sexual partners of HIV patients in Spain. A high rate of acceptability of an HIV vaccine trial in this risk group has not been reported in other countries, although one study has demonstrated WTP in an overwhelming majority of monogamous married women (Suhadev, 2006). A predisposition toward WTP is already known among homosexuals (Newman, 2010b; Li, 2010) and, more particularly, in those who report family support for participation and expect that the vaccine will protect them against HIV infection (Li, 2010).

The WTP of drug users in this study was lower than that of other studies conducted in our area and in other areas. For example, a study recently conducted in our area on 326 drug users found WTP in 83% of cases (51% would definitely participate, and 32% would probably participate) (Etcheverry, 2011). In China, a study conducted among 401 IDUs showed a rate of definite WTP of approximately 75%; the rate reached 94% if the group that indicated a probable WTP was included (Yin, 2008).

One of the findings among drug users is noteworthy: those who showed an increased risk of infection were the most likely to agree to participate in a phase III vaccine trial. A recent meta-analysis of HIV vaccine acceptability indicated a significant impact of self-identification as a member of a risk group and perceived susceptibility to HIV infection on HIV vaccine acceptability, thus suggesting potentially modifiable factors beyond vaccine characteristics that may influence uptake (Newman, 2010a). This finding may explain the high rate of WTP in this subgroup of drug users compared to the mean of this population (83.3% vs. 39.2%).

Among active drug users, women showed greater willingness to participate in a phase III vaccine trial. Greater availability and motivation of women has also been noted in other studies, although in different risk groups (Aliyu, 2010; Colfax, 2005).

The rate of HIV incidence among IDUs in our area is half that found in a similar population in Thailand (Suntharasamai, 2009; Muga, 2010). In the study by Muga et al., the proportion of IDUs admitted for substance abuse treatment had decreased considerably in recent years (Muga, 2010). When combined with the relatively low incidence of HIV infection in recently recruited IDUs, these data suggest that drug users may not be included in future studies on preventive HIV/AIDS vaccine efficacy trials.

The results from this study indicate that the prevalence of HCV in drug users and in sexual partners of HIV-positive patients is relatively high (41.6% and 8.3%, respectively). These results suggest the possibility that some of the individuals in the drug users group who self-reported as non-IDUs may have injected drugs in the past. However, the risk of sexual transmission of an HCV infection is associated with a history of multiple sexual partners and a lack of condom usage (Alter, 1990; Osmond, 1993; Rauch, 2005). Thus, the high prevalence of HCV infection in both risk groups in this study could be explained by the large number of subjects who said that they never use condoms. It was also noted that over 20% of drug users had been vaccinated for HBV. Although the percentage of people vaccinated against HBV is low globally, these results are consistent with others noting that vaccine-induced immunity to HBV infection in Spain has been increasing (Rivas, 2010).

Several limitations of this study should be mentioned. First, the survey did not include issues related to vaccine trial attributes, such as vaccine-induced infection, side effects, or false-positives on HIV tests, which are associated with lower WTP (Mills, 2004). Thus, the results of this study may overestimate WTP. In addition, self-reported data on risk behaviors related to drug use and sexual behavior could overestimate current risk behaviors. This study has a cross-sectional design and therefore cannot analyze changes in the WTP that might be seen following retention strategies and vaccine education.

This is the first study in Spain to evaluate WTP among sexual partners of HIV-positive patients. The number of people at risk who participated is high, and the study environment is appropriate because the involved facilities have the ability to implement phase I or II vaccine trials.

In the case of a phase III preventive vaccine trial in Spain, it could become necessary to recruit a large number of people at risk of infection. The stated WTP in hypothetical HIV vaccine trials was high among sexual partners of HIV-positive patients. Specific interventions are needed to increase the acceptability of vaccine trial participation among drug users at risk of HIV infection.

Recommended Sites of HIV/AIDS Vaccine Initiatives
Internacional AIDS Vaccine Initiative: http://www.iavi.org
HIV Vaccine Trials Network: http://www.hvtn.org
World Health Organization: http://www.who.int/hiv/topics/vaccines/Vaccines
AIDS Vaccine Advocacy Coalition: http://www.avac.org
Vaccine Research Center: http://www.niaid.nih.gov/about/organization/vrc

5. Acknowledgment

This work was funded by grants from Ministry of Science and Innovation, Spain (grant PI07/0342, RD06/001 and RD06/006), and the Agency for Management of University and Research Grants-AGAUR (grant 2008 BE-2 00269).

6. References

Adimora, A. A.; Schoenbach, V. J.& Doherty, I. A. (2006). HIV and African Americans in the southern United States: sexual networks and social context. *Sexually transmitted diseases,* 33, 7 Suppl, (Jul), S39-45, 0148-5717

Aliyu, G.; Mohammad, M.; Saidu, A.; Mondal, P.; Charurat, M.; Abimiku, A.; Nasidi, A.& Blattner, W. (2010). HIV infection awareness and willingness to participate in future HIV vaccine trials across different risk groups in Abuja, Nigeria. *AIDS Care,* 22, 10, (Oct), 1277-1284, 1360-0451

Alter, M. J.; Hadler, S. C.; Judson, F. N.; Mares, A.; Alexander, W. J.; Hu, P. Y.; Miller, J. K.; Moyer, L. A.; Fields, H. A.& Bradley, D. W. (1990). Risk factors for acute non-A, non-B hepatitis in the United States and association with hepatitis C virus infection. *JAMA : the journal of the American Medical Association,* 264, 17, (Nov 7), 2231-2235, 0098-7484

American Psychiatric Association. (2000).Diagnostic and statistical manual of mental disorders. 4th Ed. (DSM IV-TR).Washington DC:Government Printing Office

Baliunas, D.; Rehm, J.; Irving, H.& Shuper, P. (2010). Alcohol consumption and risk of incident human immunodeficiency virus infection: a meta-analysis. *International journal of public health,* 55, 3, (Jun), 159-166, 1661-8564

Booth, R. E.; Kwiatkowski, C. F.& Chitwood, D. D. (2000). Sex related HIV risk behaviors: differential risks among injection drug users, crack smokers, and injection drug users who smoke crack. *Drug and alcohol dependence,* 58, 3, (Mar 1), 219-226, 0376-8716

Bruandet, A.; Lucidarme, D.; Decoster, A.; Ilef, D.; Harbonnier, J.; Jacob, C.; Delamare, C.; Cyran, C.; Van Hoenacker, A. F.; Fremaux, D.; Josse, P.; Emmanuelli, J.; Le Strat, Y.; Filoche, B.& Desenclos, J. C. (2006). Incidence and risk factors of HCV infection in a cohort of intravenous drug users in the North and East of France. *Revue d'epidemiologie et de sante publique,* 54 Spec No 1, (Jul), 1S15-1S22, 0398-7620

Castilla, J.; Lorenzo, J. M.; Izquierdo, A.; Lezaun, M. E.; Lopez, I.; Moreno-Iribas, C.; Nunez, D.; Perucha, M.; R'kaina Liesfi, C.& Zulaika, D. (2006). Characteristics and trends of newly diagnosed HIV-infections, 2000-2004. *Gaceta sanitaria / S.E.S.P.A.S,* 20, 6, (Nov-Dec), 442-448, 0213-9111

Celentano, D. D.; Beyrer, C.; Natpratan, C.; Eiumtrakul, S.; Sussman, L.; Renzullo, P. O.; Khamboonruang, C.& Nelson, K. E. (1995). Willingness to participate in AIDS vaccine trials among high-risk populations in northern Thailand. *AIDS (London, England),* 9, 9, (Sep), 1079-1083, 0269-9370

Colfax, G.; Santos, G. M.; Chu, P.; Vittinghoff, E.; Pluddemann, A.; Kumar, S.& Hart, C. (2010). Amphetamine-group substances and HIV. *Lancet,* 376, 9739, (Aug 7), 458-474, 1474-547X

Colfax, G.; Buchbinder, S.; Vamshidar, G.; Celum, C.; McKirnan, D.; Neidig, J.; Koblin, B.; Gurwith, M.& Bartholow, B. (2005). Motivations for participating in an HIV vaccine efficacy trial. *Journal of acquired immune deficiency syndromes (1999),* 39, 3, (Jul 1), 359-364, 1525-4135

de Azevedo, R. C.; Botega, N. J.& Guimaraes, L. A. (2007). Crack users, sexual behavior and risk of HIV infection. *Revista brasileira de psiquiatria (Sao Paulo, Brazil : 1999),* 29, 1, (Mar), 26-30, 1516-4446

Duan, S.; Xiang, L. F.; Yang, Y. C.; Ye, R. H.; Jia, M. H.; Luo, H. B.; Fu, L. R.; Song, L. J.; Zhao, Y. X.; Yang, J. H.; Wang, B.; Liu, Z. Y.; Pu, Y. C.; Han, W. X.; Yang, Z. J.; Li, W. M.; Wang, J. B.; Zhu, W. M.& He, N. (2009). Incidence and risk factors on HIV infection among injection drug users in Dehong prefecture area of Yunnan province. *Zhonghua liu xing bing xue za zhi,* 30, 12, (Dec), 1226-1229, 0254-6450

Etcheverry, M. F.; Lum, P. J.; Evans, J. L.; Sanchez, E.; de Lazzari, E.; Mendez-Arancibia, E.; Sierra, E.; Gatell, J. M.; Page, K.& Joseph, J. (2011). HIV vaccine trial willingness among injection and non-injection drug users in two urban centres, Barcelona and San Francisco. *Vaccine,* 29, 10, (Feb 24), 1991-1996, 1873-2518

European Monitoring centre for Drugs and Drug Addiction (2009). .Drug-related infectious diseases and drug-related deaths, In: Annual Report, 1609-6150, Avaliable from: http://www.emcdda.europa.eu/publications/annual-report/2009

Golub, E. T.; Purvis, L. A.; Sapun, M.; Safaeian, M.; Beyrer, C.; Vlahov, D.& Strathdee, S. A. (2005). Changes in willingness to participate in HIV vaccine trials among HIV-negative injection drug users. *AIDS and behavior,* 9, 3, (Sep), 301-309, 1090-7165

Hallfors, D. D.; Iritani, B. J.; Miller, W. C.& Bauer, D. J. (2007). Sexual and drug behavior patterns and HIV and STD racial disparities: the need for new directions. *American Journal of Public Health,* 97, 1, (Jan), 125-132, 1541-0048

Hernandez-Aguado, I.; Avino, M. J.; Perez-Hoyos, S.; Gonzalez-Aracil, J.; Ruiz-Perez, I.; Torrella, A.; Garcia de la Hera, M.; Belda, F.; Fernandez, E.; Santos, C.; Trullen, J.& Fenosa, A. (1999). Human immunodeficiency virus (HIV) infection in parenteral drug users: evolution of the epidemic over 10 years. Valencian Epidemiology and Prevention of HIV Disease Study Group. *International journal of epidemiology,* 28, 2, (Apr), 335-340, 0300-5771

Jacobson, R. M.; Targonski, P. V.& Poland, G. A. (2007). A taxonomy of reasoning flaws in the anti-vaccine movement. *Vaccine,* 25, 16, (Apr 20), 3146-3152, 0264-410X

Kellogg, T. A.; McFarland, W.; Perlman, J. L.; Weinstock, H.; Bock, S.; Katz, M. H.; Gerberding, J. L.& Bangsberg, D. R. (2001). HIV incidence among repeat HIV testers at a county hospital, San Francisco, California, USA. *Journal of acquired immune deficiency syndromes (1999),* 28, 1, (Sep 1), 59-64, 1525-4135

Kozlov, A. P.; Shaboltas, A. V.; Toussova, O. V.; Verevochkin, S. V.; Masse, B. R.; Perdue, T.; Beauchamp, G.; Sheldon, W.; Miller, W. C.; Heimer, R.; Ryder, R. W.& Hoffman, I.

F. (2006). HIV incidence and factors associated with HIV acquisition among injection drug users in St Petersburg, Russia. *AIDS (London, England)*, 20, 6, (Apr 4), 901-906, 0269-9370

Li, Q.; Luo, F.; Zhou, Z.; Li, S.; Liu, Y.; Li, D.; Shi, W.; Raymond, H. F.; Ruan, Y.& Shao, Y. (2010). Willingness to participate in HIV vaccine clinical trials among Chinese men who have sex with men. *Vaccine*, 28, 29, (Jun 23), 4638-4643, 1873-2518

Mills, E.; Cooper, C.; Guyatt, G.; Gilchrist, A.; Rachlis, B.; Sulway, C.& Wilson, K. (2004). Barriers to participating in an HIV vaccine trial: a systematic review. *AIDS (London, England)*, 18, 17, (Nov 19), 2235-2242, 0269-9370

Ministerio de Sanidad y Política Social, Ministerio de Ciencia e Innovación. (2010). Nuevos diagnósticos de VIH en España periodo 2003-2009, Actualización 30 de Junio de 2010. Available from: http://www.emcdda.europa.eu/publications /annual-report/2009

Muga, R.; Martinez, E.; Torrens, M.; Bolao, F.; Rivas, I.; Rall, R.; Sanvisens, A.; Fuster, D.& Tor, J. (2010). Low rates of HIV seroconversion among injecting and non-injecting drug users in Barcelona, Spain. 1997-2006. *2010 NIDA Intenational Forum*, Scottsdale, Arizona, June 2010

Newman, P. A. & Logie, C. (2010a). HIV vaccine acceptability: a systematic review and meta-analysis. *AIDS (London, England)*, 24, 11, (Jul 17), 1749-1756, 1473-5571

Newman, P. A.; Roungprakhon, S.; Tepjan, S.& Yim, S. (2010b). Preventive HIV vaccine acceptability and behavioral risk compensation among high-risk men who have sex with men and transgenders in Thailand. *Vaccine*, 28, 4, (Jan 22), 958-964, 1873-2518

Osmond, D. H.; Padian, N. S.; Sheppard, H. W.; Glass, S.; Shiboski, S. C.& Reingold, A. (1993). Risk factors for hepatitis C virus seropositivity in heterosexual couples. *JAMA : the journal of the American Medical Association*, 269, 3, (Jan 20), 361-365, 0098-7484

Rauch, A.; Rickenbach, M.; Weber, R.; Hirschel, B.; Tarr, P. E.; Bucher, H. C.; Vernazza, P.; Bernasconi, E.; Zinkernagel, A. S.; Evison, J.; Furrer, H.& Swiss HIV Cohort Study. (2005). Unsafe sex and increased incidence of hepatitis C virus infection among HIV-infected men who have sex with men: the Swiss HIV Cohort Study. *Clinical infectious diseases : an official publication of the Infectious Diseases Society of America*, 41, 3, (Aug 1), 395-402, 1537-6591

Rivas, I.; Martinez, E.; Sanvisens, A.; Bolao, F.; Tor, J.; Torrens, M.; Pujol, R.; Fuster, D.; Rey-Joly, C.; Munoz, A.& Muga, R. (2010). Hepatitis B virus serum profiles in injection drug users and rates of immunization over time in Barcelona: 1987-2006. *Drug and alcohol dependence*, 110, 3, (Aug 1), 234-239, 1879-0046

Schutten, M.; de Wit, J. B.& van Steenbergen, J. E. (2002). Why do gay men want to be vaccinated against hepatitis B? An assessment of psychosocial determinants of vaccination intention. *International Journal of STD & AIDS*, 13, 2, (Feb), 86-90, 0956-4624

Staras, S. A.; Cook, R. L.& Clark, D. B. (2009). Sexual partner characteristics and sexually transmitted diseases among adolescents and young adults. *Sexually transmitted diseases*, 36, 4, (Apr), 232-238, 1537-4521

Strauss, R. P.; Sengupta, S.; Kegeles, S.; McLellan, E.; Metzger, D.; Eyre, S.; Khanani, F.; Emrick, C. B.& MacQueen, K. M. (2001). Willingness to volunteer in future preventive HIV vaccine trials: issues and perspectives from three U.S. communities. *Journal of acquired immune deficiency syndromes (1999),* 26, 1, (Jan 1), 63-71, 1525-4135

Suhadev, M.; Nyamathi, A. M.; Swaminathan, S.; Venkatesan, P.; Raja Sakthivel, M.; Shenbagavalli, R.; Suresh, A.& Fahey, J. L. (2006). A pilot study on willingness to participate in future preventive HIV vaccine trials. *The Indian journal of medical research,* 124, 6, (Dec), 631-640, 0971-5916

Suntharasamai, P.; Martin, M.; Vanichseni, S.; van Griensven, F.; Mock, P. A.; Pitisuttithum, P.; Tappero, J. W.; Sangkum, U.; Kitayaporn, D.; Gurwith, M.; Choopanya, K.& Bangkok Vaccine Evaluation Group. (2009). Factors associated with incarceration and incident human immunodeficiency virus (HIV) infection among injection drug users participating in an HIV vaccine trial in Bangkok, Thailand, 1999-2003. *Addiction (Abingdon, England),* 104, 2, (Feb), 235-242, 1360-0443

Van Tieu, H. & Koblin, B. A. (2009). HIV, alcohol, and noninjection drug use. *Current opinion in HIV and AIDS,* 4, 4, (Jul), 314-318, 1746-6318

Vanichseni, S.; Kitayaporn, D.; Mastro, T. D.; Mock, P. A.; Raktham, S.; Des Jarlais, D. C.; Sujarita, S.; Srisuwanvilai, L. O.; Young, N. L.; Wasi, C.; Subbarao, S.; Heyward, W. L.; Esparza, L.& Choopanya, K. (2001). Continued high HIV-1 incidence in a vaccine trial preparatory cohort of injection drug users in Bangkok, Thailand. *AIDS (London, England),* 15, 3, (Feb 16), 397-405, 0269-9370

Wang, B.; Li, X.; Stanton, B.; Zhang, L.& Fang, X. (2010). Alcohol Use, Unprotected Sex, and Sexually Transmitted Infections Among Female Sex Workers in China. *Sexually transmitted diseases,* 37, *10,* (Jul 1), 629-636, 1537-4521

Yin, L.; Zhang, Y.; Qian, H. Z.; Rui, B.; Zhang, L.; Zhu, J.; Guan, Y.; Wang, Y.; Li, Q.; Ruan, Y.& Shao, Y. (2008). Willingness of Chinese injection drug users to participate in HIV vaccine trials. *Vaccine,* 26, 6, (Feb 6), 762-768, 0264-410X